ADVANCES IN **SPORT** AND **EXERCISE** SCIENCE SERIES

# The
# Physiology
# of Training

I would like to dedicate this book to my wife, Penny, for her unwavering support during the production of this book and throughout my career, and to my mum and dad for all their love and support across the years.

*For Elsevier:*
*Senior Commissioning Editor*: Sarena Wolfaard
*Associate Editor*: Dinah Thom
*Project Manager*: Emma Riley
*Designer*: Stewart Larking
*Illustration Buyer*: Gillian Murray
*Illustrations:* Hardlines Studio

ADVANCES IN **SPORT** AND **EXERCISE** SCIENCE SERIES

# The
# Physiology
# of Training

Edited by

**Gregory Whyte** BSc PGCE MSc PhD FACSM
*Director of Science and Research, English Institute of Sport,*
*Bisham Abbey National Sports Centre, Buckinghamshire, UK*

**SERIES EDITORS**

**Neil Spurway** MA PhD
*Emeritus Professor of Exercise Physiology, University of Glasgow, Glasgow, UK*

**Don MacLaren** BSc MSc PhD CertEd
*Professor of Sports Nutrition, School of Sport and Exercise Sciences,*
*Liverpool John Moores University, Liverpool, UK*

Foreword by

**James Cracknell** OBE BSc MSc
*Two times Olympic Champion, six times World Champion, Rowing*

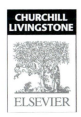

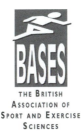

THE BRITISH
ASSOCIATION OF
SPORT AND EXERCISE
SCIENCES

EDINBURGH LONDON NEW YORK OXFORD PHILADELPHIA ST LOUIS SYDNEY TORONTO 2006

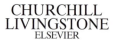

## CHURCHILL
## LIVINGSTONE
ELSEVIER

First published 2006

ISBN 0 443 10117 5
ISBN-13 978-0-443-10117-5

**British Library Cataloguing in Publication Data**
A catalogue record for this book is available from the British Library.

**Library of Congress Cataloging in Publication Data**
A catalog record for this book is available from the Library of Congress.

**Notice**
Knowledge and best practice in this field are constantly changing. As new research and experience broaden our knowledge, changes in practice, treatment and drug therapy may become necessary or appropriate. Readers are advised to check the most current information provided (i) on procedures featured or (ii) by the manufacturer of each product to be administered, to verify the recommended dose or formula, the method and duration of administration, and contraindications. It is the responsibility of the practitioner, relying on their own experience and knowledge of the patient, to make diagnoses, to determine dosages and the best treatment for each individual patient, and to take all appropriate safety precautions. To the fullest extent of the law, neither the publisher nor the editor and contributors assume any liability for any injury and/or damage to persons or property arising out of, or related to, any use of the material contained in this book.

*The Publisher*

# Contents

# Contributors

**Colin Boreham** BSc MSc PhD FACSM FECSS
*Colin Boreham is Professor of Sport and Exercise at the University of Ulster. His research interests lie in exercise and health in young people and elite sport. Colin is a former UK record holder in the high jump, and represented GB and NI at the 1984 Los Angeles Olympics as a decathlete.*

**Richard Budgett** OBE MA MBBS DipSportsMed DRCOG DCH MRCGP FFSEM FISM
*Richard is currently the Director of Medical Services to the British Olympic Association, Chief Medical Officer at the Olympic Medical Institute, and Sports Physician, English Institute of Sport South East Region. Richard has published extensively in the area of chronic fatigue in elite athletes and the overtraining syndrome. Richard was an Olympic Gold Medallist in rowing (coxed fours) at the 1984 Olympic Games.*

**Roslyn Carbon** MSc(SportsMed)Lond MBBS DipSportsMed MLCOM FACSP FFISEM
*Roslyn Carbon is a sports physician based in London, UK. She served as a medical officer with the British team and at world championships in six different sports. She was the senior lecturer and clinician at the Academic Department of Sports Medicine at the Royal London Hospital during the 1990s. Having been the inaugural Sports Medicine Fellow at the Australian Institute of Sport, she was more recently the National Medical Director of the English Institute of Sport. She is currently working in professional rugby union and is a consultant for the Irish Sports Council.*

**Nicholas Diaper** BSc MSc
*A former international swimmer, having captained the Kenyan national swimming team at the 1998 and 2002 Commonwealth Games, Nicholas holds a Masters degree in exercise physiology from Manchester Metropolitan University and at the time of writing he was a sports science intern working with the English Institute of Sport.*

**Andrew Franco** BSc
*Andrew Franco is a postgraduate student at Brunel University currently studying the influence of different types of training upon cardiac structure and function. Andrew is also an active rugby coach, currently responsible for a large inner city rugby project targeting children from ethnic minorities and low-income backgrounds.*

**Richard Godfrey** BSc PhD
*During 12 years working as a Chief Physiologist for the BOA, Richard Godfrey staffed 60 elite athlete training camps, attended two Olympic Games, and completed his PhD in growth hormone and exercise. He is currently a Senior Research Lecturer at Brunel University.*

**Stephen Ingham** BSc PhD
*During 7 years as Senior Sports Physiologist at the Olympic Medical Institute and the English Institute of Sport, Steve has supported track athletes and rowers to numerous Olympic medals. He has a BSc in sports science and a PhD in exercise physiology and is BASES accredited and holds NSCA certification. Steve is a national league sprinter.*

**Yiannis Koutedakis** BSc MA PhD
*Yiannis has attended many national, international and world championships and Olympic Games as competitor, professional coach/trainer and scientific advisor. He was one of the founders of the British Olympic Medical Centre. He is currently a Professor in Applied Physiology at the University of Thessaly (Greece) and a Visiting Professor at Wolverhampton University (UK), and has published extensively in the area of human physical fitness.*

**Alison K. McConnell** BSc MSc PhD FACSM
*Alison is Professor of Applied Physiology at Brunel University. Originally a graduate of biological sciences (physiology), she made the transition into exercise physiology after completing an MSc in human and applied physiology at King's College London, and a PhD in the Department of Thoracic Medicine at King's College Hospital. Alison's main research interest is in 'respiratory limitations to exercise', which has its roots in her competitive background in track and field and, later, rowing.*

**Giorgos S. Metsios** BSc MSc
*Giorgos has been a member of the Greek national water-polo team. He obtained his BSc in sport and exercise science from Thessaly University (Greece) and his MSc in sport science from Wolverhampton University (UK). He is currently extending his studies to PhD level in the area of exercise science.*

**Robert Shave** BSc MSc PhD
*Rob is a Reader in Sport and Exercise Physiology within the School of Sport and Education at Brunel University. Prior to his appointment at Brunel Rob was an applied physiologist at the British Olympic Medical Centre for 3 years where he provided physiological support to a number of Olympic and professional sports.*

**Antonis Stavropoulos-Kalinoglou** BSc MSc
*Antonis has been a member of the Greek national skiing team. He obtained his BSc in sport and exercise science from Thessaly University (Greece) and his MSc in sport science from Wolverhampton University (UK). He is currently extending his studies to PhD level in the area of exercise science.*

**Ken van Someren** BSc PhD
*Ken is currently the National Physiology Lead at the English Institute of Sport. He competed in four Sprint Kayaking World Championships and has supported a wide range of national and international athletes. His research interests include physiological determinants of sports performance, training techniques and exercise-induced muscle damage.*

**Gregory Whyte** BSc MSc PhD FACSM

*Formerly Director of Research for the British Olympic Association, Greg is currently the Director of Science and Research at the English Institute of Sport. He is an Associate Professor at Brunel University and has published extensively in the area of cardiovascular function in health and disease and performance physiology. Greg represented Great Britain at the 1992 and 1996 Olympic Games and is a World and European medallist in modern pentathlon.*

# Foreword

Human athletic performance continues to improve across all sporting activities. However the margins of improvement are reducing. Indeed, there are suggestions that the limits to human performance have been reached in some events. A closer examination of the determinants of performance and the optimal adaptation of those determinants is required as athletes move closer to the genetic ceiling of perform-ance. The advancement of sports science and sports medicine in recent years has created an avenue of exploration in the identification of the determinants of athletic performance and the optimization of training and health. Physiology, as a sub-discipline of sports science and sports medicine, has made a significant contribution to our understanding of athletic performance. In an attempt to understand what the human body goes through when training and competing, with an end goal of learn-ing how to make the most of mine, I studied for a Masters in Sports Science. The knowledge it gave me was invaluable, allowing me to exploit whatever ability I had.

The physiological examination of exercise was first documented in the early 1900s. However it was not until the 1960s that we observed a growing interest in exercise and, by inference, sports physiology. Since that time there has been a growing body of literature examining athletic performance, its determinants and training-induced adaptations. Despite the large volume of available research there are only a limited number of books that examine the physiological aspects of athletic performance. Indeed, those texts currently available tend to focus on single sporting disciplines. *The Physiology of Training* represents a significant contribution to the available liter-ature, offering a contemporary, across-sport account of training physiology. Opening with a detailed review and update of the principles of training, it focuses upon the key areas of periodization, specificity and tapering. Understanding the principles of training is of paramount importance in the development of effective training programmes. Having provided a comprehensive commentary on the principles of training *The Physiology of Training* examines, in detail, all facets of physiology associated with athletic performance across aerobic, anaerobic, power and strength-based sports. These chapters draw upon available knowledge to give an under-standable and concise review of each area and, underpinned by the authors' practical experience and expertise in the area, offer practical applications of the available research across sport. In contrast to the books currently available, *The Physiology of Training* goes on to examine the impact of the environment on training and offers practical solutions to common problems encountered when training in the heat, cold and at altitude. Furthermore, it explores some commonly observed health problems associated with training. Environment and health are important areas that receive little coverage in training texts.

Drawing upon the knowledge and expertise of an outstanding group of authors, this book is a 'must have' for sports scientists, coaches, personal trainers and physical educators. *The Physiology of Training* is an excellent 'one stop' resource offering a contemporary, in-depth and concise mix of theory and practice that should be found on the bookshelves of all those involved in sport, at all levels.

*James Cracknell*

# Preface

During the late 19th Century and early part of the 20th Century the Victorians imposed an amateur ethic on athletic participation that resulted in only the wealthy being able to compete in the vast majority of sports. Along with this amateur ethos came a belief that physical training was unsportsmanlike and not in the true spirit of competition. With the end of the Victorian era came an expansion of physical participation, sport and competition, leading the way to a 'professionalization' of sport with the development of training and the introduction of dedicated coaches. This period of emancipation coincided with the first attempts of scientists to describe the physiological response to exercise in man. The mid-1900s saw an acceleration of focused programmes of research designed to evaluate the result of physical training on performance. Since that time, exercise physiology has become an integral part of coaching and training science.

Despite the ever increasing library of research evidence there are very few comprehensive texts examining the physiology of training. While many books contain single chapters on the subject, often the coverage lacks depth and academic rigor. Furthermore, advances in training science have led to a large number of original research and review publications in recent years. These publications have yet to be fully reviewed and presented in a single text dedicated to the physiology of training. This book encompasses the available research evidence supported by practical examples that will provide a valuable, contemporary addition to the existing literature.

Existing texts on the physiology of training often focus on individual sports and fail to provide the breadth or depth of information necessary for undergraduate and postgraduate students, and the coaching community. The goal of this book is to offer a significant contribution to the field of training physiology by providing an in-depth explanation of coaching science using both theoretical and practical models for training, across a wide range of sporting disciplines. This book will fulfil an important role in the teaching of training science to a broad community of scientists and coaches. It is envisaged that *The Physiology of Training* will become a key element in the education of those involved in sport and exercise science, and coaching, and act as an ongoing resource to all those involved in sport and exercise physiology, coaching, teaching and the fitness industry.

The contents are arranged to allow the reader to access information in an organized and sequential fashion, covering all key areas underpinning the physiology of training. The principles of training are the focus of attention in Chapters 1, 2 and 3, examining the areas of periodization, specificity and tapering. Using these principles, Chapters 4, 5, 6 and 7 cover the physiology of endurance training, anaerobic endurance training, sprint and power training, and strength training. Chapter 8, on the environment and training, examines the impact of heat, cold and altitude on training physiology, offering practical guidelines in combating the potentially deleterious effects of such environments. Finally, Chapter 9 presents an overview of four common medical conditions associated with training – 'reproduction health in exercising women', 'the athlete's heart', 'unexplained underperformance syndrome' and 'asthma and exercise-induced asthma'.

In addition to the dedicated, contemporary coverage, *The Physiology of Training* has drawn upon high-profile authors who are proven academics in the field of coaching science and who have worked closely with high-performance athletes and coaches. Each author offers a wealth of theoretical knowledge underpinned by a proven record of application in the practical setting. The authorship team includes major championship medallists from a variety of sports, enabling them to offer a unique perspective on the physiology of training.

In summary, the expertise and experience of the authors has resulted in a unique, contemporary text examining the physiology of training that will become a key resource for sport and exercise scientists, coaches, teachers and health professionals.

In preparing this text, I would like to acknowledge the assistance I have received from **Professor Craig Sharp**; I would also like to thank him for his mentorship throughout my career.

*Buckinghamshire 2006*                                              ***Gregory Whyte***

# Chapter 1

# Periodization of exercise training in sport

Yiannis Koutedakis, Giorgos S. Metsios and Antonis Stavropoulos-Kalinoglou

## LEARNING OBJECTIVES:

This chapter is intended to ensure that the reader:

1. Appreciates the historical, theoretical and scientific background of periodization.
2. Distinguishes between fatigue due to normal training, over-reaching and over-training.
3. Understands the importance of recovery following exercise training.
4. Understands the concepts and components of periodization.

5. Structures periodized training programmes on the basis of basic principles of periodization.
6. Understands differences between training cycles.
7. Distinguishes periodization procedures for developing aerobic endurance and strength.

## SUMMARY

The necessity of superior performance in sport has impelled coaches to use increasingly effective and sophisticated training methods. This has been better served by applying the principals of periodization whereby, as levels of a particular fitness-component increase, a higher exercise stress is required to create overload and lead to specific physiological adaptations. The modern theory of periodization was advanced in the early 1960s when coaches realized that focusing on an important competition was more effective than preparing the athlete for a year-round competition programme. This has been supported by limited scientific data indicating that athletes who train using periodized models attain levels of performance superior to those who use non-periodized models. Performance improvements in most sport activities have been directly linked to changes in structures and metabolic capacities of skeletal muscle. Periodized resistance training, for instance, causes hypertrophy of muscle fibres of all types, especially those with fast-twitch characteristics. In contrast, aerobic training leads to increases in the number and volume of mitochondria (essential for energy production trough aerobic pathways), mainly in slow-twitch fibres.

## INTRODUCTION

Ever since sport began, athletes have been trying to get the most out of their training. However, it was not until the last few decades, that levels of sport performance have exhibited a spectacular increase. Records that once were imaginary can now be regularly reached. At the same time, the amount of training of modern competitors is considerably higher than that used in the past. This would not be possible without the concurrent evolution in training methodology. The necessity of superior performances in competition has impelled coaches to introduce increasingly effective and sophisticated training methods.

Several sciences have contributed to the understanding of the effects of exercise on the body, and together have formed a science of their own, the science of training. The latter focuses on sports performance and aims to understand, measure and improve the effects of exercise on the body and minimize the prevalence of injury.

During competition, the participant is expected to withstand several stressful stimuli, while performance can be influenced by numerous internal factors (e.g. physiological, biochemical, technical and tactical) and/or external factors (e.g. climatic, travelling, financial). Training has to be structured in a way that simulates these conditions and prepares for the actual event. For optimal performance, therefore, competitors must be experts in the technical side of their event, be psychologically prepared to handle the enormous stress of critical situations, and be free from injury; they must also be physically 'fit'.

Physical fitness is served by individual sciences such as paediatric and adult physiology, biochemistry, biomechanics and sports medicine (Fig. 1.1) and it can be defined as the individual's ability to meet the demands of a specific task. It primarily consists of elements of aerobic and anaerobic fitness, muscular strength and flexibility. Regardless of the performance level, sex and age, all competitors use one or more of these elements of fitness during their daily practice. For example, in an

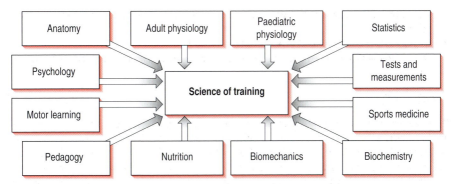

**Figure 1.1**    The science of training and selected contributing elements.

endurance event such as the marathon, aerobic capacity is the most important element for success, whereas in sprinting events, such as the 100 m, anaerobic power predominates. Consequently, training programmes have to address the most important elements of physical fitness for each individual sport.

Training planning has existed, though in a crude form, since the ancient times and was used for the Olympic Games or military purposes. The Greek athlete Milon from the city of Croton was the first known competitor who, perhaps unwittingly, implemented the principle of periodization as early as the 6th Century BC. He determined the training cycles by carrying a bull calf on his back each day until the animal reached maturity. As levels of a particular fitness component increase, a higher quality of exercise stress is needed to create overload and lead to physiological adaptations.

As early as the middle of the 19th Century appeared the first studies on human muscular performance, published in the then popular *Philosophical Magazine*. However, the modern practice of periodization can be traced to the 1950s and early 1960s when East European coaches observed that their athletes could not withstand the enormous training load to which they where subjected. In contrast, coaches observed that focusing on just a few important competitions was far more effective than preparing the athlete for a year-round competition programme. This anecdotal evidence was later supported by some scientific data, suggesting that athletes who trained using periodized models attained superior levels of performance than those who used non-periodized models (Fleck 1999). The aim of this chapter is to provide information on the appropriate planning of exercise training programmes for the purpose of enhancing performance in sports, utilizing the principle of periodization.

## EXERCISE TRAINING

### Training theories and methodologies

The human body is structured in such a way that it maintains relatively stable internal physiological conditions, or homeostasis. Blood volume, haematocrit, arterial pressure and core temperature are among the most important physiological indicators of homeostasis. When this balance is disturbed, the body reacts acutely in an attempt to preserve homeostasis and, if the 'disturbance' continues, it adapts its functions to a higher level. Physical training aims to cause such an imbalance in the body over a period of time, while training theory and methodology deals with the understanding of the cause and optimization of training results. The theoretical background of training originally comes from the work of Dr Hans Seyle, who first introduced the General Adaptation Syndrome (GAS) theory in 1956. In his model, Seyle suggested that the body responds to stress in three different stages.

The first stage, or 'shock stage', is when the source of biological stress is identified by the body, which responds to this change and tries to overcome the imbalance caused by the stressor. As the stressor persists, physical and mental performance is reduced below baseline levels. In terms of training, this stage refers to the introduction of a training programme where the individual experiences soreness, stiffness and tiredness due to the initial 'shock' caused by the exercise.

The second stage of the GAS is termed the 'resistance stage' which starts as soon as the stressor is removed. During this stage, the human body recovers from the temporary imbalance and adapts at a higher level of performance to compensate for the increased demands. These two stages are natural responses to the stressor and have positive effects on the body. The third stage is referred to as the 'exhaustion' or 'fatigue' stage, and can be reached when the stressor is of great longitude or magnitude, and the body does not have sufficient time to adapt.

Performance optimization is the result of long-term, demanding and well-structured exercise training. For the athlete to gain maximum benefits from exercise, several factors involved in the adaptation mechanism have to be considered. These factors include overload, specificity, individual differences and reversibility.

Overload refers to the intensity and duration of the training stimuli. Exercise training has to be sufficient in its intensity and duration to activate the adaptation mechanism and bring about changes in structural, physiological, neural, psychological and endocrine functions. If the training exercise does not stress the body sufficiently, no adaptation occurs. On the other hand a very high stress can lead to injury or over-training, hence, any new increase should be followed by an unloading phase during which the body relaxes, adapts and prepares for a new increase in load (Harre 1982).

Not every type of exercise is appropriate for all sports. The performed exercise has to be sport-specific and focus on the muscles and organs stressed during the actual competition. Low-intensity strength training, for example, does not prepare the muscle for the demands of competition in which high muscle forces are required, while speed increases should be possible only if training loads are low but with high-velocity muscular actions (Fig. 1.2). In general, similarities should exist between the training conditions and those required in the field during competition. Chapter 2 will examine the principles of specificity in greater detail.

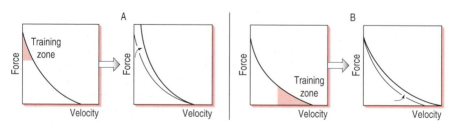

**Figure 1.2**   The force–velocity relationship (redrawn from Komi & Häkkinen 1988). If one wants to increase force levels, exercises should be characterized by high loads and low velocities (A). Alternatively, if the speed of movement is the intended adaptation, exercise-loads should be low but with high-velocity muscular actions (B).

A training programme has also to be planned according to the training principle of individuality in order to meet the needs of each athlete. Inter-individual variation in responses to exercise and adaptation rate are partially because of genetic differences. The relative predominance of fast- or slow-twitch motor units in muscles and endocrine factors determine to a great extent the level of adaptation. The competition level can also affect individual training programmes, particularly in relation to overall length, which may extend from 8 to more than 30 hours per week.

The opposite of training is detraining. When an athlete is not subjected to sufficient training over a period of time, performance deteriorates significantly. In other words, reversibility (or detraining) is a deconditioning process caused by the reduction or cessation of optimal training stimuli. As a general rule, the longer the training period the slower the detraining (Moritani & deVries 1979). The time needed for this decrease is shorter than that required by the athlete to regain the previous level of performance. In addition, much consideration has to be given for the time allowed for detraining because an unduly prolonged deconditioning period may significantly compromise the regaining of performance. For instance, it has been found that although 4 weeks of reduced training or inactivity provided no decreases in muscular strength, the ability to generate power declined dramatically (Neufer et al 1987).

## TRAINING ADAPTATION

Adaptations due to exercise training can be either acute or long-term in nature. The former includes homeostatic regulatory responses, activation of oxygen transport and use of energy reserves with the main aim being to optimize ATP resynthesis. Structural and functional changes occurring during prolonged periods of training are associated with long-term adaptations, which, in turn, are founded on adaptive protein synthesis. For instance, endurance (i.e. aerobic) training results in an increased concentration of myoglobin, mitochondrial enzyme activity, mitochondrial density, increased respiratory capacity and oxygen transport, as well as enhanced cardiac output (Viru & Viru 2001). On the other hand, strength and power training results in increased muscle cross-sectional areas, or hypertrophy. However, these training-induced adaptations at the muscle cell level are also associated with concomitant adaptations in myocardial, hepatic, renal, endocrine and other cells. Bone growth is also affected by exercise. It has been found that low- and high-intensity exercise training may respectively enhance and hinder bone growth in children (Matsuda et al 1986).

## THE SUPERCOMPENSATION CYCLE

The supercompensation cycle (SC) is the direct transposition of GAS into the theory and methodology of training and deals with the association between training load and regeneration as the biological bases for physical arousal (Bompa 1999). SC is divided in four parts: exercise, fatigue, recovery and adaptations (Fig. 1.3).

When an athlete trains, the body has to supply muscle and organs with energy at a higher rate than resting. These excess energy needs are covered by stored supplies. The drainage of energy stores as well as the accumulation of by-products, such as lactic acid, in the blood and cells leads to fatigue. This is the first phase of the SC, which is characterized by temporary decrements in performance.

Following exercise training, homeostasis has to be restored. Energy stores are replenished and by-products are removed, while tissue micro-damage is repaired to

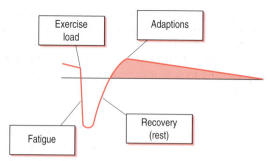

**Figure 1.3**   Supercompensation cycle. Following recovery, the tissues adapt to tolerate higher exercise load, i.e. athletes are in a higher state of fitness.

prevent further, more serious damage. These functions take place during the second phase of SC, the compensation, or recovery phase. However, the third phase of the SC, or supercompensation phase, is the most important one as the body achieves a new, higher level of homeostasis. This means – inter alia – that more energy is stored, especially in the form of glycogen, more contractile proteins are synthesized for efficient and dynamic muscular work, while oxygen is supplied to the mitochondria at a higher rate via a sufficiently developed capillary network.

For these adaptation processes to succeed, an appropriate length of time is required where little or no physical activity is involved. This appears to be about 24 hours following exercise, when glycogen stores are completely replenished and muscle protein synthesis reaches its highest rates. However, the length of recovery time depends on the intensity and duration of training, and it is influenced by the appropriateness or otherwise of nutrition. Inadequate recovery negatively affects adaptation and, therefore, levels of fitness and even health. In particular, any imbalance between training and recovery may bring about the characteristic impairment in physical performance, which is referred to as 'overtraining' (Koutedakis & Sharp 1999, Koutedakis 2000). On the other hand, if the time between two consecutive training sessions is greater than required, the supercompensation state will start to deteriorate until it reaches the original level of homeostasis. This unwelcome development, termed involution, should be avoided.

Ideally, the exercise-training stimulus should be applied when the athlete is at the phase of supercompensation, so that the new supercompensation cycle can begin at a higher level of homeostasis, which may increase the possibilities for improved performances over time (Fig. 1.4). However, most elite athletes do not

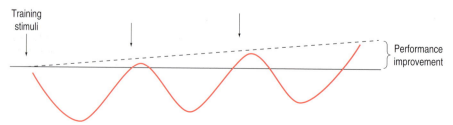

**Figure 1.4**   Accumulative effects of exercise training on performance.

have sufficient recovery time between consecutive training sessions. Coaches have to find ways to alternating high- and low-intensity training so that the different energy sources are stressed. In this way, several training sessions may result in decreases in homeostatic level for a given period of time, but eventually allow the athlete to reach the desired levels of supercompensation (Fig. 1.5).

## RECOVERY

Structural and functional changes incurred during prolonged periods of training are associated with long-term adaptations. As mentioned earlier, however, most of these changes take place during recovery periods following training. Recovery or regeneration refers to the procedures followed by the body to restore homeostasis and adapt its functions and systems at a higher level. These include increased contractile protein synthesis, elevated glycolytic and Krebs' cycle enzymes mobilization, and the return to normal function of endocrine, nerve and immune systems. In a properly structured training schedule, recovery is of equal significance to the training itself.

The time required for recovery depends on several factors and varies considerably among athletes. Physical conditioning and experience play a very important role in recovery rates. Highly conditioned individuals demonstrate higher rates of energy transfer into and removal of waste out of the cells compared to their less conditioned counterparts. Also, in general, supercompensation in athletes younger than 18 years of age requires more time to materialize, while athletes older than 25 require more recovery time.

Hormones, such as testosterone and cortisol augment or inhibit recovery respectively. Males, due to their higher levels of testosterone, exhibit faster recovery rates than females (Noakes 2001). On the other hand, high concentrations of cortisol inhibits muscle growth and repair, as well as impairing the neuromuscular co-ordination (Davis et al 2000). The type of exercise used in each training session can further affect recovery rates.

External factors, such as nutrition, environmental conditions and travelling may also affect recovery. Administration of the required nutrients soon after the training session is completed can positively influence recovery. There seems to be a 2-hour optimal window after the cessation of exercise for the ingestion of carbohydrate. Exercising at altitude, of higher than 2500 to 3000 metres, results in impaired recovery rate due to the reduced partial pressure of oxygen. Similarly, cold adversely affects the production of regenerative hormones such as testosterone and human growth hormone and in this way inhibits recovery. Human growth hormone may also be

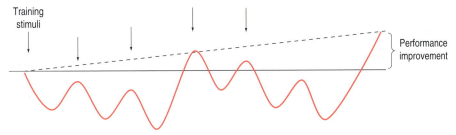

Figure 1.5  Effects of successive exercise-training sessions with different loadings.

affected chronobiologically by travel. Travelling over time zones with 3–10 hours difference affects circadian rhythms with negative effects on recovery.

Accordingly, researchers have tried to establish a time course for recovery. It has been shown that heart rate and blood pressure will return to baseline values in the hour following exercise. After intensive aerobic exercise, 10–48 hours are required for the body to replenish glycogen stores depending on intensity and duration of exercise, whereas 5–24 hours would usually be needed for glycogen replenishment after anaerobic exercise (Koutedakis & Sharp 1999). Following resistance training 24–36 hours are required for the muscle to be completely normalized (Viru & Viru 2001). Recovery of the nervous system, depending on the severity of the stimuli, may take up to 48 hours (McArdle et al 2001).

Recovery rate follows a curvilinear pattern (Fig. 1.6), divisible into three parts. In the first, almost 70% of the required recovery is completed; the rate is then reduced so that an additional 20% is accomplished and the remaining 10% occurs in the third part of the recovery curve (Bompa 1999). Depending on the energy system used during training and the required recovery, the shift from the first to the last part of the recovery curve can last from a few hours to several days, or even months in the case of overtraining (Koutedakis 2000).

## TRAINING FATIGUE AND OVER-REACHING

Training stimuli, when properly applied, result in a disturbance to the homeostatic balance. As indicated above, this imbalance may last several hours depending on the training load and the other factors discussed.

When a training stimulus exceeds the tolerance levels of the athlete, a greater disturbance in homeostasis may occur. This short, acute imbalance appears as acute fatigue and lasts for 1–2 days. Acute fatigue is usually accompanied by muscular overstrain and results in muscle soreness, insomnia and increased allergenic response. When this is followed by a second intense training session, without an appropriate intervening recovery period, a state of overload stimulus with muscular strain develops, where the same symptoms are present but last for more than 2 days.

Further engagement in intense training without adequate recovery leads to accumulation of fatigue and to the condition termed 'over-reaching'. This usually occurs slowly over the course of several weeks. Symptoms are similar to those of

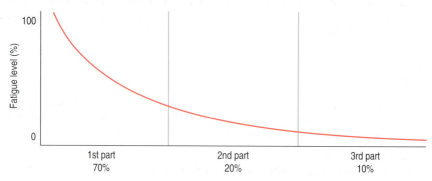

Figure 1.6   Recovery rate.

the overload stimulus, but more severe. Additionally, athletes in a state of over-reaching might observe an increased resting heart rate, increased heart rate and lactic acid concentrations during sub-maximal exercise, early fatigue during training, reduced ability to tolerate training load and increased thirst. Over-reaching is a temporary state and usually lasts from a few days to 2 weeks.

Coaches utilize training methods to voluntarily place the athlete in one of the above described states. These methods are used to achieve a greater training impact. However, such techniques have to be implemented with extreme caution and after careful planning and monitoring of the effects of training, otherwise overtraining – or the recently introduced 'unexplained underperformance syndrome' – may result (Budgett et al 2000).

## UNEXPLAINED UNDERPERFORMANCE SYNDROME (UPS)

The terms *unexplained underperformance syndrome* (UPS; also referred to as 'over-training', 'overtraining syndrome' or 'burnout'), *staleness, chronic fatigue* (or 'chronic fatigue syndrome') and *post-viral fatigue* are often used interchangeably to describe the condition in which active individuals complain of reduced physical perform-ances for no apparent medical or other obvious reasons.

Although these terms are used by many as synonyms to describe more or less the same condition – i.e. poor physical performances, coupled with chronic and unexplained fatigue and certain behavioural changes – the condition itself may have different origins or may be triggered by different chains of events.

## Aspects contributing to UPS

UPS is a clinically complex condition of indeterminate cause with a range of indi-vidually varying symptoms and signs. It tends to occur in athletes during periods of increased commitments, either in training or competition, and in individuals whose daily practices produce an imbalance between physical activity and recovery. Inadequate recovery may negatively affect adaptation and, therefore, levels of fit-ness and/or health. Steinacker (1993) has cautioned that if high volumes of exercise and training are undertaken (more than 1000 hours per year) even work at moder-ate levels may be felt as an intensive effort.

Relatively low levels of physical fitness may also contribute to the development of UPS. For the same workload, fitter athletes are working relatively more easily than their unfit counterparts. Also, 'individual' activities (e.g. cycling, swimming and dance) are more likely to induce UPS than team-events such as basketball and volleyball. External stresses, personal relationships and financial difficulties may further contribute to the development of the condition.

## Symptoms

When feelings of constant fatigue and poor performance are simultaneously pres-ent, other symptoms have to be considered. These are non-specific and may vary from individual to individual. Symptomatology may include:

- excessive sweating;
- inability to recover optimally following intensive exercise;
- loss of desire and enthusiasm for exercise training (feelings of helplessness);

- breakdown of technique;
- poor concentration;
- loss of appetite and loss of body weight;
- disturbed sleep often with nightmares or vivid dreams;
- increased susceptibility to injuries.

## Signs

As in the case of symptoms, there are no consistent signs on clinical examination or laboratory tests associated with overtraining. However, the known signs could be grouped according to those indicating acute UPS (lasting for up to 1 month) and those related to chronic UPS (lasting for many weeks or months).

## Acute UPS

Acute or short-term UPS is the result of an imbalance between exercise and recovery over a period of just a few days or weeks. However, the effects of acute UPS quickly disappear when the reasons for causing it are removed. Muscle damage is perhaps the most common outcome indicating that the work volumes exceeded the capabilities of the muscle in question. The most common signs include:

- increased normal resting heart rates by 5–10 beats per minute;
- increased resting blood pressure;
- raised resting lactic acid concentrations;
- decreased maximal lactic acid levels following intensive physical exercise;
- following specific exercise/training routines, heart rate return to resting levels may take 2–3 times longer than normal;
- decreased ability by the body to utilize oxygen during maximal exercise;
- muscle damage.

## Chronic UPS

Chronic or long-term UPS is the result of an imbalance between exercise and recovery over a period of weeks or months. When the condition is fully developed, the following signs may appear in addition to those mentioned above:

- menstrual irregularities, even cessation of menstruation;
- susceptibility to infections, especially of the skin and upper respiratory tract;
- increased rates of allergies and minor scratches may heal more slowly.

## Management of UPS

The concept 'no pain no gain' should be played down by athletes as there is normally little gain to be made by working through fatigue, illness or injury. Research has clearly demonstrated that periods of physical rest (or reduced activity) may be beneficial to underperforming elite competitors (Koutedakis et al 1990). Once a case of UPS has been diagnosed and dealt with, there is danger of relapse in about 3 months. During this period, athletes should never attempt to increase physical loads by more than 5% per week.

# PERIODIZATION

## Definition and concepts

Periodization can be defined as the purposeful variation of a training programme over time, so that the competitor will approach his/her optimal adaptive potential just prior to an important event. It is based on the principles of multilateral development, specialization, variety and long-term planning. The first three are necessary for the optimization of physiological factors, whereas long-term planning provides both the athlete and the coach with time to gradually increase physical performance. In the simplest form of periodization, competitors use a hard/easy model for daily workouts. In its more advanced form, training is arranged into blocks of time, the magnitude of which may range from days to weeks to months or even years. During each of these blocks, a particular element of physical performance (e.g. physical fitness, technique etc.) is highlighted. As a framework for structuring an athlete's training, the practice of periodization has much to offer. Although performance is allowed to decrease temporarily (i.e. over-reaching), complete recovery is ensured between each training period to avoid long-term performance decrements (i.e. UPS or overtraining).

## Scientific research

Although the structural, physiological and metabolic characteristics of athletes have been thoroughly studied over the years, the physiological mechanisms which support the efficiency of periodized training programmes remain unclear. Existing scientific data have mainly focused on observations and comparisons of periodized regimes with non-periodized training programmes.

The majority of such studies have been conducted on males and have used strength and power training interventions over periods of 7–24 weeks. Specifically, researchers have investigated the effects of systematic variation in training volume and intensity in relation to linear programmes using a constant-sets-and-repetitions approach. Results have demonstrated that both methods significantly increase strength and power compared to pre-exercise levels. However, the effects were of a greater magnitude in the groups that followed periodized programmes than their counterparts engaging in linear training programmes. Even in relatively short training regimes, periodized programmes are able to elicit significantly greater adaptations in selected performance indices than non-periodized (Fleck 1999).

The most plausible explanation for such results is the use of different types of muscle fibres, neural activation and utilization of different energy pathways resulting from the variation of training intensity and duration. Human muscle is formed of comparable proportions of slow- and fast-twitch muscle fibres within a person's body (McArdle et al 2001). The systematic variation of training duration, intensity and type of exercise used in periodized programmes acts as a sufficient overload to the targeted muscle fibre type and as a facilitator for the required recovery for the other type of muscle fibres and the neurons which activate them (Kraemer et al 1996). Moreover, this variation results in a similar alteration in the utilized energy source, which again operates as an overload or recovery drill for the energy systems. Another explanation for the supremacy of the periodized training approach may be that, compared to controls, higher training loads have been reported by groups practising these programmes, which eventually bring about significantly greater adaptations and performance improvements (Stone et al 1999).

## Types of periodization

Not all sports or athletes have the same competition calendar. For instance, several sports require their competitors to participate in just one major competition every year. The training plan that supports these needs is termed the 'monocycle' (Fig. 1.7A). A different planning approach is required for sports that need more than one performance peak each year and typically those peaks are months apart. Training programmes that incorporate two peaks in a year are termed 'bi-cycle' (Fig. 1.7B), and consist of two monocycles in a single year with a short transition phase between them. To achieve the required adaptations during bi-cycles, competitions have to be more than 4 months apart. Levels of performance might be lower in one cycle, so the most important competition of the calendar should take place in the other.

When competitors are required to participate in three competitions in the course of a single year, a triple 'tri-cycle' periodization is adopted (Fig 1.7C). An unloading phase is required following each peak for the athlete to regenerate for the following cycle. Models with more than three peaks within a year do not allow the athlete to adapt properly.

## PERIODIZATION PHASES

## Preparation phase

This is the longest phase of the annual cycle. During this phase, selected endurance, technical and tactical components should to be developed, in order to prepare the athlete for the next phase. It usually contains three training periods, each lasting 4–8 weeks. In the first period, the training mode is general and the load varies from medium to high aiming at a continuous development of performance. In the second period, special training methods have to be applied and the load must be close to the athlete's personal best. The third period requires a clear shift from general to special training, which closely resembles actual competition. The training methods are strictly sport-specific, and the load is high, necessary for adaptation and further progress in the next phase. At the end of each of the three training cycles, both coaches and athletes should monitor progress through established laboratory or field-testing.

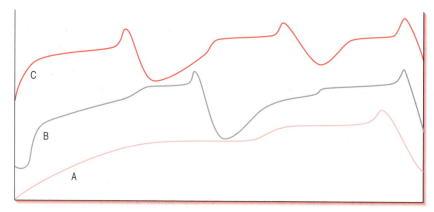

Figure 1.7   Types of periodization: monocycle (A), bi-cycle (B) and tri-cycle (C).

## Competition phase

This phase is determined from the competition dates and can be either simple or complex in nature. The former is usually divided into two periods; the first of these periods is reserved for the development of desirable fitness levels, while in the second, the acquired fitness has to be optimally maintained. The latter normally embraces three periods; the first is for minor competition, the second is a transitional cycle for regeneration, and the third is the main competitive cycle. Simple competition phases last 2–3 months, while complex ones last longer.

## Transition phase

This is a regeneration phase following a year's hard training and competition, which normally last 3–6 weeks. It is characterized by:

- decreases in training loads;
- lack of competition;
- maintenance of the acquired fitness levels;
- 'recharging of the energy batteries'.

## COMPONENTS OF PERIODIZATION – TRAINING CYCLES

Training volumes and intensities are inversely varied by cycle; increases in training volumes are accompanied by decreases in intensities and vice versa. However, the profile of each cycle depends on the competition level and on the specific demands of a given sporting event. In rowing, for instance, sustained distance and aerobic interval training in the boat make up most of the work, supplemented by some medium- to high-resistance and medium- to low-volume weight training in the gym. As rowers progress toward competition, training volumes are decreased and intensities increased. There is no evidence that periodization should be different for male and female competitors.

The longest blocks of training-time are called macrocycles; these could last from 2 months to a whole year. Smaller blocks are called mesocycles, usually 6–8 weeks' duration, and are typically incorporated within each macrocycle. The smallest training cycles, microcycles, usually last 1 week and constitute the mesocycles. In this chapter, the microcycle will be discussed first.

## Microcycle

A microcycle is a group of training units and it normally refers to a weekly training programme (Monday to Sunday). Each microcycle is constructed according to the objective of the training and can be repeated more than once in a period, for the required training elements to be improved and performance to be enhanced. There are several aspects to be considered in designing a microcycle (Ozolin 1971):

- perfect technique at submaximal and maximal intensity exercise;
- develop speed of short duration;
- develop anaerobic endurance;
- improve strength;
- develop muscular endurance at medium and low loads;
- develop muscular endurance with high and maximum intensity;
- develop cardiorespiratory endurance with maximum intensity;
- develop cardiorespiratory endurance with medium intensity.

## Structuring a microcycle

Structuring a microcycle requires two or three repeated training units of similar objectives and content. This repetitive nature is crucial for learning a technical element or developing a motor ability. This is also important for general endurance and strength purposes during the early phases of periodization, which require a training stimulus every second day. Approaching competition, specificity in training units takes place, with maximal specific endurance and strength development requiring two, and two to three training sessions per week, respectively.

Regeneration to avoid fatigue is the most important aspect of training. Therefore, after a strenuous training session, regeneration units have to be applied. The reason is that the athlete has to restore the energy lost, recuperate, and be physiological ready for the next session.

When designing a microcycle, the coach has to identify the objectives (i.e. the targeted physical component), the exact level of intensity and has to decide on the specific training methods that have to be applied. Each microcycle has to start with low- (50–70% of maximum) to moderate-intensity (70–90% of maximum) training units and to progress with subsequent intensity increases ranging from 90 to 100% of maximum. According to the period of the athlete's training programme and sport, the coach has to decide whether the athlete has to perform one or two training sessions per day. Based on low-intensity training, application of regeneration microcycles has to be considered in order to eliminate fatigue and restore energy supplies. However, a decrease in training demand facilitates supercompensation before competition and sets the body up for good performance (Bompa 1999). There are three models for the configuration of loading during the week (Fig. 1.8):

1. Low-load microcycle with only one maximum-load training session.
2. Medium-load microcycle with two maximum-load training units.
3. High-load microcycle with two maximum-load training units and a demanding exercise training programme between the two maximum-load units.

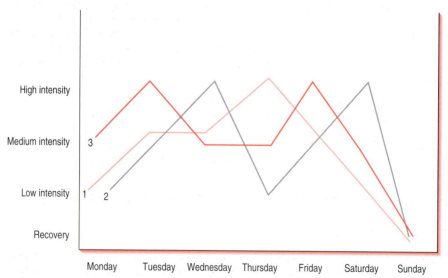

Figure 1.8   Three models for the exercise loading dynamics during training microcycles.

In general, variations in microcycle designing vary because the load in training is sport- and individual-specific. Nevertheless, based on training principles, the peak should be planned during one of the three middle days of the week. Medium- and high-load intensity or energy-demanding microcycles should be placed during the two ends of the week, always followed by one or two regeneration training sessions.

To ensure optimal training quality and quantity for a given microcycle, the following steps should be adopted. First, each day's intensity has to be planned for the whole week, to enable the athlete alternate intensities, energy systems, and the type of work. Secondly, the technical, tactical, or physical elements of training have to be separated, and decide which of them should be present at any given time. Finally, no more than two types of work, which strain the same energy system, should be applied.

## Mesocycle

Mesocycles are periods of similar objectives, content, training volumes and intensities. However, the last mesocycle before a key event normally incorporates two parts. In the first, the emphasis is on maximal intensity work specific to the endurance, strength and/or power requirements of the particular sport. The second part is reserved for the taper. This is thought to be a means of optimizing performance by allowing adequate recovery from intensive training prior to a significant competition. Evidence indicates that up to a 50% reduction of the usual training volume, in conjunction with short but intense workouts, provides the basis for optimal results (Houmard & Jones 1994).

## Macrocycle

A macrocycle consists of two or three mesocycles which are required to meet specific objective(s) and/or a desirable level of performance, although some differences exist from sport to sport. Careful consideration must be given in macrocycles longer than 8 weeks because the athletes' motivation might be reduced, a phenomenon that might compromise the adaptation processes.

Macrocycles that form the preparatory phase are usually the longest and their objectives are mainly dependent on the technical, tactical or physiological elements that need to be developed or perfected. Conversely, the competitive phase requires shorter macrocycles which end with the competition itself. Planners have to decide on the most important competition and prepare the athlete accordingly, giving less but enough attention to other athletic engagements. In general, in designing a macrocycle the following should be considered:

- objectives set for each microcycle and mesocycle;
- percentages of general, special and competition-specific training;
- number of training sessions according to the individual's available time;
- number of repetitions, sets, intervals, intensity and load-progression;
- degree of flexibility in changing the training methods when necessary.

## PERIODIZATION OF SELECTED PHYSICAL FITNESS ELEMENTS

## Aerobic endurance

Athletes exhibiting higher levels of aerobic endurance (or cardiorespiratory fitness) can exercise longer before fatigue develops and can continue exercising for more time in a state of fatigue than those with lower levels of endurance. Maximum oxygen uptake ($\dot{V}O_2$max) is a major indicator of endurance as it represents the maximum ability of an athlete to utilize oxygen. Improved aerobic endurance requires enhanced oxidative potential of muscle fibres, which is founded in an increased number and volume of mitochondria (increased mitochondrial density) and elevated activity of oxidative enzymes. Recovery rates are also highly related to endurance performance. Faster recovery allows the athlete to decrease rest intervals in and between training sessions, and to increase the overall training load.

Aerobic training brings about adaptations that influence the processes of energy transportation and use by the working muscle. Major cell and anatomical adaptations include increases in the size and number of mitochondria, density of capillaries, haemoglobin concentration, and left ventricular enlargement. These directly contribute to increments in $\dot{V}O_2$max, providing the foundation for improved physical performance. However, such increments have to take place in stages (or phases) during which the foundations for further improvements are established and the special needs of each sport are addressed. For example, on the basis of a single periodization model (monocycle), the athlete develops endurance in three phases; foundation of endurance, introduction of specific endurance, and specific endurance (see Ch. 4).

## PERIODIZATION FOR DEVELOPING ENDURANCE

### Foundation of endurance

The athlete builds or maintains the basic fitness levels required for further progression, improves general endurance and copes with fatigue. This phase lasts from 6 weeks up to more than 3 months depending on the desired level of adaptation, and takes place during the transition and preparatory phases of the annual plan (Fig. 1.9).

The most suitable training mode is that of steady-state exercise with moderate intensity for 30 minutes to more than 2 hours. As this phase progresses, adjustments in the training load must be made by primarily increasing volume and, to a lesser

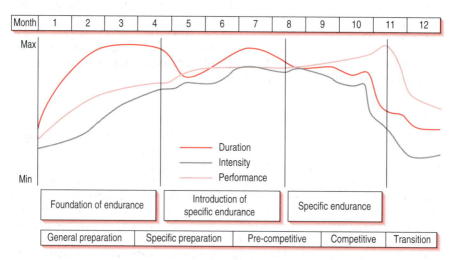

**Figure 1.9**   Duration, intensity and performance curves during each phase, for the development of endurance.

extent, intensity. This exercise mode does not place high levels of stress on the musculoskeletal or the physiological systems and the athlete trains below his/her lactate threshold (Pate & Branch 1992). Nevertheless, it does induce glycogen depletion in the muscle, increases lipid metabolism, and forces the body to maintain or enhance the acquired functional adaptations within the heart and muscle.

## Introduction of specific endurance

In this phase (Fig. 1.9), training aims to enhance the athlete's physiological adaptations and introduce aspects of sport-specific activities. Aerobic endurance is still the main component of training, although several elements of anaerobic activity are introduced into the programme. Depending on the complexity of the activity, and the adaptation rate of the athlete, this phase might last 2–4 months.

At the beginning of this phase, duration remains elevated while intensity increases progressively. After the desirable endurance levels have been reached, it is recommended that sport-specific activities during training be introduced. At this time, duration gradually decreases to eventually reach moderate levels, while the intensity of exercise is in the range of the athlete's lactate threshold. This should be applied towards the end of that period as it stresses the body to a considerable extent and may lead to negative effects if the underlying adaptations have not been achieved.

## Specific endurance

In this phase, the maximum potential performance of the athlete has to be addressed. The use of activities above the anaerobic threshold is introduced while intensity reaches the highest possible level with a concomitant decrease in duration (Fig. 1.9). Nevertheless, the duration curve remains generally higher than that of intensity to ensure that training focuses on the dominant energy system for performance (Bompa 1999). This phase lasts approximately 3 months and coincides with the precompetitive and competitive phases of the annual plan.

The most effective training mode is the intermittent interval training, which results in increased accumulation of lactic acid. Short rest intervals of up to 2 minutes are provided between the activities. This type of training allows the athlete to perform exercise of an increased total duration at an intensity that could not be tolerated for a prolonged period. At the end of this phase, and for the last week before the competition, both intensity and duration of training decrease so that the athlete supercompensates before the competition.

## STRENGTH

Strength is among the most important components for almost every sport. Strength training aims to increase the athlete's competition performance by: (a) enhancing the neural component of muscle contraction, and (b) augmenting the muscle-fibre size (Fig. 1.10). The latter has been based on the hypothesis that exercise training causes an accumulation of metabolites which specifically induce the adaptive synthesis of structural and enzyme proteins resulting in larger and more efficient muscle (Viru & Viru 2001). Consequently, muscle hypertrophy is the result of a cumulative effect of several training sessions arranged in particular training cycles.

Resistance training induces hypertrophy in muscle fibres of all types, particularly those designated as fast-twitch or type II fibres, the area occupied by which may increase by as much as 90%, mainly due to increased rates of protein synthesis and

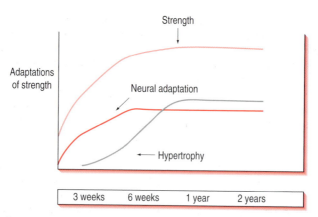

Figure 1.10  Strength training adaptations.

the associated augmentation in myofibrilar size (see Ch. 7). However, speed or power training results in a selective hypertrophy of fast-twitch glycolytic (type IIb) or fast-twitch oxidative (type IIa) fibres (see Ch. 6). It should be stressed here that stretching exercise can increase protein synthesis in the exercised muscle through a chain of events which involve satellite cell multiplication.

## Periodization for developing strength

Following the principles of periodization, a strength-training programme requires the arrangement of the annual plan into different phases, each having specific goals and objectives (Fig. 1.11). The first phase is reserved for neural adaptations; strength training should involve most muscle groups to prepare the athlete for the next phases and for future increases in strength load. A very important aspect during this first phase is the strengthening of the antagonist muscles, which will help to balance the musculature surrounding joints. Its duration depends on the athlete's strength-training background and it is sport-specific. For instance, in young athletes this phase lasts 8–10 weeks, whereas for athletes involved in strength-dependent sports it takes 3–5 weeks (Kraemer 1998).

The neural-adaptation phase is followed by the maximum strength training phase, which aims at developing the highest level of strength. This phase lasts 1–3 months depending on the sport's requirements and athlete's needs. Exercises are at intensities

| | Preparation | | Competition | | Transition |
|---|---|---|---|---|---|
| Strength training | General training | Specific training | Pre-competition training | Main competition training | Transition training |
| | **Anatomical adaptations** | **Maximum strength** | **Strength endurance & power** | **Maintenance** | **Active rest** |

Figure 1.11  Periodization of strength training: goals and objectives.

above 75% of maximum; this appears to be the most effective loading as it brings about the larger accumulation of non-protein nitrogen in the blood compared to lower exercise intensities.

This is followed by the 'conversion phase' (or third phase) that aims to convert the benefits gained during the previous phase into sport-specific strength (i.e. strength endurance, or power), and which normally lasts 4–8 weeks. The fourth phase is for maintenance, as the athlete approaches the competition. Strength training at this stage enters a very sport-specific phase which is short and intensive, and which must not generally exceed 45 minutes to 1 hour. The maintenance phase has to end 1 week prior to competition.

The last phase is for an 'active rest' characterized by a considerable reduction in the training intensity and volume. For the elite athlete, this 'rest' lasts between 4 and 6 weeks, which can be extended up to 10 weeks in competitors of lower calibre.

Ideally, strength training should be part of the athlete's plan to excel in every phase of the yearly plan. However, given that muscle utilizes glycogen as its main fuel, strength training has to be conducted during days on which the total energy demands are kept low. Following a demanding strength-training session, glycogen stores can be restored within 24 hours. Additional intensive exercise, along with strength-training, may extend glycogen restoration by up to 48 hours. To circumvent these difficulties, strength training microcycles should be arranged according to whether the aims are for low, medium or high training loads (Fig. 1.12). It should be noted here that the weekly frequency of strength sessions is higher during the preparatory (four or five sessions) compared to competition (two or three sessions) period.

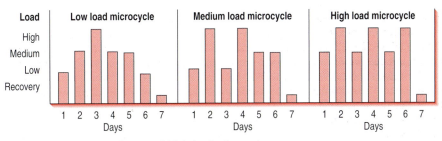

Figure 1.12   Low-, medium- and high-load microcycles.

## KEY POINTS

1. The human body responds to exercise-stress in three stages, i.e. shock, resistance and exhaustion or fatigue. Exercise training with the use of periodization procedures stresses the body's systems and factions to adapt at a higher level without causing prolonged fatigue. Thus, periodization is the purposeful variation of a training programme over time, so that the competitor will approach his/her optimal adaptive potential just prior to an important event.

2. Not all sports or athletes have the same competition calendar. For instance, several sports require their competitors to participate in just one major competition every year. Training plans that support these needs are different from those serving more than one performance peak each year. An unloading phase is required following each peak for the athlete to regenerate and to be ready for the following cycle. Models with more than three peaks within a year do not allow the athlete to adapt properly.

3. Using the principles of periodization, each annual training cycle normally consists of three phases (preparation, competition and transition) with different aims and training context.
4. Based on time-lengths, annual training cycles can also be divided into smaller sections. The longest section (macrocycle) could last from 2 months to a whole year. Smaller sections (mesocycles) usually are 6–8 weeks long. The smallest training cycle (microcycle) usually lasts for just 1 week.
5. Periodization of aerobic power and muscular strength involve incremental work in stages (or phases) during which the foundations for further improvements are established and the special needs of each sport are addressed.

## References

Bompa TD 1999 Periodization: theory and methodology of training, 4th edn. Human Kinetics. Champaign IL

Budgett R, Newsholme E, Lehmann M et al 2000 Redefining the overtraining syndrome as the unexplained underperformance syndrome. British Journal of Sports Medicine, 34:67–68.

Davis SN, Galassetti P, Wasserman DH, Tate D 2000 Effects of gender on neuroendocrine and metabolic counterregulatory responses to exercise in normal man. Journal of Clinical Endocrinology and Metabolism 85:224–230

Fleck SJ 1999 Periodized strength training: A critical review. Journal of Strength and Conditioning Research 13:82–89

Harre D (ed.) 1982 Trainingslehre. Sportverlag, Berlin

Houmard JA, Jones RA 1994 Effects of taper on swim performance. Practical implications. Sports Medicine 17:224–232

Komi PV, Hakkinen K 1988 Strength and power. In Dirix A, Knuttgen HG, Tittel K (eds) The encyclopaedia of sports medicine: The Olympic book of sports medicine, vol 1. Blackwell, Oxford, p 181–193

Koutedakis Y 2000 Burnout in dance: the physiological viewpoint. Journal of Dance Medicine and Science 4:122–127

Koutedakis Y, Sharp NCC 1999 The fit and healthy dancer. John Wiley, Chichester

Koutedakis Y, Budgett R, Faulmann L 1990 Rest in underperforming elite competitors. British Journal of Sports Medicine 24:248–252

Kraemer WJ 1998 Periodization in resistance training. IDEA Personal Trainer 9:27–34

Kraemer WJ, Fleck SJ, Evans WJ 1996 Strength and power training: physiological mechanisms of adaptation. Exercise and Sports Science Reviews 24:363–397

McArdle WD, Katch FI, Katch VL 2001 Exercise physiology. Energy, nutrition and human performance. Lippincott, Williams & Wilkins; Baltimore

Matsuda J, Zernicke R, Vailas A et al 1986 Structural and mechanical adaptation. Journal of Applied Physiology 60:2028–2034

Moritani T, deVries HA 1979 Neural factors versus hypertrophy in the time course of muscle strength gain. American Journal of Physical Medicine 58:115–130

Neufer PD, Costill DL, Fielding RA et al 1987 Effect of reduced training on muscular strength and endurance in competitive swimmers. Medicine and Science in Sports and Exercise 19:486–490

Noakes T 2001 Lore of running. Oxford University Press, Oxford

Ozolin NG 1971 Athlete's training system for competition. Phyzkultura I sports, Moscow

Pate RR, Branch JD 1992 Training for endurance sport. Medicine and Science in Sports and Exercise 24:340–343

Steinacker JM 1993 Physiological aspects of training in rowing. International Journal of Sports Medicine 14:3–10

Stone MH, O'Bryant HS, Schilling BK et al 1999 Periodization: effects of manipulating volume and intensity. Journal of Strength and Conditioning 21:54–60

Viru A, Viru M 2001 Biochemical monitoring of sport training. Human Kinetics, Champaign IL

## Further reading

Åstrand PO, Rodahl K 2003 Textbook of work physiology, 4th edn. Human Kinetics, Champaign IL

Bompa T 1999 Periodization. Theory and methodology of training. Human Kinetics, Champaign IL

Dick FW 2002 Sports training principles, 4th edn. A & C Black, UK

# Chapter 2

# Training specificity

Richard Godfrey and Gregory Whyte

## LEARNING OBJECTIVES:

This chapter is intended to ensure that the reader:

1. Understands the concept of specificity.
2. Appreciates the physiological adaptations associated with specific types of training.
3. Appreciates the meaning of specificity within the context of some selected sports.
4. Understands the role of cross-training in athletic performance.
5. Appreciates the importance, practical applications and limitations of specificity in the field and laboratory based testing of athletes.

## INTRODUCTION

Within the context of sports performance there are a number of basic principles which, when appropriately applied, can aid optimal adaptation. Collectively these are known as the 'training principles' and they include: individuality, reversibility, progression, overload (progressive overload), periodization and specificity. Chapter 1 examined the principles of progressive overload, reversibility and periodization. It is the aim of this chapter to focus on the principle of specificity with reference to individuality of training prescription, and its relationship to the other key principles of training.

Training specificity is encapsulated by the acronym 'SAID' – specific adaptations to imposed demands – and is defined as:

'A basic training principle which states that in order to improve a particular component of physical fitness, a person must emphasise that component in training. A training programme must stress the physiological systems used to perform a particular activity in order to achieve specific training adaptations' (Kent 1998, p 402).

In order to optimally stress the physiological systems associated with performance, three components of specificity exist: (i) skill specificity, (ii) muscle group specificity, and (iii) energy system specificity. Often athletes and coaches interpret the definition of specificity as the requirement to replicate performance in terms of the mode of exercise and pace in all training sessions. Indeed, there are numerous examples of coaches and athletes who think that the only way to train is at race pace as that is the pace they must specifically learn to cope with. One example of the folly of this is the marathon runner who only ever runs at race pace. The athlete may be unaware that the best training pace to improve the body's ability to minimize depletion of carbohydrate stores and lactate production, and hence reduce the onset of fatigue, is to work at a pace associated with 'lactate threshold', a pace that is generally faster than marathon pace (see Ch. 4). Indeed, there are often a number of physiological factors underpinning performance that must all be addressed if performance is to be optimized. Thus, specificity is best addressed when considering those stimuli leading to adaptations that allow the individual to best cope with the physiological demands of the 'target' activity. Accordingly, there is no single intensity, duration or frequency to prepare the individual for all of the physiological demands of a given sport or event. Hence, training will always require a range of intensities and durations. The elements of training prescription are specific to the individual and his/her current level of conditioning. Further, the role of supplemental training, in the form of cross training, may enhance the adaptive response and avoid the potential for over use injuries and possible overtraining resulting in underperformance (see Ch. 9).

Knowledge of the underpinning physiology associated with training adaptation is crucial to an understanding of specificity. This underpinning physiology knowledge will also assist in understanding the secondary and even tertiary adaptations that are possible as a result of a training stimulus. In this chapter specificity of training will be examined by first selecting a number of individual attributes (strength and power, flexibility, speed, endurance). Second, the effects of some selected, commonly applied, training sessions on tissues and on physiological systems will be explored. Third, a few individual sports will be examined. In this way there will first be a reductionist view of training specificity, leading through to the effects of training type and ending with a reintegration of information such that a whole systems/whole person perspective is achieved. This will allow greater ease of application to 'real-world' performance. Finally, the chapter will end with a brief examination of the importance of specificity when testing athletes in the field and laboratory.

## Summary box 2.1

Specificity is best addressed when considering those stimuli that result in adaptations allowing the individual to best cope with the physiological demands of the 'target' activity. Specificity addresses the three key areas of skill, muscle group and energy system. There is no single intensity, duration or frequency to prepare the individual for all of the physiological demands of a given sport or event. Training, therefore, requires a range of intensities, durations and frequencies to optimize training adaptation and, therefore, performance.

# SPECIFICITY

A specific stimulus results in specific adaptation. If the stimulus is reduced or removed reversibility or detraining begins. In every biological system there is a tendency to revert to the lowest 'energy state' for that individual. This is largely pre-programmed; in other words, it is dependent on heredity and such a state exists as a result of evolution. In our ancient past humans evolved as hunter gatherers with developed systems that protected the organism against times when food was in short supply. A good example of this is the muscle growth inhibitor myostatin. Muscle is extremely energy costly and so it makes sense that there should be a limit to the development of muscle beyond that required for normal function. The genotype of the organism is the result of genetic heritability that is further influenced by environmental pressures. The result is 'phenotype': the function and/or appearance. Remove the environmental pressure and the organism will revert to 'type' (i.e. genotype). Let's take an example. Aerobic power ($\dot{V}O_2$max) has a large genetic component but it can also be influenced by environmental factors (e.g. training). Hence your genetic 'pre-programming' may mean that at 25 years of age, without any training, your $\dot{V}O_2$max might be 60 mL.kg$^{-1}$.min$^{-1}$. With training this might improve by 20% to 72 mL.kg$^{-1}$.min$^{-1}$. Remove training and you revert to your genotype of 60 mL.kg$^{-1}$.min$^{-1}$. Accordingly, to maintain a given trained state requires regular application of the stimulus that created it. Research has demonstrated that detraining can begin between 2 and 6 weeks after cessation of the exercise stimulus (Mujika & Padilla 2000). To prevent detraining an appropriate regular stimulus is required. Clearly, it is not possible to achieve optimal conditioning of every physiological parameter or system at once. Hence a cycling of stimuli is required and so specificity, and preventing detraining, forms the basis for the rationale behind the development of periodization (see Ch. 1).

# BIOCHEMISTRY AND MOLECULAR EXERCISE PHYSIOLOGY

There is a growing trend throughout sport and exercise science towards examination and elucidation of the molecular processes that operate as a result of the exercise stimulus. This is a reflection of the same trend operating throughout the life sciences. Although this has been ongoing for almost 15 years, the early completion of the human genome project in 2003 has accelerated interest and research into molecular, cell and genetic biology. Much of the research in this field in exercise science has focused on two major areas: strength and endurance; however, research into other areas is expanding. In broad terms, the general principle is that exercise represents a broad class of differing stimuli each of which initiates adaptation signalling and gene regulation. The nature of that signalling, the gene regulated, the subsequent cascade of events, and ongoing modification of an initiated cascade, are all entirely dependent on a specific stimulus. So, again, specificity plays a key role.

Exercise can activate signal transduction pathways in a number of specific ways through growth factors and hormones binding to membrane and nuclear receptors (as discussed below), through changes such as a flux in the concentration of $Ca^{2+}$, mechanical stretch or tension, energy status, hypoxia and cell damage. Any one of these examples (from a vast array of possible stimuli) will each, in isolation or in combination, initiate a specific response or pathway activation. As one pathway is initiated, crosstalk between transduction proteins can occur, mainly, by covalent phosphorylation. As the final step in the pathway, a nuclear transduction signal is activated and translocated into the cell's nucleus. This can then act as a transcription factor (to aid the copying of a transcript of the relevant portion of the cell's DNA) or activate existing nucleus-dwelling transcription factors. Depending on the tissue and the nature of the stimulus (mode, duration, intensity) exercise stimulates: (i) expression of growth factors, (ii) synthesis of contractile proteins, enzymes and other functional proteins, (iii) satellite cell proliferation and donation of nuclei to skeletal muscle fibres, (iv) mitochondrial biogenesis, and (v) apoptosis (i.e. programmed cell death) (Wackerhage & Woods 2002).

---

**Summary box 2.2**

Specificity is key at the molecular level. Depending on the tissue and the nature of the stimulus (mode, duration, intensity) exercise stimulates expression of (i) growth factors, (ii) contractile proteins, enzymes and other functional proteins, (iii) satellite cell proliferation and donation of nuclei to skeletal muscle fibres, (iv) mitochondrial biogenesis, and (v) apoptosis (programmed cell death).

---

## TRAINING FOR STRENGTH AND POWER

### Strength

Improvements in strength occur initially as a result of neuromuscular adaptations associated with an improved recruitment of motor units (Sale 1988). Although changes in muscle cross-sectional area also begin in the initial stages of a strength-specific training programme this only begins to contribute to strength as hypertrophy becomes more observable. There is a direct relationship between muscle cross-sectional area and the force it is capable of generating. Fast-twitch (type II) fibres have larger cross-sectional area and generate more force than slow-twitch (type I) fibres. Hypertrophy is dependent on increased myofibrillar protein synthesis and translocation of nuclei from satellite cells. These two parameters are regulated by a number of factors. For many years the main explanation for muscle hypertrophy was believed to be encapsulated in the 'somatomedin hypothesis' in which, originally, somatic growth was believed to be controlled by growth hormone (hGH) and mediated by circulating insulin-like growth factor (IGF-1) of hepatic origin.

A number of studies over the last 10–15 years have, however, demonstrated a wider distribution of IGF-1 and it is now accepted that many tissues have their own IGFs which effect their actions by autocrine or paracrine means. ('Autocrine' means that the tissue releases the substance which then acts on the tissue of origin; 'paracrine' refers to a substance which acts close to the point of secretion – as opposed to 'endocrine', which refers to a substance released into the general circulation and which has effects on tissues distal to the point of secretion.) Indeed, many specific tissue IGFs are increasingly being renamed; in particular, there is a suggestion that muscle-specific IGF should be renamed MGF (mechano growth factor) (Yang et al 1996). This term also recognizes that this growth factor can be released in response to muscle contraction per se (in a similar way that muscle contraction per se can facilitate the peripheral uptake of glucose in the absence of insulin).

Recent evidence suggests that growth hormone (GH) has a more direct role in increases in muscle strength and hypertrophy than previously believed. It is already widely accepted that exercise, particularly high-intensity resistance exercise, stimulates GH secretion. As a result, increases in muscle strength and size are likely to be the combined effect of the somatomedin hypothesis coupled with the direct action of GH on myostatin (Liu et al 2003). The normal function of myostatin is to 'switch off' muscle growth and so mutations of the gene for myostatin generally result in individuals that have greater muscle hypertrophy and, coincidently, a lower fat mass.

Because heavy resistance exercise tends to target the fast-twitch motor units it is primarily these that undergo major adaptation with increases in myofibrillar protein synthesis. Strength training specifically targets fast-twitch fibres, leading to an increased cross-sectional area further differentiating force production and cross-sectional area between slow- and fast-twitch motor units. While fast-twitch motor units generate much more force than slow-twitch motor units, they also fatigue more rapidly.

One non-specific and perhaps surprising benefit of training for strength is an attendant increase in local muscular endurance. Improved muscular endurance is linked to an increased strength of individual motor units and so when working with a standardized, sub-maximal load, once strength is improved through appropriate training, the load represents a lesser stress on the muscle. This reduced stress is primarily associated with the need to recruit fewer motor units for the same sub-maximal load and hence as working motor units become fatigued other motor units can be brought into play.

Specificity exists in a number of areas when considering resistance training; strength will, in general, only be increased in those muscle groups which are activated during the exercise. Movement pattern is also important because, particularly in the initial stages of strength development, adaptation is largely via neural activation (see Ch. 7). Neural feedback from joint proprioceptors also ensures the joint angles at which training occurs will specifically relate to strength improvements at those same joint angles. It is therefore important, where safety and injury prevention allow, that resistance training reflects the specific range of motion of the target activity.

### Summary box 2.3

Originally the mechanism for hypertrophy was described solely by the somatomedin hypothesis. Somatic growth was believed to be stimulated by the action of growth hormone (GH) and mediated by circulating IGF-1 of hepatic origin. It is now known, however, that local IGF-1 (renamed mechano-growth factor, MGF) is probably a more important mediator of muscle growth. In addition, MGF can be stimulated by muscle contraction per se. A more direct role for GH is also recognized in muscle hypertrophy in targeting and inhibiting myostatin, the factor that normally inhibits muscle growth.

## Local muscular endurance

'Local muscular endurance is the degree to which specific muscle groups can continue contracting against a given load in a given period of time or for a given number of repetitions. It is determined by the type of muscular contraction, the speed of contraction, the cadence of repetitions, and the magnitude of the resistance. The limiting factors to muscular endurance exist within the muscle groups being exercised and their neuromuscular control, and are not associated with cardiorespiratory/cardiovascular factors' (Jenkins 1997, p 154).

Local muscular endurance is usually a mix of both aerobic and anaerobic endurance and once the demands of the sport or activity are identified training should be structured to address these demands.

Training to improve local muscular endurance generally requires the imposition of fatigue, but in a controlled manner, as fatigue often acts as a powerful stimulus to adaptation. Changes in energy substrates (fuels) within cells act as a gauge in this instance and increasingly the enzyme adenosine monophosphate kinase (AMPK) is recognized as an energy sensor initiating cell signalling that effects adaptation. Fatigue can be better controlled by using interval training where intervals of work are separated by periods of active or passive recovery. Circuit training is traditionally a more general way of addressing improvements in local muscular endurance, which also has some benefits for cardiovascular conditioning, and will be covered in detail later in the chapter.

It is clear that strength training results in specific adaptations of fast-twitch motor units that are joint angle specific. What is also apparent, however, is that strength training can lead to non-specific adaptation of local muscular endurance leading to a broader role for strength training than may be immediately obvious.

## Power

In the context of muscle, power can be described as the force produced per unit time and so is largely the result of entraining the motor unit to recruit muscle fibres rapidly. Accordingly, this is largely a neuromuscular phenomenon where strength is a prerequisite and speed is an important cofactor. Power cannot be considered without reference to the interaction between tendon and muscle (i.e. the tendon–muscle complex) and the specific training which can optimize this interaction to allow maximal power generation. The relationship between muscle and tendon can be complex but in many movements can be described as muscle causing the tendon to stretch (storage of potential energy) prior to recoil of the tendon (kinetic energy/energy return). Designing strength training programmes therefore requires an understanding of the movement pattern and how muscle and tendon behave during that movement. At certain times of year it is important to improve muscle strength and power and at other times improvement of tendon elasticity is the aim. Hence periodization is again demonstrated to be intimately linked to specificity, in this case in attempting to optimize force generation (see Ch. 6).

Specific training focusing on power has led to the development of specialist training techniques involving explosive movements in which adaptation relies on the rapid switch from an eccentric (muscle lengthening during contraction) to a concentric contraction (muscle shortening during contraction) i.e. plyometrics. Typically, this type of training comprises the use of hopping, bounding and jumping performed with maximal effort. The emphasis is on very short foot–ground contact times when training explosive power in the legs for example. Exercises can also be used to develop explosive power in the upper body in a similar way. For legs another means of improving explosive power is by using drop jumping from a height of 1.10 m as demonstrated by Verhoshansky (1986). In drop jumping the individual drops from a platform 1.10 m high and, immediately following landing, jumps up as high as possible. In general, plyometric training has been suggested as being particularly useful in sports demanding high anaerobic power or explosive movements. This includes sports such as basketball, volleyball, weightlifting and sprinting or athletic events requiring jumping or throwing (see Ch. 6). In theory the benefits in such training are derived from adaptations in the central nervous system (CNS) and the muscle. The extreme transient stretch may facilitate neural adaptation while the extremely high tension, derived as the combined result of several times body weight landing and muscle contracting to overcome this and lift the body off the ground, results in muscle adaptation. Counter-intuitive to this, as it provides an argument which does not appear to support specificity, is the recent use of plyometric training in middle distance running, which is discussed further below.

The highly explosive nature of plyometric activity is in stark contrast to rhythmic aerobic activity; however, research evidence suggests plyometrics training may be of value in middle distance running. Paavolainen et al (1999) examined the effect of substituting 32% of training volume for explosive strength training in the training programmes of elite cross-country runners and demonstrated a significant improvement in 5 km running time and in running economy. Hence, again we can see that the issue of specificity is less straightforward than might be, at first, supposed.

## Training for speed

In terms of whole body displacement (movement from one place to another) speed is the distance travelled per unit time. Speed, however, can also refer to the ability to move, not just the whole body but body segments fast. With respect to specificity, training for speed requires attempts to move as fast as possible. There is however, a proviso to this and that is where accuracy of movement is also required. Fitts law states that accuracy is related to the inverse of speed. In other words there is a trade-off between speed and accuracy. This is particularly important in racket and combat sports, especially when learning a new skill, but becomes less important once the skill is overlearned. Accordingly, new skills are practiced at slow speeds and speed built up gradually as the skill becomes 'engrained'.

Speed drills generally involve short duration maximal speed efforts with long-duration recoveries so that fatigue does not interfere with speed development. Those individuals with a higher genetic predisposition for fast-twitch muscle fibres will have faster speed and speed of movement but everyone can improve speed with specific training. In general, increased force of muscle contraction is required for greater speed. This requires more myofibrillar protein and hence, in general, increases in speed are accompanied by muscle hypertrophy as fast-twitch fibres are targeted: those with inherently larger cross-sectional area (CSA). Type IIa fibres become more like type IIx fibres by increasing their glycolytic capacity, and type IIx fibres become more glycolytic. Thus, both are more able to produce power rapidly. With respect to rapid limb movement there are a number of techniques that can be employed. Simply attempting to move the limb fast, using the desired movement pattern, can improve speed. The use of heavy or weighted objects used in the sports-specific movement are often used to improve the amount of energy required of the muscle. Thus, it is common to use weighted balls in ball games, weighted rackets in racket sports and weighted boxing gloves for boxing training. All of these will improve the muscle's ability to generate force. However, after a few minutes of use if these are substituted for the non-weighted (lighter) implements, and the individual asked to move the limb as fast as possible, training speed is improved. Much of this improvement is a result of improved kinesthetics as propriceptor feedback is facilitated and the sensation of speed is enhanced associated with a reduction of the normal process of neuromuscular inhibition. Carrying out such drills regularly can result in a chronic improvement in limb speed. Care is warranted to focus training on sports-specific movements as adaptations are skill- and joint-angle-specific.

## TRAINING FOR ENDURANCE PERFORMANCE

### Cardiopulmonary endurance

Cardiopulmonary, cardiovascular or cardiorespiratory endurance are the terms used, often interchangeably, when referring to the endurance developed in the cardiovascular and respiratory systems, a necessity for improving endurance in whole-body rhythmic exercise. This, for example, includes running, cycling, swimming, rowing and cross-country skiing.

In whole-body activity, improvements in endurance can reflect changes in aerobic power, lactate threshold, lactate production and clearance, lactate tolerance, acid–base balance in muscle and systemically, fractional utilization, muscle temperature, human stress proteins, mitochondria, structural proteins, globular 'enzymatic' proteins, gene activation, trainability (genetic factors) and so on.

---

**Summary box 2.4**

Endurance involves both local muscular endurance and 'whole body endurance' or cardiopulmonary endurance. For improving local muscular endurance, training centres around adaptations which will limit future fatigue of specific muscle groups. This generally involves exercises using high numbers of repetitions and low loads. For improved cardiopulmonary endurance, whole-body rhythmic exercise utilizing large muscle groups for periods of 30–90 minutes is generally required. In many sports with a high endurance requirement specific physiological prerequisites and determinants can be identified. In general, these include $\dot{V}O_2$max, fractional utilization, lactate threshold (LT), oxygen and movement economy and power or speed at LT and at maximal intensity. The relative importance of each of these depends on the intensity and duration of competition. Hence the fraction of a training programme dedicated to each should be specific to the demands of the activity and the current conditioned state of the athlete.

---

## SPECIFICITY AND TRIATHLON

Triathlon is comprised of three events completed back to back and continuously. These are swimming, cycling and running, usually performed in that order. The main distances are Ironman distance (swim 3 km, cycle 180 km and run 42 km), Olympic distance (swim 1500 m, cycle 40 km, run 10 km) and sprint distances which can vary considerably (one example is swim 600 m, cycle 25 km, run 5 km). The main elite distances tend to be those of Ironman and Olympic distance, with sprint distances largely contested by recreational or club-level triathletes. Physiologically triathlon provides a very good example of the importance of specificity with respect to the level of conditioning found in each discipline. The rapid change from one discipline to another, i.e. from swimming to cycling and cycling to running, is known as transition. In recognition of the physiological impact of transition it has often been referred to as the 'fourth discipline'. With this in mind many triathletes undertake 'brick' sessions involving the combination of swimming and cycling and/or cycling and running in a single session. In general, most triathletes practice and train for the transition from cycling to running. Relatively few, however, train the transition from swimming to cycling because generally it is quite impractical to do so. The change from supine, predominantly upper body exercise to upright, predominantly lower body exercise, together with the removal of hydrostatic pressure associated with water submersion in swimming, results in a significant physiological strain during the swim to bike transition. The inclusion of swim to bike transitions should, therefore, form a key part of triathlon training.

Swimming exercise elicits specific physiological responses which are imposed as a result of the body being horizontal, submerged in cool/cold water and using the arm musculature as the primary means of locomotion. Hence, for the same relative intensity of work, heart-rate is lower while stroke volume, blood pressure and blood lactate are all higher. After working in this way for periods lasting 4 minutes (sprint distance) to 1 hour (Ironman distance) a steady state is achieved with all physiological systems responding to the specific stress of swimming exercise. The rapid change in modality to cycling, where the body mass is supported, the body is upright and the primary muscles of locomotion are in the lower body, represents a considerable functional stress. Similarly, to then change to running where, although the body is still upright, the body mass is no longer supported and the primary muscles of locomotion are in the lower leg, again causes functional stress.

Novice triathletes often report feeling fatigued when leaving the swim and trying to cycle with perception of exertion being focused in the chest and legs. When switching from cycling to running the legs can feel heavy and the joints 'stiff'. Brick training; alternating between swimming and cycling and between cycling and running, appears to result in positive adaptations. The primary adaptations following brick sessions are probably associated with a more rapid shift in blood flow to the working musculature combined with an improved pacing strategy and experience. Further, the skill development accrued during brick sessions will result in a reduction in the transition times between disciplines. Accordingly, as a result of brick sessions, athletes report that during competition they adjust from one discipline to the other more quickly, resulting in performance enhancement. Examples of brick sessions:

    5 × (400 m swim/10 minutes cycling)
    3-mile run, 10-mile cycle, 3-mile run
    3 × (10 minutes cycling/10 minutes running)

Establishing all factors underpinning performance is crucial to allow specific training prescription. This may not be a simple task, particularly in those sports in which physiological, environmental or skill demands of the sport change throughout performance. Specific testing and monitoring of athletes in the field and laboratory allows an interrogation of the factors underpinning performance, together with profiling of athletes and the monitoring of training adaptation across time.

## CROSS-TRAINING

The advent of triathlon has led to a popularization of cross-training in recent years. Cross-training, however, has been employed by coaches and athletes for decades in an attempt to optimize the training stimulus and enhance performance. Despite the fact that cross-training is not a new approach for improving performance, limited scientific evidence exists examining the transfer of training effects.

Cross-training can be defined in a number of ways: (i) the simultaneous training for two or more events (i.e. triathlon); (ii) the cross-transfer of training effects from one sport to another; (iii) the conveyance of training effects from one one limb to the contralateral or ipsilateral limb (Tanaka 1994). Irrespective of the definition the primary goal of cross-training is performance enhancement or maintenance. Anecdotally performance enhancement from cross-training may be obtained through a number of mechanisms: (i) direct improvement in performance from an alternative mode of exercise; (ii) improved training compliance associated with a more interesting/diverse training programme; (iii) reduced incidence of overuse injury; (d) maintained training stimulus during rehabilitation from injury.

Studies examining cross-training have focused on the transfer effects of: (i) dissimilar modes of exercise i.e. swimming and running; (ii) modes of exercise employing similar muscle groups i.e. running and cycling; (iii) simultaneous strength and endurance training (Loy et al 1995). The vast majority of studies have used $\dot{V}O_2$max as the criterion measure in the absence of performance measures. Thus, the conclusions drawn from these studies should be viewed with caution as changes in $\dot{V}O_2$max do not necessarily confer changes in performance.

The findings of studies examining cross-training using dissimilar modes of exercise in highly trained athletes suggest that limited benefit is gained from the combination of exercise modes whose principle locomotor muscle groups are different, i.e. swimming and running. While the benefit of this type of cross-training in highly trained individuals is of limited value, enhanced performance may be observed in less conditioned individuals. Further, this type of cross-training may improve long-term training compliance in recreational athletes. Despite the absence of performance changes for the highly trained athlete, cross-training using dissimilar modes of exercise may be valuable during rehabilitation where participation in sport-specific exercise is limited.

The majority of studies examining cross-training using similar modes of exercise have focused on cycling versus running training. This type of training has received increasing support based upon anecdotal evidence. Indeed, there is an increasing trend in elite sport to use cross-training of similar modes during the off-season. Rowers and canoeists often use cross-country skiing during the winter phase of training, and skiers use cycling as a training tool during the summer months. The use of similar muscle groups and energy systems (aerobic and anaerobic) has underpinned the belief that cross-training may be beneficial. While running and cycling use major muscles in the lower body, cycling predominantly uses the quadriceps muscle group, whereas running uses the plantar flexors. Further, neuromuscular adaptations associated with the acquisition of skill will be limited between different exercise modalities. Indeed, even within a particular mode of training, some training conditions, such as posture (e.g. upright versus supine cycling) and training terrain (uphill versus flat running), result in specific adaptations.

The benefits of cross-training using similar modes of exercise appear to be more closely linked with improved performance in highly trained athletes than those observed with dissimilar modes of exercise. Data suggest, however, that the greater the level of conditioning to begin with the smaller the relative improvement observed.

Cross-training is a commonly used training tool. Evidence supporting the efficacy of cross-training, however, is limited. For the highly trained athlete, cross-training may be beneficial during rehabilitation to maintain general conditioning or as a means of reducing the potential for overuse injury and boredom associated with a single sport focus. It is clear, however, that cross-training effects never exceed those induced by specific training.

## CIRCUIT TRAINING

Circuit training is composed of a number of specific exercises targeted at muscle groups (and often skills) involved in the target activity. In order to stress muscular endurance optimally, recovery periods between exercises are often relatively short to allow only partial recovery.

There are a large number of formats that can be used with circuit training; the following is one example of many. On the first circuit the individual must attempt to complete the greatest number of repetitions possible in a selected time interval. Enough rest is given between exercises to allow full recovery. The number of reps achieved for each exercise is halved and on the second occasion each exercise, with the calculated number of reps, is completed one after the other without a break. This is one circuit and any number of circuits can be programmed but the whole is conducted continuously, without breaks, against the clock. Improvement over weeks is determined as a faster time for a given number of circuits. After a number of weeks the individual can be re-tested as on the first occasion or the exercises can be changed and the whole process re-commenced. While generally adopted for improved muscular endurance, circuit training can be employed to target a variety of performance variables by altering the number of sets, number of repetitions, and recovery duration. Table 2.1 suggests the number of repetitions generally used for specific aims.

## TRAINING FOR FLEXIBILITY

Many coaches question the need for specific training to address improvements in flexibility or range of movement. Their argument is that the athlete should not have too much flexibility as this could impair performance. To some degree this is true, as we have seen above in training for strength and power if the muscle does not provide enough stiffness then less energy can be stored in the tendon leading to a reduction in force generation. Some coaches also insist that the athlete need only be flexible enough to meet the demands of their sport and hence performing the sports-specific movements will adequately address these flexibility needs. This may be perfectly true for distance running and other closed sports where there is little or no challenge to the range of movement a joint must work through. This could, however, be further debated for open sports where the nature of the event or the nature of play is unpredictable and may force a joint to attempt a range of movement for which it is not adequately prepared. In sports and activities where more extreme

Table 2.1   The number of repetitions usually associated with development of specific conditioning

| Development of | Repetitions |
| --- | --- |
| Strength | 4–8 |
| Strength-endurance | 8–12 |
| Local muscular endurance | 14–25 |
| Endurance | 30–40 |

ranges of movements are required, such as martial arts, gymnastics and dance, additional supplementary training is required which specifically addresses flexibility. Where flexibility training is agreed as necessary for a given activity two forms should be addressed: static and dynamic flexibility.

Static flexibility represents the range that a joint or muscle can achieve and is limited by the structure of bones, joints and muscles and by muscle tone. Improving static flexibility involves holding the joint at the limit of its range for a minimum of 7 seconds. The reason for this is that, when stretched, the muscle proprioceptor, the muscle spindle, is stretched, causing a train of afferent signalling to the spinal cord. The resulting efferent signal causes the muscle to contract, resisting the stretch. Holding the stretch for at least 7 seconds allows the golgi tendon organ (GTO) to be activated, inhibiting the stretch reflex and allowing a reflex relaxation and subsequently the muscle/joint can be stretched further. This process, whereby the GTO inhibits the muscle spindle, is known as autogenic inhibition. All of the joints requiring greater flexibility must be stretched in this way. Where movement is required at the limit to the range of movement, however, dynamic flexibility is also required.

Dynamic flexibility refers to the range of movement through which a muscle/joint can act when in motion and, as such, it can be described as the limit of active range of movement of the joint. Dynamic flexibility is limited by static flexibility and by nervous system function and co-ordination. Static flexibility limits dynamic flexibility to limit joint excursions beyond the maximum range of static flexibility during movement that could result in injury. Improvements in dynamic flexibility are extremely important in high-speed movement and so should be a major goal for many sports. A session which aims to work on improvements in dynamic flexibility should begin with sports-specific movement patterns performed at low speed where the limits to range of movement are not explored. Throughout the session the speed and range of movement pattern should be increased until full-speed movements are being performed to the limit of the range of movement.

In sports where flexibility is a key component, increasing flexibility should typically involve three to five stretching sessions per week. Because flexibility is significantly affected by the temperature of soft-tissue structures, sessions are most effective when the target tissue temperature is increased. Accordingly, stretching for improving long-term flexibility is best performed at the end of a training session. Any stretching conducted as part of the warm-up should be 'non-aggressive' and should only aim to have joints and muscles feel comfortable when approaching the limits to the joint's current range of movement (Popov 2001).

### Summary box 2.5

Depending on the sport, improvements in both static and dynamic flexibility should be considered. Static flexibility improvement requires the joint to be taken to the limit of its range of movement and the stretch held for a minimum of 7 seconds. Active static stretching, including PNF stretching, can involve a partner who helps to fix the stretch at the limit of the range of movement while the athlete exerts a maximal contraction, for 7 seconds, resisting the stretch. This can help to stretch antagonist muscle groups and may potentiate stretching of the agonists. A dynamic flexibility session should begin with gentle movements in which the range of movement is only just challenged and over the course of the session very gradually build until at the end range of movement is severely challenged and in an explosive fashion.

# SPECIFICITY IN THE PHYSIOLOGICAL ASSESSMENT OF ATHLETES

Laboratory- and field-based physiological assessments of the athlete are fundamental elements in training prescription. Physiological assessment is used to: (i) identify physiological parameters underpinning performance, (ii) profile athletes, and (iii) assess training adaptation and programme efficacy. A detailed examination of physiological testing protocols is beyond the scope of this text; however, a brief overview of the role of laboratory- and field-based testing is presented here. For a more detailed review of sports-specific testing protocols the reader is directed to the work of the Australian Institute of Sport (Australian Sports Commission 2000) and the British Association of Sport and Exercise Science (BASES 1997). The following section examines the method of establishing the physiological factors underpinning performance, and the use of laboratory- and field-based physiological assessments for training prescription and monitoring, using rowing as an example.

## Identifying the physiological factors underpinning performance

The physiological determinants of performance are event-specific and are multifactorial, depending on a number of factors. Establishing the physiological factors underpinning performance is crucial in training prescription if optimal adaptation is to be achieved. Further, by identifying the determinants of performance, specific testing protocols can be designed to profile athletes, establishing strengths and weaknesses, and focusing training on specific areas leading to an enhanced training stimulus. Continuous and targeted testing can be used to monitor training adaptation or maladaptation, allowing training programmes to be modified specifically to the requirements of the athlete. Therefore, establishing the determinants of performance is crucial for the efficacy of training prescription.

Determining the physiological factors underpinning performance is often a difficult task, particularly in those sports that have a significant 'open-skill' contribution to performance, for example, football. For this reason, the majority of studies examining the physiological factors underpinning performance have focused on 'closed skill', cyclic events such as running, cycling, swimming and rowing. Recent attempts have been made to establish the physiological determinants of performance in 'open skill' events and the reader is directed to these studies for further reading (e.g. Ingham et al 2002). Case study 2.1 outlines the methods employed to establish the physiological factors underpinning performance in rowing. Having established the physiological determinants of performance, specific testing protocols can be designed to profile and monitor athletes, enhancing the specificity of training prescription.

## Laboratory-based testing

The demand from coaches for greater amounts of field-based testing and, at the same time, for reducing the amount of laboratory-based testing is increasing. To a large degree this demand is justified and justifiable. The limitations of laboratory-based testing and benefits of field-based testing can be largely encapsulated in the concept of specificity. It can be very difficult to recreate the exact movement patterns and limb velocities and to utilize exactly the same muscle groups using laboratory-based ergometers compared to the actual sport performance. The argument for increased field testing, which centres around the need for greater specificity,

## Case study 2.1

Ingham S, Whyte G, Jones K & Nevill A 2002 Determinants of rowing performance in elite rowers. *European Journal of Applied Physiology* 88:243–246.

This study examined physiological determinants of 2000-m ergometer rowing performance in rowing or sculling World Championship finalists from all competitive categories of rowing (19 male and 13 female heavyweight; 4 male and 5 female lightweight). Discontinuous incremental rowing to exhaustion established lactate threshold, maximum oxygen consumption ($\dot{V}O_2max$) and power at $\dot{V}O_2max$; five maximal strokes assessed maximum force, maximum power and stroke length. Results were compared to maximal 2000-m ergometer time trial speed. The strongest correlations were for power at $\dot{V}O_2max$, maximum power and maximum force ($r = 0.95$; $P < 0.001$). Correlations were also observed for $\dot{V}O_2max$ ($r = 0.88$, $P < 0.001$) and $\dot{V}O_2$ at lactate threshold ($r = 0.87$, $P = 0.001$). Physiological variables were included in a stepwise regression analysis to predict performance speed (m.s$^{-1}$). The resultant model included power at $\dot{V}O_2max$, $\dot{V}O_2$ at lactate threshold, power at 4 mM blood lactate and maximum power that explained 98% of the variance in 2000-m ergometer rowing performance. The model was validated in 18 elite rowers, producing limits of agreement of −0.006 to 0.098 m.s$^{-1}$ for 2000-m rowing ergometer speed, equivalent to times of −1.5 to 6.9 s (−0.41% to 1.85%). Together, power at $\dot{V}O_2max$, $\dot{V}O_2$ at lactate threshold, power at 4 mM blood lactate and maximum power could be used to predict rowing performance.

undoubtedly has some merit. The benefits, and even necessity, to retain laboratory-based testing, however, may be overlooked or, more commonly, not well understood by coaches. Although field-based testing always provides information and data that are more ecologically valid, it may lack control and, therefore, often lacks reliability. Field testing is far more subject to the vaguaries of the weather and to the idiosyncracies of location and topography and to the presence or absence of others. The best exercise-testing programme will, of course, utilize both occasional laboratory testing with more frequent field testing.

While laboratory-based testing may reduce the ecological validity it enhances reliability and allows measurements to be taken that would otherwise be impossible in field settings. In the laboratory, the environment can be far better standardized such that on successive occasions any change in the values obtained can be more readily interpreted as reflecting a change in the conditioned state of the athlete. In an appropriately equipped exercise physiology laboratory, temperature and air-flow can be standardized and the flow of people controlled to limit the Hawthorne effect (audience effect).

To ensure greater specificity in the laboratory, appropriate selection of sports-specific ergometers is fundamental. Ergometry is the use of an exercise device which can provide information on the rate of work performed for a mode of exercise similar to the target activity. The specificity of the ergometer in replicating the movement patterns of the chosen sport is crucial in optimizing the validity of data collection. Hence, if the aim is to exercise-test a rower, then, in a laboratory setting, a rowing ergometer is best; a canoe ergometer is best for canoeing, a treadmill for running and a cycle ergometer is used for cycling. Once the appropriate ergometer is selected the exercise protocol design should aim to elicit information that will allow the current conditioned state of the athlete to be ascertained. This must be performed with reference to the specific performance determinants of the sport (see above).

Taking distance running as an example, the physiological parameters important for distance running performance have been reported to be $\dot{V}O_2$max, fractional utilization, running economy and lactate tolerance (Berg 2003). A treadmill test which uses 4-minute stages of increasing exercise intensity to maximal exercise will allow measurement of most of the above. In addition, if re-applied in exactly the same way, and under exactly the same conditions, each time such a test will provide a 'snap-shot' of the athlete's changing state of conditioning. This allows the design of a more specific training programme and ensures that training is more precisely customized to the individual.

## Designing a laboratory test for an elite distance runner

Figure 2.1 demonstrates a typical laboratory-based treadmill protocol that is employed to obtain information appropriate to the needs of the elite distance runners (marathon or 10 km).

The testing protocol employs $5 \times 4$-minute stages with each stage being faster than the previous stage (0.6 $km.h^{-1}$ per stage). A 30-second rest interval exists between stages for collection of an earlobe blood sample and subsequent lactate analysis. Establishing the velocity of each stage begins with the conversion of a recent best time for 10 km to a treadmill speed. Using the example of an athlete with a best time of 37 minutes 30 seconds for 10 km, 16.0 $km.h^{-1}$ is used as the reference velocity. The third stage is then set at the 10 km race velocity (16.0 $km.h^{-1}$) and the velocities for stages 1, 2, 4 and 5 are calculated by subtracting or adding 0.6 $km.h^{-1}$. Hence, the protocol will begin with stage 1 at 14.8 $km.h^{-1}$, stage 2 at 15.4 $km.h^{-1}$, stage 3 at 16.0 $km.h^{-1}$, stage 4 at 16.6 $km.h^{-1}$ and stage 5 at 17.2 $km.h^{-1}$. To improve the validity of the assessment, the treadmill gradient is set at 1% as this more accurately reflects the energy cost of outdoor running at the same velocity (Jones & Doust 1996a).

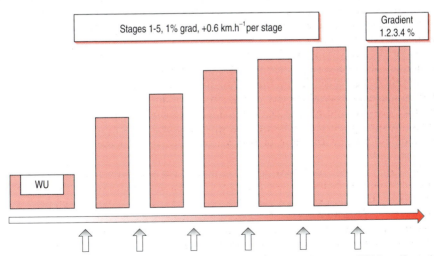

Stages 1-5, 1% grad, +0.6 $km.h^{-1}$ per stage

Gradient 1.2.3.4 %

WU

**Figure 2.1** An example of a treadmill protocol to test a distance runner. WU is self-paced 10-minute warm-up. In the case of the example chosen here, a distance runner with a 10 km pb of 37.5 minutes stages 1–5 are 14.8, 15.4, 16.0, 16.6 and 17.2 $km.h^{-1}$ respectively. The arrows represent earlobe blood samples taken after each 4-minute stage, during 30-second rest interval.

Following the completion of stage 5, and immediately after the 30-second rest interval, the athlete remounts the treadmill with the belt moving at the same speed as in stage 5 and the rest of the test is conducted at that speed. After 60 seconds the gradient is increased by 1% and likewise every subsequent 60 seconds until the athlete can no longer continue (volitional exhaustion).

Heart rate, preferably using ECG (alternatively telemetry, i.e. Polar), and oxygen consumption, using indirect calorimetry, are measured continuously throughout the test, with the collection of a capillary blood sample at the end of each 4-minute stage, analysed for blood lactate concentration.

## Derivation of $\dot{V}O_2$max and fractional utilization

Maximum oxygen consumption ($\dot{V}O_2$max) is established from a test lasting between 9 and 16 minutes. The type of test described above will take about 25 minutes and hence in this instance maximal oxygen uptake is referred to as '$\dot{V}O_2$peak'. $\dot{V}O_2$peak has been demonstrated to be within 3% of $\dot{V}O_2$max (Jones & Doust 1996b). When testing athletes, precision rather than accuracy is the more important issue and, where athletes have limited time, one test rather than two is considered better, providing better compliance and so on.

Fractional utilization is the volume of oxygen consumed at lactate threshold expressed as a percentage of $\dot{V}O_2$max (%$\dot{V}O_2$max). It is also sometimes used, however, to describe $\dot{V}O_2$ as a percentage of $\dot{V}O_2$max (or $\dot{V}O_2$peak) at a specified intensity. For example the %$\dot{V}O_2$max at marathon or 10 km velocity in running or at 16 km.h$^{-1}$ on the treadmill or at 330 watts on the rowing ergometer.

## Derivation of economy

In exercise physiology the term 'economy' is generally used to refer to oxygen economy or movement economy. Oxygen economy refers to the volume of oxygen taken up by active muscle at a given sub-maximal exercise intensity. During running on the treadmill the standard velocity selected, to compare oxygen uptake on successive occasions, is 16 km.h$^{-1}$. Reduced volume of oxygen consumed at this sub-maximal pace is interpreted as an improved oxygen economy. Movement economy, for example, 'running economy', differs from oxygen economy by virtue of the fact that it concerns not just the physiological measure of oxygen consumption. Appropriate assessment of movement economy, either acutely or longitudinally, requires the use of biomechanics, psychology and physiology. Biomechanics is crucial as technique is a key component in the assessment of movement economy. For example, in running, subtle changes in distance per stride and stride rate at the same velocity will change the volume of oxygen consumed. Psychology is important because skill acquisition or changes in acquired skill has a psychological basis.

## Derivation of lactate threshold

Lactate threshold (LT) is a complex phenomenon that has received significant attention in recent years. While a debate exists as to whether an inflection in blood lactate occurs during incremental exercise, the issue of defining LT remains a key discussion both in the literature and between scientists and coach. The term 'lactate threshold' has been used to describe a number of different physiological points associated with a sustained increase in blood lactate above resting levels including: (i) a non-linear increase in blood lactate of at least 1 mmol.L$^{-1}$ (Coyle 1995); (ii) a workload preceding a non-linear rise in blood lactate during progressive exercise (Ivy et al 1980); (iii) the point of deflection in the logged blood lactate versus logged $\dot{V}O_2$ transformation (Beaver et al 1985). Others have suggested a second breakpoint further along the lactate transition curve associated with a workload at which blood lactate begins to accumulate rapidly, and as such represents the highest work intensity at which blood lactate can equilibrate. This breakpoint has also been defined by a number of terms: (i) anaerobic threshold (AT; Kindermann et al 1979); (ii) the onset of blood lactate accumulation (OBLA; Sjodin & Jacobs 1981); (iii) maximum lactate steady state (MLSS); (iv) critical velocity (CV). While debate regarding the presence and definition of LT persists, the concept of lactate breakpoints and their identification is central to many scientific support programmes. It is key that physiologists work closely with coaches and athletes to accurately define LT and standardize its identification.

Figure 2.2 illustrates the lactate and heart rate profile for the sample endurance athlete discussed above. From the graph it can be seen that the breakpoint occurs at 16.0 km.h$^{-1}$ and the heart rate corresponding to this speed is 140 beats.min$^{-1}$. Giving a single heart rate value to an athlete would not provide useful training information as a range of training intensities is fundamental in targeting the physiological mechanisms underpinning performance. Thus, providing a heart rate range based on the test information is far more practical. Accordingly, for training outdoors the athlete would be advised to use a 10-beat range, in this case 135–145 beats.min$^{-1}$. If training on the treadmill indoors, where weather and terrain do not change, a 5-beat range of 137–142 beats.min$^{-1}$ can be given. Because the athlete's LT heart rate is now known, heart rates for base endurance training (long slow distance, LSD) is calculated at 120–130 beats.min$^{-1}$ (i.e. staying 5 beats below the LT range). The test will also have provided an estimate for maximal heart rate and in this athlete it is assumed to be 180 beats.min$^{-1}$. As a result, for high-intensity training (of 2–4 minutes) heart rate should be above 90% of maximum heart rate (162 beats.min$^{-1}$). In this way three training zones are identified (see Ch. 4).

Following a number of weeks training, re-testing would reveal changes in $\dot{V}O_2$peak, fractional utilization, economy and lactate threshold. As previously stated an index of improved endurance is characterized by a rightward shift in the work rate–lactate curve, as can be seen in Figure 2.3. If training goes particularly well and

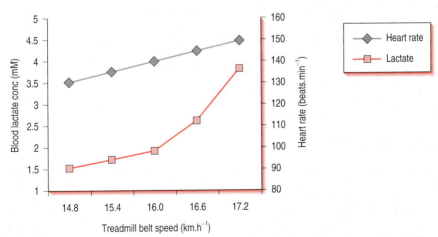

**Figure 2.2** Heart-rate and blood lactate concentration during a discontinuous treadmill running protocol.

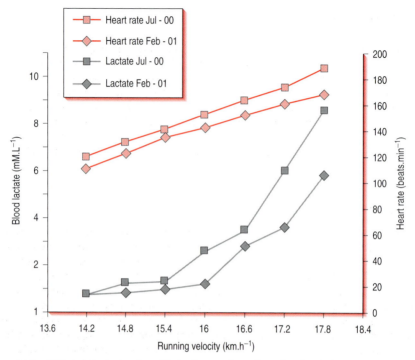

**Figure 2.3** This demonstrates the effect of a number of weeks of training on the work rate–blood lactate profile in an endurance runner. Note the downward and rightward shift of both the heart rate and blood lactate curves following training.

the prescribed heart-rate zone proves to be ideal for the individual at that time it may be possible to see an increase in the intensity at which LT occurs. This is seen in Figure 2.3 where on the first occasion LT pace is 16.0 km.h$^{-1}$. On the second occasion after a number of weeks of LT specific training, the entire curve has shifted to the right and the velocity at LT intensity has increased to 16.6 km.h$^{-1}$, demonstrating a training-induced physiological adaptation and therefore conferring confidence in the efficacy of the training programme.

The prescription of training using individual heart rate zones allows specific, targeted training prescription that can have a profound effect on training adaptation. Establishing laboratory- and field-based tests to identify training intensities for all underpinning physiological parameters of performance is fundamental in optimizing training prescription.

## Field–based testing

Field-based testing is generally said to have good ecological validity. In other words it is more sports-specific than laboratory-based testing. However, because it is very difficult to standardize the test environment from one occasion to the next it can lack construct validity and test–retest reliability. In short, it tends to be far more subjective. Laboratory-based testing does allow standardization of the test environment, is more objective and provides better construct validity and test–retest reliability. Hence, it is clear that a combination of both field- and laboratory-based testing is best for providing an optimal service to the high-level or elite athlete in any sport.

## Summary box 2.6

Field-based testing provides more sport-specific data but is often subjective. Laboratory-based testing provides objective data which can be less sport-specific; however, it can provide a good measure of the current conditioning of the athlete and allows the identification of specific areas that require work. The best physiological support programme is one which incorporates both field- and laboratory-based support and achieves the appropriate balance between the two methods of assessment. For laboratory-based testing, specificity requires the selection of sport-specific ergometers and the design of exercise protocols which examine the primary demands of the activity.

## CONCLUSION

Specificity is a key component in the design of any sports training programme. Physiological adaptation is specific to the imposed stimulus and as such training should closely mimic the skill, muscle group(s) and energy system(s) required during competition. Knowledge of the physiological mechanisms underlying performance is fundamental in the design of training programmes. Specific laboratory- and field-based testing allow a thorough interrogation of the physiological mechanisms underlying performance and the monitoring of adaptations across the training cycle. Cross-training lacks specificity and is unlikely to enhance training adaptations; however, cross-training may be valuable for the rehabilitating athlete and to add variety to prolonged training periods. Specificity is a complex concept and only a sound underlying knowledge of physiology will allow appropriate application of this training principle.

## KEY POINTS

1. Specificity is one of the training principles.
2. Physiological adaptation is specific to the stimulus imposed.
3. Specificity should address the three key areas of: skill, muscle group and energy system.
4. Understanding the physiological mechanisms underlying performance is fundamental in the prescription of specific training programmes.
5. Cross-training is unlikely to enhance performance.
6. Cross-training may be efficacious in the treatment of the rehabilitating athlete.
7. To provide the best physiological support to the athlete requires the integrated use of both field- and laboratory-based assessment.

## References

Australian Sports Commission 2000 Physiological tests for elite athletes. CJ Gore (ed). Human Kinetics, Champaign IL

BASES 1997 Physiological testing guidelines, 3rd edn, Bird S & Davison R (eds)

Beaver WL, Wasserman K, Whip BJ 1985 Improved detection of lactate threshold during exercise using a log-log transformation. Journal of Applied Physiology 59(6):1936–1940

Berg K 2003 Endurance training and performance in runners: research limitations and unanswered questions. Sports Medicine 33(1):59–73

Brooks GA, Fahey TD, White TP 1996 Exercise physiology. Human bioenergetics and its applications. Mayfield Publishing Company, California

Costill DL, Thomas R, Robergs RA et al 1991 Adaptations to swimming training: influence of training volume. Medicine and Science in Sports and Exercise 23:371–377

Coyle EF 1995 Integration of the physiological factors determining endurance performance ability. Exercise and Sport Science Reviews 23:25–63

Dubouchaud H, Butterfield GE, Wolfel EE et al 2000 Endurance training, expression, and physiology of LDH, MCT1, and MCT4 in human skeletal muscle. 278(4). American Journal of Physiology and Endocrinology Metabolism E571-E579

Hoh JF 1975 Neural regulation of mammalian fast and slow muscle myosins: an electrophoretic analysis. Biochemistry 14(4):742–747

Ingham S, Whyte G, Jones K, Nevill A 2002 Determinants of rowing performance in elite rowers. European Journal of Applied Physiology 88:243–246

Ivy JL, Withers RT, Van Handel PJ et al 1980 Muscle respiratory capacity and fiber type as determinants of the lactate threshold. Journal of Applied Physiology 48(3):523–527

Jenkins S 1997 Sports science handbook, 3rd edn. Sunningdale Publications, Berkshire, England

Jones AM, Doust JH 1996a A 1% treadmill grade most accurately reflects the energetic cost of outdoor running. Journal of Sports Sciences 14:321–327

Jones AM, Doust JH 1996b A comparison of three protocols for the determination of maximal aerobic power in runners. Journal of Sports Sciences 14:89

Kent M 1998 Oxford dictionary of sports science and medicine. Oxford University Press, Oxford

Kinderman W, Simon G, Keul J 1979 The significance of the aerobic-anaerobic transition for the determination of work load intensities during endurance training. European Journal of Applied Physiology and Occupational Physiology 42(1):25–34

Liu W, Thomas SG, Asa SL et al 2003 Myostatin is a skeletal muscle target of growth hormone anabolic action. Journal of Clinical Endocrinology and Metabolism 88(11):5490–5496

Loy SF, Hoffmann JJ, Holland GJ 1995 Benefits and practical use of cross-training in sports. Sports Medicine 19(1):1–8

Mujika I, Padilla S 2000 Detraining: loss of training-induced physiological and performance adaptations. Part 1. Sports Medicine 30(2):79–87

Paavolainen L, Hakkinen K, Hamalainen I et al 1999 Explosive-strength training improves 5-km running time by improving running economy and muscle power. Journal of Applied Physiology 86(5):1527–1533

Popov V 2001 Flexibility training. In: Pyke FS (ed), Better coaching, 2nd edn, Australian Coaching Council, Canberra, pp 137–138.

Sale DG 1988 Neural adaptation to resistance training. Medicine and Science in Sports and Exercise 20:S135-S145

Sjodin B, Jacobs I 1981 Onset of blood lactate accumulation and marathon running performance. International Journal of Sports Medicine 2(1):23–26

Tanaka H 1994 Effects of cross-training. Transfer of training effects on $\dot{V}O_2$max between cycling, running and swimming. Sports Medicine 8(5):330–339

Verhoshansky Y 1986 Speed–strength preparation and development of atrength endurance of athletes in various specializations (part 1). Soviet Sports Review 21(2):82–85.

Wackerhage H, Woods NM 2002 Exercise-induced signal transduction and gene regulation in skeletal muscle. Journal of Sports Science and Medicine 1:103–114

Wasserman K, Hansen JE, Sue DY, Whipp BJ 1987 Principles of exercise testing and interpretation. Lea and Febiger, Philadelphia

Yang SY, Alnaqeeb M, Simpson H, Goldspink G 1996 Cloning and characterisation of an IGF-1 isoform expressed in skeletal muscle subjected to stretch. Journal of Muscle Research and Cell Motility 17:487–495

## Further reading

Astrand P-O, Rodahl K, Dahl HA, Strømme SB 2003 Textbook of work physiology. physiological bases of exercise, 4th edn. Human Kinetics, Champaign IL

Bosch F, Klomp R 2005 Running. Biomechanics and physiology applied in practice. Elsevier Ltd, Edinburgh

Foran B (ed) 2001 High-performance sports conditioning. Human Kinetics, Champaign IL

Gore CJ (ed) 2000 Physiological tests for elite athletes. Australian Sports Commission. Human Kinetics, Champaign IL

Kraemer WJ, Häkkinen K (eds) 2002 Strength training for sport. An IOC Medical Commission Publication. Blackwell Science Ltd, Oxford

Chapter **3**

# The physiology of tapering

Gregory Whyte and Nicholas Diaper

## LEARNING OBJECTIVES:

This chapter is intended to ensure that the reader:

1. Gains an appreciation of the various types of tapering.
2. Gains an understanding of the physiological adaptations that occur in response to the different tapering modalities employed by athletes.
3. Appreciates the performance changes observed as a result of effective tapering.
4. Understands the impact of travel on performance and strategies employed to reduce travel fatigue and jet lag.
5. Understands the role of glycogen loading during taper.
6. Appreciates the need for individually tailored tapering programmes.

## INTRODUCTION

Tapering can be defined as a specialized exercise training technique designed to reverse training-induced fatigue without a loss of the training adaptations (Neary et al 1992). It is the final phase of training prior to competition and involves a reduction in training load that can elicit improvements in physiological, psychological and performance indices. A successful taper phase requires careful planning and should aim to optimize all the determinants of performance at a single point in time. This amalgamation is often termed 'peaking' and is used synonymously with tapering as the taper period allows an athlete to attain peak performance at important events.

Tapering is complex and subtle, requiring an in-depth knowledge of sports performance, including physiological, psychological, nutritional and technical aspects. Psychological aspects of tapering are beyond the scope of this chapter. The reader is directed to the large number of published reviews examining this crucial element of tapering (Hooper et al 1999).

The purpose of tapering is to bring about a peak in performance by the manipulation of training volume (intensity, frequency, duration). The period of time required for an optimal taper may vary dependant on how training volume is manipulated. The balance between the reduction of training volume and the period of time employed to elicit a peak is crucial if optimal tapering is to be achieved. A taper period that is too long, or reduces training volume too rapidly, may not provide sufficient training stimulus to prevent a detraining effect, whereas a taper period that is too short or fails to reduce training volume sufficiently will not allow sufficient time for full physiological and psychological recovery. Each of these situations may result in athletes 'missing their peaks', thus compromising optimal performance and undoing an otherwise well designed training programme. It is no surprise therefore that the taper period is a critical period for coaches, sports scientists and athletes alike. This chapter will attempt to unravel some of the complexities of peaking and tapering and offer some guidelines on how best to optimize performance.

## TYPES OF TAPER

As training load or volume is the product of intensity, duration and frequency, one or more of these aspects of training must be manipulated in order to reduce the training load. The most potent stimulus to training load is intensity and therefore any increase in this aspect will significantly increase training load. The primary goal of tapering, however, is to elicit a performance peak, i.e. velocity, power. Successful tapers are, therefore, high intensity in nature and as such, duration and/or frequency should be lowered if volume is to be reduced. This is paramount if sufficient rest and recovery between or within sessions is to be attained.

Four main types of taper (Fig. 3.1) have been described, each of which reduce the training volume at varying rates (Mujika & Padilla 2003). Exponential tapers can be either slow- or fast-decay, with the latter consisting of a lower training load. The linear taper has the slowest rate of decline and therefore comprises a greater training load than either of the exponential tapers. These are true tapers by definition of the word as the work load is gradually 'tapered' off in the days leading up to competition. In contrast, the step taper constitutes a sudden drop in training load that is then maintained through to competition without a progressive reduction in work load.

## PHYSIOLOGICAL RESPONSES

Despite the relatively short period of time employed during tapering, a number of physiological adaptations take place during the taper period, some of which are better understood than others.

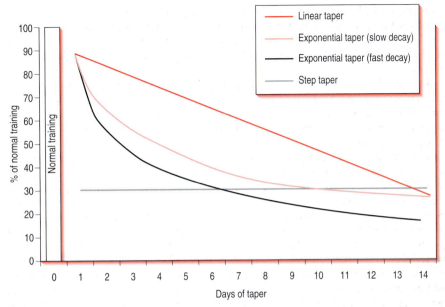

**Figure 3.1**  Types of taper.

## Cardiorespiratory adaptations

### Heart rate

Resting and sub-maximal heart rates (HR) appear to be unaffected by the taper phase, except when athletes may be in an over-reached state prior to the taper phase. Over-reaching is often employed by coaches to elicit an enhanced super-compensation following a reduction in training volume (see Ch. 1). Distinct differences exist between over-reaching and over-training and as such these terms should not be confused. Over-reaching is characterized by a transient decline in performance as a result of a short term heavy training (Busso et al 2002) and can be easily recovered with a few days of reduced training such as a taper phase. Over-training (often termed over-training syndrome, unexplained underperformance syndrome or burn out) on the other hand is characterized in athletes by reduced capacity to train and perform over long periods and generally weeks or months are required to recover normal training capacity (see Ch. 9). In an over-reached state resting heart rate may be increased and maximum exercise capacity is often reduced due to accumulated fatigue leading to a reduced maximum heart rate. Jeukendrup et al (1992) described a reduction in sleeping HR of 3 beats.min$^{-1}$ after tapering in a group of cyclists that were intentionally over-reached during the period preceding the taper phase.

Results from studies investigating the effects of tapering on maximal HR have demonstrated inconsistent findings (see Mujika et al 2004). Houmard et al (1994) observed no change in maximal HR during taper in runners performing a progressive treadmill run to exhaustion. Likewise, Rietjens et al (2001) also reported no change in maximal HR following taper in a group of cyclists during an incremental cycling test to exhaustion. In contrast to these studies, slight increases in maximal

HR have been observed following 1 week of taper in cyclists (Martin & Anderson 2000) and 2 weeks of taper in swimmers (Hooper et al 1999). Jeukendrup et al (1992) observed a 3% increase in maximal HR after a taper period in a group of male competitive cyclists that had intentionally been over-reached prior to the taper phase. However, the post-taper value was similar to that measured before the over-reaching phase.

The opposite effects on maximal HR of blood volume expansion and the level of catecholamine depletion that may have occurred due to the intense training phase preceding the taper may account for these inconsistent findings (Mujika et al 2004).

## Maximal oxygen uptake

Maximal oxygen uptake ($\dot{V}O_2$max) is a fundamental aspect of fitness for a number of sports, particularly those that are predominantly aerobic in nature or performed at intensities at or near $\dot{V}O_2$max. A number of studies have reported significant increases in laboratory assessed $\dot{V}O_2$max scores in the range of 2.5–9.1% following a taper period. Neary et al (2003a) demonstrated a 2.4% increase in $\dot{V}O_2$max for seven male endurance-trained cyclists who maintained training intensity (85–90% maximum heart rate), while lowering training duration over 7 days. In the same study, the group that progressively reduced exercise intensity (85–55% maximum heart rate) but maintained duration demonstrated no significant improvement in $\dot{V}O_2$max. Others have shown greater increases in $\dot{V}O_2$max of 4.5% in cyclists (Jeukendrup et al 1992) and 9.1% in triathletes (Zarkadas et al 1995).

Increases in $\dot{V}O_2$max are not always evident following a taper phase (Houmard et al 1994, Shepley et al 1992). Shepley et al (1992) reported a 22% increase in running time to fatigue following a high-intensity 7-day taper in the presence of an unchanged $\dot{V}O_2$max. Likewise, Houmard et al (1994) observed a 3% improvement in 5-km running time with no accompanying increase in $\dot{V}O_2$max in a group of well trained distance runners. Performance improvements independent of changes in $\dot{V}O_2$max are commonly associated with adaptations at the skeletal muscle level as opposed to oxygen delivery (Houmard et al 1994, Shepley et al 1992).

While evidence supports enhanced performance in the absence of an improved $\dot{V}O_2$max, investigations such as these demonstrate that a well planned and structured taper phase should not result in a detraining effect with regard to $\dot{V}O_2$max. Training intensity appears to be the key component in ensuring that $\dot{V}O_2$max is either enhanced or maintained during the taper period.

# Muscle fibres

Trappe et al (2000) reported an 11% increase in the diameter and 24% increase in the cross-sectional area of type IIa muscle fibres in a group of highly trained swimmers following a 21-day taper. Type I fibre diameter and cross-sectional area remained unaltered. Further type IIa fibres also produced greater peak force, contracted faster and were more powerful following the taper whereas no change was observed for type I fibres. These data imply that fast-twitch (type IIa) fibres are more responsive to tapers following periods of high-volume training. The authors suggest that the intense high volume of training preceding the taper phase in this group of swimmers was responsible for inducing negative changes in type IIa fibres relating to their size which did not influence type I fibres. Indeed, type IIa fibres have been shown to decrease 15% in size following a two-fold increase in training volume for 10 days (Fitts et al 1989).

The contention that type IIa fibres are more responsive to tapers has recently received more support. Neary et al (2003a) demonstrated a 14.2% increase in cross-sectional area of type II fibres in seven endurance-trained cyclists performing a high-intensity taper with reducing duration for 7 days with no significant changes in type I fibres. No significant changes in type IIa fibres were observed in the group employing a low-intensity, longer duration taper over 7 days, suggesting that successful tapers should be high intensity in nature.

Examining the metabolic adaptations that occurred at the single fibre level, Neary et al (2003a) reported significant and differential effects being observed in type I and IIa fibres. Following a 7-day high-intensity low-volume taper, type IIa fibres demonstrated an increase of approximately 14% in myofibrillar ATPase (mATPase), cytochrome oxidase (CYTOX), beta-hydroxyacyl coenzyme A dehydrogenase (β-HOAD) and succinate dehydrogenase (SDH). In contrast, type I fibres demonstrated increases of only 10–11% in mATPase and SDH with no change in CYTOX or β-HOAD. The only increases in enzyme activity in the high-volume low-intensity taper were a similar increase in β-HOAD (15%) in type IIa fibres, and increases of 9% and 15% in CYTOX and β-HOAD respectively for type I fibres. It is important to note, however, that such changes in enzyme activity and fibre size must be considered only an estimate of the exercising musculature due to the nature and limitations of muscle biopsies. Furthermore, it should be stressed that single cell measurements are conducted under considerably different conditions than the normal physiological environment in which whole muscles perform – and therefore direct comparisons from single cell to whole muscle performance should be viewed with caution. It does seem reasonable, however, to conclude that changes in contractile function at the single muscle fibre level contribute to enhance whole muscle function and improved performance.

It is clear from this evidence that the intensity of exercise during endurance-based tapers determines the nature and extent of muscle fibre adaptation and that type IIa fibres are more responsive to such training compared to type I fibres.

## Muscle glycogen

Muscle glycogen stores can be depleted during periods of heavy training as is often the case in the training phase preceding the taper. A number of reports have demonstrated that muscle glycogen concentration is increased following a Taper (Neary et al 1992, 2003a, Riggs et al 1983, Shepley et al 1992, Walker et al 2000). Neary et al (1992) reported a 17% increase in muscle glycogen stores after 4 days of taper and a 25% increase following an 8-day taper. In a more recent study, Neary et al (2003a) compared muscle glycogen levels in three groups of male endurance cyclists undergoing different 7-day taper strategies. A 26% increase in muscle glycogen concentration was reported for the group that maintained training intensity at 85–90% of maximum HR with a progressive reduction in exercise duration. A 22% increase was observed in the group that maintained training duration but lowered exercise intensity.

Shepley et al (1992) observed a 15% increase in muscle glycogen stores in a group of highly trained cross-country and middle-distance runners following 7 days of high-intensity taper. In the same study, glycogen stores were unaffected by a low-intensity taper and were 8% higher after a rest-only taper. The cessation of training together with a high-carbohydrate diet may have stimulated this overshoot in glycogen synthesis following the rest-only taper, although this does not explain why a similar effect was not seen after the low-intensity taper (Shepley et al 1992).

Increases in stored muscle glycogen result in a greater endogenous store of energy and are particularly beneficial for events where substrate availability can limit performance. The extent to which this supercompensation effect takes place is largely governed by the dietary intake of carbohydrates. Indeed, dietary intake is a crucial factor in the successful taper and this will be covered in more detail later.

## STRENGTH AND POWER

It is well documented that taper programmes elicit increases in strength and power (Johns et al. 1992, Martin et al 1994, Shepley et al 1992, Trappe et al 2000). In line with other components of fitness, strength and power are often suppressed by long periods of heavy training and the taper period allows the recovery of these components to levels above baseline (supercompensation).

Trappe et al (2000) investigated the effects of a 21-day, high-intensity, low-volume taper on swim bench and tethered swimming power in highly trained swimmers. The authors reported a 7–20% improvement. Swim bench power was dependent on the isokinetic velocity employed with consistently higher power outputs for each velocity ranging from 1.4 m.s$^{-1}$ to 3.28 m.s$^{-1}$. In an earlier study Johns et al (1992) reported that tethered swimming power, measured in the water, improved by 13% following the taper. Further, the authors observed improvements in tethered swimming power of 5% following a taper of 10–14 days in intercollegiate swimmers.

In a study involving cross-country and middle distance runners, Shepley et al (1992) reported an increased maximal voluntary isometric strength of the knee extensors following a 7-day taper of high-intensity and low-volume, low-intensity and moderate-volume, or rest only. It should be noted that running time to fatigue decreased by 3% in the rest-only taper whereas the low-intensity and moderate-volume intervention showed no effect and the high-intensity taper resulted in a 22% improvement in time to fatigue.

Gibala et al (1994) performed one of the few studies to date dealing with strength-trained athletes. The authors examined voluntary strength of the elbow flexors over a 10-day rest-only or reduced-volume taper in resistance-trained males. Maximum isometric peak torque increased by 7.5% at day 6 and 6.8% at day 10 of the taper in the reduced-volume taper and the authors attributed this to enhanced contractile performance and/or to an increase in neural activation. In contrast, maximum isometric peak torque did not increase in the rest-only condition. Improvements in strength during a taper phase have also been documented in cyclists, whereby Martin et al (1994) reported an increase in quadriceps strength of 8–9% following a 2-week step taper.

The mechanisms responsible for these taper-induced improvements in muscular strength and power may be related to alterations in local enzymatic activity and single muscle fibre characteristics which, in turn, may positively affect neuromuscular, biomechanical and metabolic efficiency (Mujika et al 2004).

## LACTATE

In a study by Jeukendrup et al (1992) a group of competitive male cyclists were subjected to three consecutive periods of training; moderate standardized training, heavy training (high-intensity intervals) and reduced training. Each period lasted for 2 weeks with the aim of the heavy training phase to intentionally over-reach the participants. Peak blood lactate levels as measured after a maximal cycle ergometer test were reduced by 50% during the heavy training phase. The subsequent taper period resulted in a 78% increase in peak lactate levels. Sub-maximal blood lactate values were also lower during over-reaching and higher following the taper period. Such findings may be the result of a decreased glycolysis due to depleted glycogen stores which have been observed following heavy training (see section above).

In contrast, Shepley et al (1992) observed no significant increases in post-exercise plasma lactate concentrations following three different tapers (high-intensity, low-intensity and rest-only) in highly trained runners. Inconsistencies regarding peak and sub-maximal blood lactate values (see Mujika et al 2004) make it difficult to categorically state whether lactate is affected by tapering. It may be that changes in blood lactate are dependent on whether or not athletes are in an over-reached state prior to the taper phase. The fact that lactate values may be influenced by a taper period has important implications for the coach and exercise scientist regarding lactate testing at these times.

## PERFORMANCE CHANGES

The improvements in performance following a taper period are associated with physiological, psychological and technical changes that take place over this relatively short training phase. The following section aims to highlight some of the performance improvements that have been observed as a result of successful tapering. The vast majority of the literature investigating performance enhancement through tapering has focused on endurance performance in swimming, running and cycling where the performance outcome is easily measured by means of time. In contrast, team and skill based events have received little attention, mainly due to the non-linear nature of such sports and the difficulties of subjectively measuring performance in these disciplines.

Trappe et al (2000) demonstrated an improvement of 3–4.7% in swimming times in a group of highly trained swimmers following a 21-day taper. Unlike some studies, performance measures were taken from actual competitive races before and after the taper period. The taper period involved a progressive reduction in training volume accompanied by an increase in training intensity (80–120% aerobic capacity) in an attempt to replicate race speeds. Mujika et al (2002a) reported similar results in swimming race times before (3 weeks) and during the Sydney 2000 Olympic Games, with performance improvements between 1.1% and 6.0% (mean 2.2%) during the 3-week taper period.

Following a 7-day taper in a group of distance runners where total training volume was reduced to 15% of previous training volume, Houmard et al (1994) observed a 3% improvement in 5-km treadmill time. Training during the taper phase consisted mainly of high-intensity, 400-m intervals at 5-km race pace or faster. Mujika et al (2002b) observed a 2% improvement in competition performance in a group of 800 m runners assigned to a high-frequency taper (training daily) for 6 days. In comparison a group that performed a moderate frequency taper (resting every third day) demonstrated no improvements. These data suggest that training frequency should also be regarded as an important aspect of tapering together with intensity.

In a simulated 40-km cycling time trial a 4.3% improvement following a 7-day taper was reported in a group of endurance cyclists whose taper phase involved maintaining intensity with a progressive reduction in exercise duration (Neary et al 2003a). In the same study the group that maintained exercise duration but progressively reduced exercise intensity demonstrated no improvements. In a shorter time trial (20 km) a 5.4% improvement in performance was observed in a group of cyclists whose 7-day taper involved a 50% reduction in baseline training volume with intensity maintained at 85% $\dot{V}O_2max$ (Neary et al 2003b). In comparison, two other groups who reduced training volume to 30 and 80% of baseline, while maintaining the same intensity, showed no improvements.

In a study investigating the effects of three different tapers (high-intensity, low-intensity and rest-only), a group of highly trained runners performed a timed run to exhaustion on a level treadmill at a constant velocity equivalent to each athlete's best 1500 m race time (Shepley et al 1992). After the high-intensity taper, running time to exhaustion increased significantly by 22%, whereas no differences were observed for the low-intensity or rest-only tapers. This further strengthens the notion that training intensity is the key variable in terms of a successful taper.

Based on the results of the studies outlined above it may be suggested that performance improvements following an effective taper are generally in the range of 1–6%, but may be as high as 22%. Although the range of 1–6% may seem like a relatively minimal change, such improvements could result in substantial differences in race placing.

## ADDITIONAL CONSIDERATIONS DURING THE TAPER PHASE

Planning of the taper phase should take place well in advanced of the proposed taper. Care must be taken to avoid 'panic' changes during the taper to avoid excessive (or rarely insufficient) training volumes possibly resulting in poor performance. There are a number of factors that can affect performance in the period immediately (< 7 days) prior to competition. Two key factors that should be addressed to optimize the taper and resultant performance are travel and nutrition. The following sections will examine the impact of these two factors on taper and performance and offer guidelines to optimize performance.

## TAPERING AND TRAVEL

International travel for training and competition is a key factor in any tapering process and there are a number of key areas that need to be addressed to reduce the impact of travel on subsequent performance.

### Prior to travel

The travelling athlete should address any medical issues prior to departure, including prescriptions for ongoing medication; the need for immunization; and a dental check-up. Ensuring that passports are up to date and whether a visa is required to enter the country of destination will reduce any undue to anxiety and delay at the airport/port. When flying, the airline should be informed in advance if the athlete is a vegetarian or has other special dietary requirements.

### During travel

Rarely does travel go smoothly. Athletes should be prepared for problems, including delays, by taking their own entertainment, for example books/magazines, handheld computer games, music. For the journey, athletes should take something comfortable to change into on long-haul flights and something warm in case the inflight temperature drops. Additional food and drinks are important to ensure optimal fluid and food intake while travelling. Alcoholic and caffeinated drinks should be avoided during travel as these will increase the chances of becoming dehydrated. Ear plugs and eye masks can assist rest, relaxation and sleep during travel. Eyes may become sore on long flights if lenses are not removed. Contact lenses should be removed on long-haul flights to avoid undue discomfort. During long-haul flights athletes should walk about, stretch and exercise occasionally to avoid ankle oedema. There may be an increased risk of deep vein thrombosis (DVT) and subsequent pulmonary embolus following long-haul flights, often termed 'economy class syndrome', associated with long periods of seated inactivity (Brown et al 2001). The risk of DVT is increased in the elderly and in those using hormonal treatment, such as the oral contraceptive pill or HRT. A number of airlines now produce literature, available on flights, giving advice on reducing the side effects of prolonged air travel. Regular stretching and exercise will reduce this risk of DVT. The ingestion of a paediatric aspirin (75 mg) may reduce the risk but should not be taken if the athlete has a history of stomach ulcers and medical advice should be sought if you have a history of asthma. Wearing support stockings during the flight may also be beneficial (Belcaro et al 2001).

## Travel fatigue and jet lag

There are two key issues that can significantly affect performance when travelling from home to training and competition venues: travel fatigue and jet lag. Travel fatigue is characterized by a group of transient negative effects associated with prolonged periods of time spent in transit, irrespective of time zone changes. Travel fatigue generally lasts 1–2 days. Factors associated with travel fatigue include sleep loss due to early departures and late arrivals; long periods of unusual activity, including carrying of heavy bags and equipment; reduced or absent periods of recovery; and disrupted eating and drinking patterns. Table 3.1 summarizes strategies for dealing with travel fatigue.

When crossing a large number of time zones the body's natural biological rhythms (circadian rhythms) are disrupted, leading to a condition termed 'jet lag'. Jet lag is simply a lack of synchrony between the body clock and the outside world (Reilly et al 1997, Waterhouse et al 1992). In addition to a general feeling of fatigue, symptoms of jet lag include loss of concentration, loss of appetite, headache, dizziness, nausea and constipation. A decline in performance of activities involving complex mental activity, reduced hand grip and leg strength, reduced maximum performance, and a general loss of motivation, are observed in athletes in the short-term following multiple time zone changes (Reilly et al 1997, Reilly & Mellor 1988).

It may be some days before the body adapts to the new cycle of day and night, depending on the number of time zones crossed. Arriving well in advance of competition will allow time to fully adjust to the new time zone and reduce the impact of jet lag on performance. In order to fully adjust, 1 day for every 1 hour time zone change is optimal.

There are a number of strategies that can be employed to reduce the impact of jet lag. Pharmacological interventions including sleeping pills and melatonin have been used successfully to accelerate recovery from jet lag. The most important factor controlling circadian rhythms are the light–dark cycle and the associated release of melatonin by the pineal gland (Arendt 1992) during the hours of darkness. Ingestion of melatonin can also advance or delay the body clock, according to the time of ingestion (Lewy et al 1998); however, melatonin is not licensed or available in the United Kingdom. The British Olympic Association Acclimatization Working Party advises great caution in the use of drugs such as hypnotics (sleeping pills) or melatonin to help overcome jet lag (Reilly et al 1998). Caffeine, which has recently

**Table 3.1**   Check list for travel fatigue (based on: Waterhouse J et al 1992 The stress of travel. Journal of Sports Science 22:946–966)

---

*Symptoms*
Fatigue
Disorientation
Headaches


*Causes*
Disruption of normal routine
Hassles associated with travel (checking in/baggage claim/customs clearance)
Dehydration due to dry cabin air
Restricted movement


*Advice*
*Before the journey*:
Plan the journey well in advance
Try to arrange for any stop-over to be comfortable
Make sure about documentation, inoculations, visas
Make arrangements at your destination

*On the plane*:
Drink plenty of water or fruit juice (rather than tea/coffee/alcohol)
Perform stretching and isometric exercises if possible
Sleep only if it is night at the destination; if not, read, watch the movie or listen to music

*On reaching the destination*:
Take a *brief* nap, if required
Take a shower
Relax with a non-alcoholic drink

---

been removed from the World Anti-Doping Authority (WADA) list of banned substances, has been employed to enhance alertness following long-haul flights, and studies suggest that caffeine enhances grip strength following long-haul flights (Lagarde et al 2001). Caution is warranted, however, as these drugs have unpredictable effects and may result in a slowing of the adjustment to the new time zone.

There are a number of practical strategies that can be used to accelerate the recovery from jet lag (see Table 3.2). Adapting to the local time immediately on arrival and adopting a local sleep/wake pattern and meal time schedule can accelerate the recovery from jet lag. Avoiding prolonged (>1 hour) daytime napping and large meals and caffeinated beverages late at night can assist with quality of sleep. The circadian rhythm is set by alternating periods of light and dark. Therefore, staying in daylight or bright artificial light during the day and maintaining a darkened room during sleeping hours will help to accelerate recovery from jet lag.

Training intensity and duration should be reduced for the first few days following travel across multiple time zones. Reduced levels of performance should be anticipated by the coach as well as the athlete during the period of adjustment.

The effects of travel fatigue and jet lag can have a profound effect upon performance. The main objective for the travelling athlete is to reduce the stress of travel and promote rapid adjustment of the body clock to the new time zone. A successful taper is more likely to be achieved by eliminating/minimizing the impact of travel.

**Table 3.2**   Check list for dealing with jet lag (based on: Waterhouse J et al 1992 The stress of travel. Journal of Sports Science 22:946–966)

1. Check to see whether the journey is across sufficient time zones for jet lag to be a problem. If it is not, then it is necessary only to refer to advice on overcoming travel fatigue (Table 3.1)
2. If jet lag is likely, then consider whether the stay is too short for adjustment of the body clock to take place (a stay of less than 3 days). If it is too short, then remain on home time, and attempt to arrange sleep and activities to coincide with this as much as possible
3. If the stay is not too short (3 days or more) and it is wished to promote adjustment, then consider ways of reducing jet lag. Advice relates to: before, during and after the flight. The most important advice relates to after the flight
4. Advice for promoting adjustment concentrates on: sleep and melatonin; exposure to, and avoidance of, bright light; behavioral factors

## CARBOHYDRATE LOADING (GLYCOGEN SUPERCOMPENSATION)

Previous sections in this chapter have demonstrated an increase in muscle glycogen stores following the taper phase. Because of the importance of glycogen during exercise a considerable amount of research has been conducted examining techniques to further increase muscle glycogen stores prior to exercise and examine the impact on performance. As a result, several carbohydrate loading regimes have been developed since the late 1960s to enable athletes to store supranormal amounts of muscle glycogen, 'glycogen supercompensation'. The original protocol proposed by Bergstom et al (1967) involves a 6-day period divided into two 3-day periods. During the first 3-day period the athlete is required to undertake two episodes of glycogen-depleting exercise separated by 3 days whilst on a high-fat/low-carbohydrate (CHO) diet. During the following 3-day period the athlete reduces training as part of a normal taper (see above), and increased CHO intake to about 70–80% of total energy intake. Early findings suggested that this regime resulted in significantly elevated muscle glycogen concentrations and improved performance in time trials lasting longer than 90 minutes (Hawley et al 1997). Sherman et al (1981) proposed a modification to this protocol whereby the athlete consumed a low CHO diet, equating to 50% of total energy intake for 3 days, followed by 3 days of high CHO, equating to 70–80% of total energy intake, in the absence of glycogen-depleting exercise. This regime was as successful in increasing muscle glycogen stores and enhancing prolonged (> 90 minutes) endurance performance. Further, this modified protocol was better accepted by athletes and coaches as it did not require glycogen-depleting exercise during the taper phase. Subsequently, this protocol has been modified to a 3-day protocol eliminating the initial 3 days with similar results (Hawley et al 1997).

A number of recent attempts have been made to reduce the period required to induce supranormal muscle stores of glycogen. Fairchild et al (2002) proposed a 1-day protocol that included a near-maximal intensity episode of exercise (150 seconds at 130% $\dot{V}O_2$max followed by 30 seconds of all out cycling) followed by a 24-hour period of high CHO ingestion (10.3 g.kg$^{-1}$.day$^{-1}$). Results from this study demonstrated significantly increased levels of muscle glycogen. Care is warranted, however, as few athletes or coaches are willing to exercise for 3 minutes at near-maximal intensities on the day prior to competition. As such, the use of high-intensity exercise to induce glycogen supercompensation in the final stages of a taper are unlikely to be of practical use.

A recent study examining the time course of muscle glycogen supercompensation employed the 3-day protocol of increased CHO intake combined with a taper (Bussau et al 2002). Endurance-trained male athletes consumed a high-CHO diet ($10 \text{ g.kg}^{-1}.\text{day}^{-1}$) for 3 days while remaining physically inactive. Results demonstrated that muscle glycogen content was significantly increased after 1 day of the high-CHO diet and remained stable over the following 2 days. These data suggest that a single day of a high-CHO diet may be sufficient to induce muscle glycogen supercompensation.

Glycogen loading can increase muscle glycogen stores to levels of 160–200 $\text{mmol.kg}^{-1}$ wet muscle mass. In order to achieve these levels the ingestion of 8–10 $\text{g.kg}^{-1}.\text{day}^{-1}$ of CHO is required, accounting for 70–80% of total energy intake (Ivy 1991). The observed increase in muscle glycogen content appears to persist for at least 3 days in resting athletes when a moderate-CHO diet (60% of total energy intake) is consumed (Goforth et al 1997).

During exercise women tend to use greater levels of lipids as a substrate for energy production. Observed gender differences may be due to differences in the distribution and/or activation of $\alpha$- and $\beta$-adrenergic receptors, aerobic capacity and/or fitness level, exercise intensity, and lack of sufficient ingestion of CHO prior to exercise. It appears, however, that it is likely to be endocrine differences, and in particular the female sex hormone 17-$\beta$-estradiol that mediates the gender differences observed (Tarnapolsky et al 2001).

The increased reliance on lipids during exercise led to the suggestion that CHO loading would be less effective in female compared with male athletes. A number of studies support this contention, reporting no increases in muscle glycogen content or performance enhancement in response to CHO loading in highly trained female athletes (Andrews et al 2003). Two key factors underpinning the absence of improvement in muscle glycogen content and performance observed in these studies, however, are the phase of the menstrual cycle and quantity of CHO consumed during the loading period.

The menstrual cycle phase appears to be a critical factor in the efficacy of carbohydrate loading. The rate of glycogen re-synthesis is greater during the luteal phase compared with the follicular phase. In particular, glycogen loading during the 5–10 days following the first day of menses reduces the impact of gonadotrophic hormones and enhances glycogen loading. Thus, the equivocal findings reported from studies examining female athletes are probably due to testing during the follicular phase of the menstrual cycle (Andrews et al 2003). In addition to menstrual cycle phase, insufficient quantities of CHO ($<8.0 \text{ g.kg}^{-1}.\text{day}^{-1}$) are often ingested by female athletes in studies reporting no changes in muscle glycogen content and performance enhancement following glycogen loading (Andrews et al 2003). Indeed, in those studies conducted during the luteal phase with CHO consumption $<8.0 \text{ g.kg}^{-1}.\text{day}^{-1}$ female athletes exhibited similar levels of muscle glycogen and performance enhancement to their male counterparts (Tarnapolsky et al 2001).

It is generally accepted that increasing muscle glycogen content to supranormal levels is only valuable for sub-maximal endurance exercise lasting longer than 90 minutes, with improvements in performance of up to 20% (Hawley et al 1997). Indeed, the majority of studies examining short duration (<5 minutes) high-intensity exercise, and moderate-intensity exercise lasting 60–90 minutes have failed to demonstrate performance gains following glycogen loading. A small number of studies, however, examining the role of carbohydrate loading on short duration, high-intensity exercise have reported improved performances (Pizza et al 1995). Therefore, in addition to sub-maximal exercise lasting longer than 90 minutes, the nature of exercise observed in team games, with intermittent, high-intensity efforts over a prolonged period of time (>60 minutes), may lend itself to a CHO-loading regime.

As with all forms of training, the use of glycogen supercompensation should be carefully planned prior to the taper phase. Previous studies have demonstrated that specific instructions and knowledge of food compositions are required if athletes are to attain the required CHO intake to optimize muscle glycogen stores. The role of the performance nutritionist in this process is fundamental.

## SUMMARY

It should be noted that there is a significant psychological and technical component to successful athletic performance following a taper, and that not all of the performance improvements highlighted above are purely physiological. There is no doubt that psychological peaking can have an influence on performance (Hooper et al 1999) and coaches, athletes and exercise physiologists alike should take note of this.

Despite the recent scientific advances in this area, there still remain a number of physiological adaptations to tapering and their performance implications that are yet to be addressed. What is clear, however, is that there are significant performance gains to be achieved by incorporating taper periods into training programmes. Tapering will remain a subtle and complex technique that requires precise planning, monitoring and evaluation. A number of key components to successful tapers are now becoming better understood. Table 3.3 summarizes the components of optimal tapering strategies that may help increase the chances of achieving peak performance. Training intensity appears to be a key 'ingredient' for effective tapering and should either be maintained or increased during the taper, together with a decrease in training volume so as to allow for sufficient rest and recovery. The primary goal of the taper should be to minimize accumulated fatigue from the previous training phase rather than achieve additional physiological adaptations. It should always be remembered that training is individual-specific and therefore the duration and type of taper will depend largely on the individual athlete as well as on the nature of the sport.

**Table 3.3**   Summary of optimal tapering strategies

Ensure precise planning and monitoring
Maintain or increase training intensity to greater than or equal to competition intensity (i.e. 80–100%)
Reduce training volume by 60–90%
Maintain training frequency at > 80%
Employ exponential taper designs between 4 and 28 days
Increase recovery between sets and/or reps
Ensure that training is race/event-specific
Remember to optimize psychological and technical aspects
Individualize taper programmes whenever possible
Perform post-competition evaluation/assessments so as to inform future tapering strategies

Although much of the scientific literature regarding tapering is traditionally associated with endurance sports such as swimming, cycling and running there is no reason why such a technique should not be practiced within other sports such as those that are team, skill or strength based. The physiological adaptations that occur as a result of the taper phase including increases in glycogen stores and strength and power will be beneficial to a wide range of sports. The use of nutritional strategies to further increase glycogen storage (glycogen supercompensation) may also be of value for a number of sports and should be considered as part of the taper phase.

Finally, it should be noted that a number of external factors can affect the taper period which, if not controlled for, can negatively affect performance. This is particularly true for long-haul flights and when competition takes place in unfamiliar environments such as in the heat, cold or at altitude (see Ch. 8).

## KEY POINTS

1. Tapering is a specialized exercise training technique designed to reverse training-induced fatigue without a loss of the training adaptations.
2. A successful taper phase requires careful planning and should aim to optimize all the determinants of performance at a single point in time.
3. There are four types of taper: fast and slow exponential taper, linear taper and step taper.
4. Physiological adaptations during a taper include an increase in $\dot{V}O_2$max, type II fibre size and glycolytic enzyme function, muscle glycogen content, strength and power, and performance.
5. External factors, including travel fatigue and jet lag, can have profound effects on an effective taper.
6. Nutritional interventions, including glycogen supercompensation, during the taper increase muscle glycogen content and may enhance performance.

## References

Andrews J, Sedlock D, Flynn M et al 2003 Carbohydrate loading and supplementation in endurance-trained women runners. Journal of Applied Physiology 95:584–590

Arendt J 1992 The pineal. In: Touitou Y, Haus E (eds) Biological rhythms in clinical and laboratory medicine. Springer-Verlag, Berlin, p 348–362

Belcaro G, Geroulakos G, Nicolaides A et al 2001 Venous thromboembolism from air travel: the LONFLIT study. Angiology 52:369–374

Bergstrom J, Hermansen L, Hultman E, Saltin B 1967 Diet, muscle glycogen and physical performance. Acta Physiologica Scandinavica 71:140–150

Brown T, Shuker L, Rushton L et al 2001 The possible effects on health, comfort and safety of aircraft cabin environments. Journal of the Royal Society for the Promotion of Health 121:177–184

Bussau V, Fairchild T, Rao A et al 2002 Carbohydrate loading in human muscle: an improved 1 day protocol. European Journal of Applied Physiology 87:290–295

Busso T, Benoit H, Bonnefoy R et al 2002 Effects of training frequency on the dynamics of performance response to a single training bout. Journal of Applied Physiology 92:572–580

Fairchild T, Fletcher S, Steele P et al 2002 Rapid carbohydrate loading after a short bout of near maximal-intensity exercise. Medicine and Science in Sport and Exercise 34:980–986

Fits RH, Costill DL, Gardetto PR 1989 Effect of swim exercise training on human muscle fiber function. Journal of Applied Physiology 66:465–475

Gibala MJ, MacDougall JD, Sale DG 1994 The effects of tapering on strength performance in trained athletes. International Journal of Sports Medicine 15(8):492–497

Goforth H, Arnall D, Bennett B, Law P 1997 Persistence of supercompensated muscle glycogen in trained subjects after carbohydrate loading. Journal of Applied Physiology 82:342–347

Hawley J, Schabort E, Noakes T, Dennis C 1997 Carbohydrate loading and exercise performance: an update. Sports Medicine 24:73–81

Hooper SL, Mackinnon LT, Howard A 1999 Physiological and psychometric variables for monitoring recovery during tapering for major competition. Medical Science in Sport and Exercise 31:1205–1210

Houmard JA, Scott BK, Justice CL, Chenier TC 1994 The effects of taper on performance in distance runners. Medical Science in Sport and Exercise 26(5):624–631

Ivy J 1991 Muscle glycogen synthesis before and after exercise. Sports Medicine 11:6–19

Jeukenfrup AE, Hesselink MKC, Snyder AC et al 1992 Physiological changes in male competitive cyclists after two weeks of intensified training. International Journal of Sports Medicine 13(7):534–541

Johns RA, Houmard JA, Kobe RW et al 1992 Effects of taper on swim power, stroke distance and performance. Medical Science in Sport and Exercise 24(10):1141–1146

Lagarde D, Chappuis B, Billaud P et al 2001 Evaluation of pharmacological aids on physical performance after a transmeridian flight. Medical Science in Sport and Exercise 33:628–634

Lewy A, Bauer V, Ahmed S et al 1998 The human phase response curve (PRC) to melatonin is about 12 hours out of phase with the PRC to light. Chronobiology International 15:71–83

Martin D, Anderson M 2000 Heart rate-perceived exertion relationship during training and taper. Journal of Sports Medicine and Physical Fitness 40:201–208

Martin DT, Scifres JC, Zimmerman SD, Wilkinson JG 1994 Effects of interval training on cycling performance and isokinetic leg strength. International Journal of Sports Medicine 15(8):485–491

Mujika I, Padilla S, Pyne D 2002a Swimming performance changes during the final 3 weeks of training leading to the Sydney 2000 Olympic Games. International Journal of Sports Medicine 23(8):582–587

Mujika I, Goya, A, Ruiz E et al 2002b Physiological and performance responses to a 6-day taper in middle-distance runners: influence of training frequency. International Journal of Sports Medicine 23(5):367–373

Mujika I, Padilla S 2003 Scientific bases for precompetition tapering strategies. Medicine and Science in Sports and Exercise 35(7):1182–1187

Mujika I, Padilla, S, Pyne D, Busso T 2004 Physiological changes associated with the pre-event taper in athletes. Sports Medicine 34(13):891–927

Neary JP, Martin TP, Reid DC et al 1992 The effects of a reduced exercise duration taper programme on performance and muscle enzymes of endurance cyclists. European Journal of Applied Physiology 65(1):30–36

Neary JP, Martin, TP, Quinney HA 2003a Effects of taper on endurance cycling capacity and single muscle fiber properties. Medicine and Science in Sports and Exercise 35(11):1875–1881

Neary JP, Bhambhani YN, McKenzie DC 2003b Effects of different stepwise reduction taper protocols on cycling performance. Canadian Journal of Applied Physiology 28(4):576–587

Pizza F, Flynn M, Duscha B et al 1995 A carbohydrate loading regimen improves high intensity, short duration exercise performance. International Journal of Sports Nutrition 5:110–116

Reilly T, Mellor S 1988 Jet-lag in student Rugby League players following a near maximal time-zone shift. In: Reilly A et al (eds) Science and football. Spon, London, p 249–256

Reilly T, Atkinson G, Waterhouse J 1997 Biological rhythms and exercise. Oxford University Press, Oxford

Reilly T, Maughan R, Budgett R 1998 Melatonin: a position statement of the British Olympic Association. British Journal of Sports Medicine 32:99–100

Rietjens GJ, Keizer HA, Kuipers H, Saris WH 2001 A reduction in training volume and intensity for 21 days does not impair performance in cyclists. British Journal of Sports Medicine 35(6):431–434

Riggs CE, Kilgour RD, Belowich D 1983 Muscle glycogen storage and effects of tapered training. Journal of Sports Medicine 23:131–135

Shepley B, MacDougall JD, Cipriano N et al 1992 Physiological effects of tapering in highly trained athletes. Journal of Applied Physiology 72(2):706–711

Sherman W, Costill D, Fink W, Miller M 1981 Effect of exercise-diet manipulation on muscle glycogen and its subsequent utilization during performance. International Journal of Sports Medicine 2:114–118

Tarnapolsky M, Zawada C, Richmond L et al 2001 Gender differences in carbohydrate loading are related to energy intake. Journal of Applied Physiology 91:225–230

The travelling athlete document 1999 The British Olympic Medical Centre

Trappe S, Costill D, Thomas R 2000 Effect of swim taper on whole muscle and single muscle fiber contractile properties. Medicine and Science in Sports and Exercise 32(12):48–56

Walker JL, Heigenhauser GJF, Hultman E, Spriet LL 2000 Dietary carbohydrate, muscle glycogen content, and endurance performance in well-trained women. Journal of Applied Physiology 88:2151–2158

Waterhouse J, Reilly T, Edwards B 1992 The stress of travel. Journal of Sports Science 22:946–966

Zarkadas PC, Carter, JB, Banister EW 1995 Modelling the effect of taper on performance, maximal oxygen uptake, and the anaerobic threshold in endurance triathletes. Advances in Experimental Medical Biology 393:179–186

## Further reading

Bompa T 1999 Periodization. Theory and methodology of training. Human Kinetics, Champaign IL

Elliot B 1999 Training in sport: applying sports science. John Wiley, Chichester

Muller E, Zallinger G 1999 Science in elite sport. Spon Press.

Reilly T, Williams M 2002 Science and soccer. Routledge, London

# Chapter **4**

# The physiology of endurance training

Robert Shave and Andrew Franco

## CHAPTER CONTENTS

## LEARNING OBJECTIVES:

This chapter is intended to ensure that the reader:

1. Gains an understanding of the physiological determinants of endurance performance.
2. Gains an appreciation of the various training modalities that endurance athletes may use.
3. Gains an understanding of the physiological adaptations that occur in response to the different training modalities employed by endurance athletes.
4. Understands the multi-factorial nature of endurance training.

5. Appreciates that differences exist between highly trained and sedentary individuals in terms of physiological adaptations to training.
6. Appreciates the need for individually tailored training programmes.

## INTRODUCTION

At the outset of this chapter it is appropriate to define what is meant by endurance performance. A continuum of performance exists with ultra-endurance exercise (such as the Ironman triathlon) at one end and very rapid sprint events (such as the 100 m sprint) at the other. Between these two extremes there is a myriad of events within the sporting field whose energy requirements are met by different contributions of the anaerobic and aerobic energy pathways. For the purposes of this chapter, endurance performance will be defined as continuous activity beyond 5 minutes, but less than 4 hours, in duration. Events shorter than this depend largely upon the anaerobic re-synthesis of ATP (see Ch. 5). While ultra-endurance events such as those lasting longer than 5 hours are likely to be affected by additional athlete-specific factors, including nutrition and psychological state, and, as such, aerobic endurance may not be the principal determinant of performance. From this definition it is clear that endurance performance covers a wide variety of events ranging from competitive rowing (~6 minutes) through to marathon competitions (~2–3 hours), and beyond to some cycle stage races (~4 hours). Although the duration of these events is different the predominant source of ATP is via aerobic processes, and thus much of the endurance training completed by these athletes is comparable in nature.

Many researchers to date have attempted to identify the specific physiological determinants of endurance performance (Ingham et al 2002). In a similar fashion, coaches and athletes have endeavoured, largely through a process of trial and error, to identify appropriate training techniques to elicit the greatest improvements in performance. The purpose of this chapter is to examine these two aspects of endurance performance by addressing the physiological determinants of endurance performance and the optimum training techniques to enhance these physiological attributes. To date, much of the research examining aerobic endurance has employed sedentary or moderately active individuals. Recent studies, however, have attempted to examine the impact of different training techniques upon aerobic endurance in highly trained individuals. Wherever possible the information presented in this chapter will be drawn from the literature examining the highly trained athlete.

A large number of studies have examined the relationship between a variety of physiological variables and endurance performance. Authors have contended that certain physiological factors may be of greater importance than others; however, it is clear from the literature that endurance performance is not governed by a single physiological variable. Rather, endurance performance is dependent upon a number of variables all of which display varying degrees of trainability. Maximal oxygen uptake ($\dot{V}O_2max$), lactate threshold, economy, fractional utilization and fuel supply all affect endurance performance (see Fig. 4.1). Discussion of each of these variables is provided in the following chapter prior to investigation of how they may be specifically targeted through training.

## MAXIMAL OXYGEN UPTAKE

Maximal oxygen uptake ($\dot{V}O_2max$) may be defined as the highest rate at which oxygen can be extracted, transported and consumed in the process of aerobic ATP

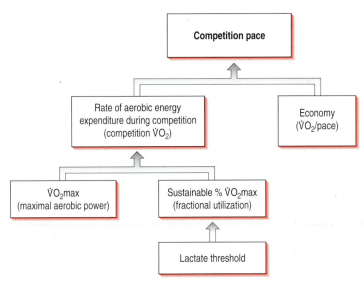

**Figure 4.1**  Physiological model outlining the major physiological determinants of endurance performance.

synthesis. Typically, $\dot{V}O_2$max is expressed in millilitres of oxygen per kilogram of body weight per unit of time (i.e. $mL.kg^{-1}.min^{-1}$). Numerous studies suggest that $\dot{V}O_2$max is highly related to endurance performance. It should be noted, however, that these relationships are based largely upon the study of heterogeneous samples, and when the relationship between $\dot{V}O_2$max and marathon performance is examined within a homogeneous group of highly trained runners (with similar performance times) there appears to be little relationship between $\dot{V}O_2$max and performance. Despite the observed lack of relationship between $\dot{V}O_2$max and performance, however, it is clear that a well developed aerobic capacity ($\dot{V}O_2$max) is a prerequisite for endurance performance. It would appear, however, that physiological parameters other than $\dot{V}O_2$max may be more important in determining endurance performance, especially within truly elite individuals.

## LACTATE THRESHOLD

It is well recognized that an exercise intensity exists beyond which muscle glycogenolysis is markedly increased, thus facilitating the exponential accumulation of lactate within the active muscles and blood (Coyle 1995). Numerous terms have been used to describe this phenomenon, including lactate threshold (LT), anaerobic threshold and 'onset of blood lactate accumulation' (OBLA). Discussion regarding the correct definition persists; further, scientists have also proposed many methods and exercise protocols of identifying the specific point at which blood lactate begins to accumulate. Some have gone so far as to suggest the use of a fixed blood lactate concentration to represent the point of accumulation. Typically, LT (as the phenomenon will be referred to within this chapter) is defined as a speed, heart rate, or $\%\dot{V}O_2$max relative to the point of lactate accumulation. Despite the contention surrounding lactate threshold, its definition, and its measurement, it is clear that a strong relationship exists between LT and endurance performance. Sjodin & Svedenhag (1985) reported correlations between 0.88 and 0.99 for the relationship between LT and performance times in endurance events of varying durations. Further, studies examining marathon running suggest that the speed associated with LT closely equates to the natural race pace selected by marathon runners.

## ECONOMY

Exercise economy can be defined as the oxygen uptake required to produce a specific power output or speed. Considerable variations in exercise economy exist between individuals, even in athletes with comparable aerobic capacities. An improvement in exercise economy manifest by a lower $\dot{V}O_2$ for the same absolute power output or speed is advantageous to endurance performance, as it will result in a lower percentage of $\dot{V}O_2$max being utilized during exercise. Further, in relation to a lower percentage of $\dot{V}O_2$max, greater economy is also associated with a lower rate of fuel consumption for a given speed or power output. Thus, improving exercise economy will preserve glycogen stores during endurance performance, favouring the more economical athlete. Although improved exercise economy may result in improved performance, in a similar fashion to $\dot{V}O_2$max, groups of highly trained individuals with similar performance times exhibit different exercise economies. Economy is velocity/power output specific and highly trained athletes will exhibit high levels of economy at their specialist race distance. It is noteworthy that athletes who participate in long-duration events tend to possess better exercise economy at slower velocities than athletes who partake in shorter duration endurance events who posses better economy at higher velocities (e.g. marathon versus 5-km runners).

## FRACTIONAL UTILIZATION

Fractional utilization refers to the percentage of $\dot{V}O_2$max that an athlete can sustain while exercising at race pace, and is dependent upon both the training status and the exercise duration. Figure 4.2 demonstrates the relationship between fractional utilization, exercise duration and training status (Bassett & Howley 2000).

Running velocity at $\dot{V}O_2$max closely corresponds to the velocity that an elite runner can sustain for 3000 m (approximately 8 minutes). Given that most endurance events last longer than 8 minutes, the majority of endurance athletes are required to work at an intensity below their $\dot{V}O_2$max. In reality, during competition athletes perform at the highest possible power output, this being the maximal exercise intensity that does not result in the debilitating effects associated with the accumulation of metabolic waste products. Fractional utilization is therefore dependent upon the %$\dot{V}O_2$max associated with LT. Within highly trained athletes who have largely maximized their $\dot{V}O_2$max, improving fractional utilization is critical in improving performance. A highly trained individual may demonstrate a fractional utilization of approximately 85% of $\dot{V}O_2$max while an untrained individual may be able to sustain only 50% $\dot{V}O_2$max.

## FUEL SUPPLY

Prolonged endurance exercise requires substantial expenditure of energy. Estimates of total energy requirement for a marathon range from 9000 to 12 000 kJ. During high-intensity exercise, muscle glycogen is utilized more readily than blood glucose and fatty acids, and is therefore preferentially used to generate the required energy.

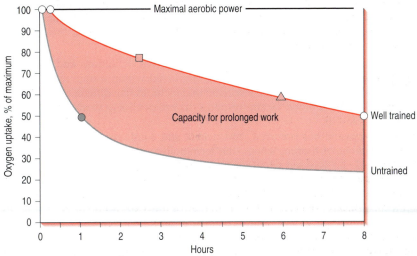

**Figure 4.2**   Percentage of $\dot{V}O_2$max that can be sustained for different durations of exercise pre- and post-training (Bassett & Howley 2000).

With training, however, athletes can improve their ability to oxidize fats at submaximal exercise intensities. Thus, highly trained athletes develop the physiological ability to spare muscle glycogen during prolonged exercise. The increased reliance on fat metabolism subsequent to training results in the delayed onset of fatigue associated with the depletion of glycogen stores. In practical terms, the ability to spare glycogen during performance enhances glycogen availability towards the end of an endurance event when an increase in exercise intensity (the sprint finish) may be critical to success.

All of the physiological variables discussed above will affect endurance performance; furthermore, they all demonstrate degrees of trainability. Coaches, athletes and support scientists aim to design training programmes to capitalize on an athlete's strengths and ameliorate the physiological weaknesses. Training modalities may be employed to specifically target certain physiological parameters; however, it is more likely that a training programme will be devised to employ numerous different training modalities, resulting in the adaptation of a number of the physiological determinants of endurance performance. In light of this typical training approach, researchers examining elite athletes have struggled to delineate the different physiological adaptations to the various training modalities employed.

The concept of training specificity was addressed earlier within this text (see Ch. 2), and although specificity needs to be at the forefront when considering training programmes, coaches and athletes should be cognisant of supplementary training sessions that initially may not appear to comply with specificity. Hence, specificity does not mean that all training should be completed at race pace. It should be remembered that each of the physiological determinants of endurance performance are multi-factorial, and thus require multiple stimuli to manifest the desired adaptations. Accordingly, aerobic, anaerobic, interval, strength, power, speed and flexibility training all have a place within a well designed training programme of an endurance athlete.

# TRAINING FOR ENDURANCE PERFORMANCE

## Training intensity

Over the years different sports have adopted different definitions and terminology to categorize the various types of training employed within a training programme. For example, rowing has adopted a scheme that includes five different training zones, based largely on the blood lactate response to progressively harder exercise intensities (see Table 4.1).

Much discussion has occurred, and debate still continues, regarding the definition and number of training zones, the terminology used, the physiological markers that should be assessed while monitoring training intensity and the appropriate periodization of training zones. Many sports have attempted to identify training zones in a very similar fashion to that described for rowing. On inspection of the scientific literature, however, it is apparent that this process may be a little optimistic. Wide-reaching review articles (Pate & Branch 1992) broadly categorize training associated with endurance performance into three distinct zones:

- Long slow distance;
- Moderate-duration, high-intensity training;
- Short-duration, very high-intensity training.

In addition to the basic training zones, a proportion of an endurance athlete's time will be devoted to strength training and flexibility. The following sections of this chapter aim to examine each of these training methods in turn, and to assess the physiological impact and importance associated with each specific training modality. In the first instance, however, a brief overview of each of the training modalities is presented.

## LONG SLOW DISTANCE (LSD)

Prolonged bouts of moderately intense exercise have become the staple training modality for the vast majority of athletes competing in a variety of endurance sports, and normally provide the largest volume to any training programme. Typical LSD sessions require the athlete to train for between 60 and 120 minutes at an intensity that equates to approximately 60–70% $\dot{V}O_2$max. Such exercise intensity probably results in a minimal blood lactate concentration well below that observed during competition, and certainly represents an intensity well below that which would be considered 'race pace'.

**Table 4.1** The system of training prescription that has been adopted by the sport of rowing

| Code | Name | Heart rate reserve (%) | Blood lactate (mmol/L) |
|------|------|------------------------|------------------------|
| UT2 | Basic oxygen utilization training | 59–67 | 0–2 |
| UT1 | Oxygen utilization training | 67–75 | 2–3.5 |
| AT | Anaerobic threshold training | 75–85 | 3.6–4.5 |
| TR | Oxygen transport training | 85–100 | 4.5–6 |
| AC | Anaerobic capacity training | | >6 |

## MODERATE-DURATION, HIGH-INTENSITY TRAINING (THRESHOLD TRAINING)

This type of training has typically been performed around an individual's lactate threshold (LT). Much discussion has taken place regarding the concept of LT: how it may be defined, the appropriate protocols to employ in order to assess LT, and even whether a threshold exists. For a comprehensive review of the LT concept readers are directed to the work of Bourdon (2000). For clarity it is, however, pertinent to understand some of the definitions employed in the literature to describe lactate breakpoints. The term 'lactate threshold' has been used to describe a number of distinct physiological phenomena; for example, a non-linear increase in blood lactate of at least 1 mmol/L (Coyle 1995), a workload preceding a non-linear rise in blood lactate during progressive exercise (Ivy et al 1980), or, the point of deflection in the logged blood lactate versus logged $\dot{V}O_2$ transformation (Beaver et al 1985). In effect, all of these definitions attempt to identify the workload at which there is a sustained increase in blood lactate above baseline values. In recent times this point has also been referred to as lactate breakpoint 1. Further along the lactate transition curve associated with incremental exercise a second breakpoint may also be identified. This second point relates to the workload at which blood lactate begins to rapidly accumulate, and as such represents the highest work intensity that blood lactate can equilibrate. This breakpoint has also been defined by a number of terms; Kindermann et al (1979) suggested that this point represented the anaerobic threshold (AT) and was demonstrated by the steep part of the exponential increase in blood lactate concentration. The onset of blood lactate accumulation (OBLA) has also been used within the literature (Sjodin & Jacobs 1981), as has a fixed blood lactate concentration of 4 mmol/L, and the term maximum lactate steady state. Although discussion of appropriate definition and terminology persists, the concept of lactate breakpoints and their identification is central to many scientific support programmes.

Notwithstanding the contentious issues surrounding LT, a training zone appears to exist that coincides with a number of the suggested definitions of LT, which is sensitive to training and results in improved performance. This type of training is performed at an intensity that equates to the point at which blood lactate begins to rise exponentially, and typically lasts in the region of 30–60 minutes.

## SHORT-DURATION, VERY-HIGH-INTENSITY TRAINING

High-intensity-interval training (HIT) involves periods of intense exercise interspersed with periods of recovery. Exercise intensity is typically above an athlete's $\dot{V}O_2$max, and due to the intense nature of this training modality, the duration of the repetitions is relatively short (30 seconds to 5 minutes), with rest intervals typically lasting 15–120 seconds. Coaches attempt to optimize the training stimulus via manipulation of the duration and intensity of both the repetition and recovery phase. Such optimization depends upon the specific event in which the athlete performs.

## RESISTANCE TRAINING

The umbrella term of resistance training encompasses a number of different training techniques (e.g. weight training and power training). Typically, however, weight training involves exercises performed against a resistance to enhance strength and muscular endurance. Exercises are usually split into repetitions and sets and are separated by periods of recovery. Similar to HIT, optimization of weight training sessions is dependent upon the manipulation of the training stimulus via weight, sets, repetitions and recovery. The period within the athletes training cycle, the athlete's specific event and the ultimate goal of the training session will influence the design of the resistance sessions (see Ch. 7). Plyometric exercises may also be included within this subset of training modalities, which typically involves bounding and jumping-type exercises, emphasizing the speed of movement and limited ground contact time principally used in the development of power (see Ch. 6).

## FLEXIBILITY

Athletes devote considerable time to improving and maintaining their flexibility. Flexibility may be defined as the ability to move a joint smoothly through its entire range of motion. It has been suggested that improved flexibility reduces the risk of injury and enhances the economy of movement, and thus may facilitate an improved performance. While there are obvious benefits for improving flexibility in certain sports, such as gymnastics, the performance benefits of increased flexibility in endurance sport are less clear. A limited number of studies have examined the relationship between flexibility and performance; those that exist will be discussed later in this chapter.

## THE PHYSIOLOGY OF LONG SLOW DISTANCE (LSD) TRAINING

Typical LSD training sessions are performed at very conservative intensities ($< 70\%$ $\dot{V}O_2max$), for prolonged periods of time that greatly exceed the duration of exercise performed during competition. Because of the mismatch between performance and LSD training it is often difficult to reconcile the reliance upon this type of training with the 'cornerstone' training principle of specificity.

Closer inspection of the physiological adaptations associated with LSD training, and a re-examination of the determinants of endurance performance reveal a number of adaptations associated with LSD training that are critical in the improvement of endurance performance. LSD training facilitates the adaptation of a number of physiological variables – including blood volume, mitochondrial size and density, fat mobilization, the ability to thermoregulate and the development of neuromuscular patterns. In addition, LSD training may benefit the athlete via the development of muscular endurance in the supporting musculature, and assist in preparing both psychological and nutritional strategies. A further benefit associated with LSD training is that although the volume of training is high, the forces placed upon the musculoskeletal system are relatively low. Due to this relatively modest intensity, athletes are able to complete a large volume of modality specific training while minimizing the risk of overuse or high-impact injuries.

## Blood volume

Much data has been generated examining the impact of training upon blood volume (BV). Cross-sectional studies have demonstrated a 20–25% greater BV in endurance athletes when compared to their sedentary counterparts. The observed increases in BV occur independently of sex and age (Convertino 1991). Longitudinal studies, however, suggest that endurance training may lead to a more conservative rise in BV of 7%. Methodological issues might explain the discrepancies between cross-sectional and longitudinal studies, specifically the training status of the participants studied. Young trained individuals with already relatively well developed BVs do not appear to be able to further enhance BV. Thus, BV expansion subsequent to LSD training may be limited by training status, or even by genetic endowment.

The expansion of BV observed during endurance training involves an initial increase in plasma volume within the first 10 days of the training programme. The proliferation of red blood cells lags behind the preliminary increase in plasma volume and may not rise appreciably until 4 weeks of training have been completed. Convertino et al (1980) report an 8% increase in BV following 8 consecutive days of LSD training (2 hours at 65% $\dot{V}O_2$max). The observed hypervolaemia in this study was a function of a 12% increase in plasma volume and no change in red cell volume. Data from the same study demonstrated that plasma osmolality and protein concentration also remained constant, hence, homeostatic control of both the osmotic gradient and electrochemical properties of fluids within the vascular space appears to be effective in maintaining a normal functional physiological environment. The rapid increase in BV in response to endurance training is matched by an equally rapid return to baseline values following 7 days of de-training. Such a rapid return demonstrates the importance of maintaining the training stimulus in order to sustain an enhanced BV.

Blood volume expansion appears to be related to an initial protein and fluid shift from the extravascular to the intravascular space followed by a sustained increase in total body water. This two-phase process results in an increased blood volume while also maintaining interstitial fluid, which is critical in terms of heat dissipation via increased sweat gland activity (an additional adaptation to endurance training). The hypervolaemia associated with endurance training benefits the athlete through three mechanisms: (i) an enhanced ability to cope with increased thermal stress (which will be discussed later), (ii) an improved cardiac function and (iii) an increased oxygen-carrying capacity.

Prolonged engagement in LSD training precipitates an enhanced stroke volume and a concomitant bradycardia, both of which probably occur as a function of the hypervolaemia propagated by endurance training. Studies have reported a 1% reduction in exercise heart rate with every 1% increase in plasma volume (Convertino 1991). Such adaptations in heart rate and stroke volume may be explained by the Frank-Starling mechanism. Hypervolaemia leads to an enhanced central venous pressure both at rest and during exercise, hence, end diastolic volume is increased (cardiac preload). It is this increase in cardiac preload that will augment stroke volume via the Frank-Starling mechanism. A greater stroke volume will result in a lower heart rate for the same absolute workload. If we remember that cardiac output (Q) is the product of heart rate and stroke volume (Q = HR * SV), the mechanisms for a reduction in heart rate at sub-maximal exercise subsequent to a training induced hypervolaemia becomes clear. During maximal exercise, an augmented blood volume results in an increased maximal cardiac output (Qmax). As cardiac output is a major factor in determining $\dot{V}O_2$max ($\dot{V}O_2$max = Qmax * a-v$O_2$diff max) any improvement in Qmax will probably result in an augmented maximal aerobic capacity.

In addition to the increased SV and resultant Qmax following a prolonged LSD training programme, the absolute haemoglobin concentration is also enhanced. As already stated, the increase in red blood cell mass is not as immediate as the increase in plasma volume; however, following prolonged training, an increased oxygen-carrying capacity is observed concomitant to an improved capacity to remove the metabolic waste associated with the production of ATP. Capillary density of the working musculature is also enhanced in response to LSD training. The main advantage associated with an increased capillary density is not an upgrading of blood flow but rather an increase in the mean transit time. Thus, even at high rates of blood flow, as observed during intense exercise, oxygen extraction (a-vO$_2$ difference) at the muscle bed is maintained. Further, during sub-maximal exercise the muscle may require a lower blood supply for the same absolute workload due to the enhanced ability to extract oxygen. Results from Tesch and associates (1984) demonstrate the difference in capillary density between endurance-trained and strength-trained athletes, endurance athletes demonstrating a 102% greater capillary density than their strength-trained counterparts. Although the study does not differentiate LSD training from other forms of endurance training, it does provide evidence for the differential capilarization between training methods employed by endurance- and strength-based athletes.

## Mitochondrial size and density

LSD training results in an enhanced size and density of mitochondria. Whether this increase will be apparent in all types of muscle fibre is dependent upon the recruitment of each type of fibre during exercise training. As LSD training probably recruits predominantly 'slow-twitch' type I fibres, it is likely that the greatest improvement in mitochondrial size and density will be observed within these fibres. Coupled with an increase in mitochondrial volume is a concomitant increase in the enzymes of the Krebs cycle, electron transport chain and malate–aspartate shuttle. It is the increase in these enzymes subsequent to training that facilitates an increased capacity of aerobic re-synthesis of ATP. These adaptations allow the athlete to exercise at a higher percentage of $\dot{V}O_2$max and hence may promote improvements in endurance performance. An improved oxidative capacity within type I fibres may delay the recruitment of type II fibres. Further, type II fibres depending on their recruitment within training (intensity dependent) may also experience an increased oxidative capacity. Both of these adaptations will reduce the contribution of anaerobic glycolysis to the total energy yield during endurance exercise and as such enhance fatigue resistance within the athlete.

## Fat mobilization

Muscle glycogen depletion and an increased rate of fat oxidation – both of which are encountered within endurance performance – are inherent to LSD training. Prolonged training in a glycogen-depleted state results in an enhanced ability to both mobilize and subsequently oxidize fatty acids from adipose tissue. Such adaptation will result in a sparing of glycogen and ultimately defer the accumulation of metabolic waste products associated with ATP production from glycolysis.

## Thermoregulation

LSD training may also facilitate improvements in performance via adaptations associated with improved heat toleration and heat dissipation. A strong relationship between elevations in core temperature ($T_c$) and endurance performance has been demonstrated within the literature (Gonzalez-Alonso et al 1999) and is anecdotally supported by the vast majority of athletes. An improved capacity to cope with rises in $T_c$ is probably a function of adaptations associated with LSD training. An enhanced plasma volume together with improved cutaneous blood flow and an improved sweat response all assist in the dissipation of heat generated during exercise. Although true heat acclimatization requires environmental exposure, high-intensity exercise may promote $T_c$ in excess of 40°C which, in turn, may facilitate a level of physiological adaptation. Thus, an improved ability to tolerate rises in $T_c$ may be the result of a combination of the adaptations to LSD and high-intensity training.

## Development of neuromuscular patterns

The development of neuromuscular patterns has also been lauded as a possible benefit derived from LSD training. It should be noted that developing neuromuscular patterns during low-intensity exercise does not necessarily reflect the neuromuscular requirements of competition pace. It is, therefore, important that endurance athletes train over a range of intensities so as to facilitate adaptations in the neuromuscular patterns recruited during race pace activity.

Many of the adaptations observed in response to LSD training plateau relatively early in an athlete's career. Subsequent to this plateau any increase in LSD training volume is unlikely to lead to improvements in performance; a study by Costill et al (1988) clearly demonstrates this issue. Costill et al (1988) examined a group of highly trained swimmers, increasing their training distance by approximately 50% for a period of 10 days while maintaining training intensity over the same period. Following the increase in training volume no change was observed in either aerobic capacity or swim performance (see Ch. 3). A recent meta-analysis suggests that once an athlete has achieved a $\dot{V}O_2$max of >60 mL.kg.min$^{-1}$ further improvements in endurance performance are not related to increases in training volume (Londeree 1997). Thus, simply increasing the volume of LSD training completed by highly trained individuals does not appear to be productive as further improvements in either physiological characteristics or endurance performance do not occur.

In light of the limitations associated with LSD training it is essential for endurance athletes and coaches to diversify the training modalities employed to elicit further physiological adaptations that will result in an enhanced performance. Fortunately, the training stimulus required to maintain the positive adaptations brought about via LSD training is considerably less than that required to initially foster them. Therefore, time is available within a training programme to employ additional training techniques to aid athlete development while still being able to sustain the adaptations stimulated by LSD work with a minimal number of LSD maintenance sessions each week.

## THE PHYSIOLOGY OF MODERATE-DURATION, HIGH-INTENSITY (LACTATE THRESHOLD) TRAINING

Moderate-duration high-intensity training may also be referred to as 'threshold', 'tempo' or 'pace' training. As outlined earlier, this type of training is conducted around an intensity that equates to an athlete's individual lactate threshold (LT). Despite the considerable discussion within the literature regarding the appropriate definition of LT (Bourdon 2000), it is clear from anecdotal case study and empirical study data that an effective training intensity exists that can be equated with the concept of a lactate threshold. Further, numerous studies have suggested that LT is an excellent predictor of endurance performance in both trained and untrained individuals. It is therefore not surprising that training at an exercise intensity equivalent to LT is related to both favourable physiological adaptations and improvements in performance.

Threshold training is typically performed at a pace, workload or heart rate similar to that observed at LT. It is a logical suggestion that improvements in performance stimulated by this type of training are related to an improved LT and probably an improved fractional utilization. Improvements in LT are demonstrated by a rightward shift in the blood lactate/workload relationship (see Fig. 4.3). In practical terms a shift such as that presented in Figure 4.3 enables the athlete to perform at a higher intensity prior to the onset of the debilitating effects associated with the accumulation of blood lactate. The example in Figure 4.3 demonstrates an improvement of approximately 20 W in LT following training.

The prescription of 'threshold' training classically involves a training zone that encompasses workloads just below and just above the LT. Such prescription usually follows the completion of an incremental exercise test that identifies the power output, speed and/or heart rate associated with LT. For a thorough discussion of the appropriate means by which to identify LT readers are directed to Bourdon (2000). Typically, LT tests involve five or six stages of between 3 and 5 minutes. Each stage is physiologically more demanding than the last (in heavyweight rowing the increments may represent a 25 W increase in work, in endurance running the stage increments may equate to a 0.6 km.h$^{-1}$ increase in running speed, and in cycling 20 W stage increments are often used). Following completion of each stage a capillary blood sample is obtained (from the earlobe or finger tip), from which blood lactate concentration is measured. Heart rate is also recorded (usually taking the mean HR for the last 30 seconds of each stage) (see Ch. 2). The data harvested during such a test may be employed to construct a lactate profile similar to that depicted in Figure 4.3. From such a lactate profile it is possible to calculate a training zone (HR or power output) that equates to LT.

A meta-analysis study completed by Londeree (1997) combined the results of 34 studies that had assessed the impact of training below, above or at an intensity equivalent to LT. The combined results of the 34 studies enabled Londeree (1997) to suggest that training at an intensity equivalent to LT is an adequate stimulus to

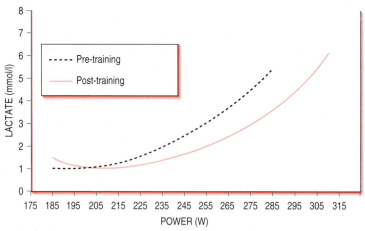

Figure 4.3    Blood lactate response to an incremental exercise test (in this case the data applies to an incremental rowing test performed on a Concept II model C ergometer), pre- and post-training.

improve the LT in sedentary subjects. The combined data, however, revealed that highly trained individuals require a more intense stimulus to improve LT. It is therefore suggested that highly trained individuals perform a significant proportion of their 'threshold' training slightly above the intensity associated with their LT.

The classic rightward shift in the lactate profile observed following a training programme incorporating LT training might be explained by one of two physiological adaptations. Firstly, improvements in LT may be a function of either a reduced rate of lactate production, an enhanced removal system or indeed a combination of these two adaptations. It is possible that lactate production may be diminished due to a lower reliance upon anaerobic glycolysis at the same relative intensity, propagated by an increased ability to generate ATP via aerobic processes. Such improvements are possible due to an increased size and density of mitochondria concomitant with an increase in the key enzymes involved in the Krebs cycle and electron transport chain. Ultimately, the increase in size and density of mitochondria facilitate a greater aerobic contribution to energy production, and subsequently reduce the production of lactate.

An enhanced ability to transport lactate out of the muscle has also been suggested as a possible mechanism for an enhanced performance following training at LT. The transport of lactate out of the muscle is dependent upon both diffusion across the cellular membrane, and more importantly the concentration of monocarboxylate transporters (MCTs). MCTs are responsible for the facilitated transport of lactate both into and out of the active muscles. It has been established that the concentration of MCTs is enhanced following intensive training, and thus the ability to remove lactate from the working muscle is enhanced in sedentary individuals following a training programme. Less information is available regarding the effect of training upon MCTs in already well-trained individuals. A recent study by Evertsen et al (2001) does, however, provide some insight into the issue. Evertsen et al examined a group of highly trained cross-country skiers following either 5 months of a moderate intensity training programme (86% training volume 60–70% $\dot{V}O_2$max, i.e. predominantly LSD training) or 5 months of a high-intensity training programme (83% training volume at 80–90% $\dot{V}O_2$max, i.e. predominantly LT training). Results from this study suggest that 5 months of high-intensity training did not increase the concentration of MCTs; however, in the moderate intensity group the concentration of MCT decreased. This suggests that high-intensity exercise (i.e. around LT) is critical in maintaining the ability to remove lactate from the working muscles. Despite no change in MCTs, the high-intensity training group demonstrated improvements in the lactate threshold and running performance. As these improvements could not be related to an improved efflux capacity of lactate the authors suggest that a reduced rate of lactate production is the likely mechanism for an improved performance.

Within an untrained population it appears that improvements in performance subsequent to a period of LT training are associated with improvements in both the rate of lactate removal and a reduction in lactate production. Within highly trained athletes, however, LT training may be critical in maintaining the concentration of MCTs and thus the ability to transport lactate rather than continuously enhancing the efflux capability. Improvements in performance in highly trained individuals following LT training may be explained by a lower lactate production, possibly stimulated by improved aerobic capabilities.

Improvements in endurance performance following LT training may also be associated with an enhanced economy. Franch et al (1998) demonstrated a 3% improvement in running economy following the implementation of higher intensity distance training into previous LSD programmes. Such improvements in economy may be explained by a reduction in submaximal $\dot{V}E$, and hence a reduction in the oxygen cost of breathing. Other mechanisms have also been suggested as possible mediators of an enhanced economy subsequent to LT training; conversion of type II fibres to type I, in addition to a general stiffening of the musculo-tendon apparatus involved with movement resulting in a greater elastic return.

## THE PHYSIOLOGY OF HIGH–INTENSITY–INTERVAL TRAINING (HIT)

Coaches and endurance athletes have long recognized the importance of high-intensity-interval training (HIT) in enhancing endurance performance. HIT may be defined as repeated bouts of short- to moderate-duration exercise (30 seconds to 5 minutes) completed at a 'high' intensity. Recovery between efforts may be active or passive, but not of sufficient duration to facilitate full recovery. The underpinning rationale for HIT is to continually stress the specific physiological components employed within an athlete's event, above and beyond the level that is required during competition, in order to bring about adaptation.

Despite the importance attributed to HIT within an endurance programme, the scientific study of the area has until relatively recently been largely unexplored. In addition, apart from a few notable exceptions (Acevedo & Goldfarb 1989, Laursen et al 2002, Stepto et al 1999) the limited work that has been completed in the area of HIT has employed recreationally active individuals. Thus, scant data are available regarding the optimization of HIT programmes for highly trained endurance athletes. The optimum duration, intensity, and recovery periods are presently not known.

Although scant data are available, the anecdotal and the limited empirical evidence examining highly trained individuals suggest that HIT will result in significant improvements in endurance performance. Acevedo & Goldfarb (1989) demonstrated an increase in 10-km running performance of approximately 3% in seven highly trained endurance runners following an 8-week programme of HIT at 90–95% peak heart rate. Stepto et al (1999) and Laursen et al (2002) stimulated an increase in 40-km cycling time trial performance in different groups of highly trained cyclists using HIT programmes. Although the benefits of HIT are marked, the underpinning physiology is not clear.

It is possible that the improvement in endurance performance observed following HIT is related to a reduction in carbohydrate oxidation and lactate accumulation at the same absolute intensity. Studies have demonstrated that following a period of HIT, athletes oxidize carbohydrate and produce lactate at lower rates for the same absolute workload. When the workload reflects the same relative workload, however, both carbohydrate oxidation and lactate accumulation are similar. The shift away from carbohydrate metabolism following HIT in highly trained athletes does not appear to be related to an increase in mitochondria size and density, such as that observed following LSD or LT training. Within sedentary individuals, increases in both oxidative and glycolytic enzyme activity coupled with an increased expression of type I muscle fibres have been shown following HIT (for a full review see Laursen & Jenkins 2002). In highly trained individuals, however, this does not appear to be the case. Weston et al (1997) demonstrated no change in a number of key oxidative and glycolytic enzymes following six HIT sessions, which consisted of six to eight, 5-minute repetitions completed at an intensity equivalent to 80% of the subjects peak power output. Despite no change in the subject's enzymatic capabilities, significant improvements in 40-km cycling time trial performance and time to exhaustion at 150% peak power were observed. Other studies have demonstrated similar findings regarding muscle enzyme activity following HIT based around other exercise modalities such as running. Thus, the improvement in performance observed in highly trained individuals is not explained by the same adaptations observed in sedentary individuals. Recent studies have attempted to further elucidate the mechanisms for such performance improvements following HIT programmes in highly trained individuals.

Despite well established improvement in endurance performance following HIT programmes $\dot{V}O_2$max remains unchanged. The lack of change in $\dot{V}O_2$max following HIT suggests that the improvements in endurance performance subsequent to HIT are probably not a reflection of central adaptations. Thus, enhanced endurance performance following HIT may therefore be related to adaptations in the periphery.

The capacity of skeletal muscle to buffer hydrogen ions ($H^+$) is a likely determinant of endurance performance as demonstrated by the significant relationship previously observed between buffering capacity and 40-km cycling time trial performance (Weston et al 1997). A limited number of studies have demonstrated an enhanced buffering capacity following HIT, for example Weston et al (1997) observed a 16% increase in buffering capacity in well trained cyclists following HIT. An enhanced capacity to buffer $H^+$ may enhance performance by abating the negative influence of $H^+$ upon muscular force production associated with $Ca^{2+}$ sequestration, ATPase activity and cross-bridge formation. Additionally, the inhibition of key glycolytic enzymes, including phosphofructokinase (PFK) and phosphorylase, that typically occurs with $H^+$ accumulation may also be reduced following HIT due to the enhanced buffering capacity leading to a higher glycolytic ATP yield. At present the data available regarding HIT, buffering capacity and enhanced endurance performance are limited, and as such continued scientific study is required to fully understand this relationship. The data available to date do provide some evidence that an enhanced buffering capacity might explain some of the improvements in endurance performance following HIT.

It is also possible that improved endurance performance subsequent to HIT may also be related to an enhanced heat tolerance. The significant alteration in $T_{core}$ observed during HIT may lead to adaptations in thermoregulation and heat tolerance resulting in an improved performance. Psychological factors should also not be discarded; completing repeated bouts of exercise above that typically performed in competition is likely to familiarize the athlete with the sensations associated with maximal exercise and may improve 'mental toughness'.

While it is widely accepted that HIT is an important component to the training programme of an endurance athlete, the optimal make up of HIT sessions is far from clear. The studies of Laursen et al (2002) and Stepto et al (1999) offer some guidance regarding HIT optimization, but both studies employed highly trained endurance cyclists and therefore generalizations to other sports are difficult. Stepto et al (1999) concluded that eight high-intensity intervals of 4-minute duration with 1.5-minute recovery completed at race pace resulted in the greatest improvement in 40-km time trial performance, while Laursen et al (2002) suggest that power at $\dot{V}O_2$max (Pmax) should be used as the exercise intensity, and 60% of time to exhaustion at Pmax should be employed as the duration of repetition within HIT for highly trained endurance cyclists. The dearth of scientific knowledge regarding the optimization of HIT programmes demonstrates a real need for further work. Notwithstanding the need for additional scientific study, interdisciplinary discussion between coaches, athletes and scientists will probably facilitate the adoption of effective protocols of HIT.

## STRENGTH TRAINING FOR ENDURANCE PERFORMANCE

At face value, training for endurance performance and training for improvements in strength represent different ends of the training spectrum. Endurance training is typically based around high-volume low-intensity muscular activity, while typical resistance training involves relatively short duration high-intensity muscular activity. Further, the muscular adaptations stimulated by the two types of training are disparate: resistance training stimulates muscular hypertrophy in all types of fibre (I, IIa and IIb), while endurance training results in a reduction in cross-sectional area of type II muscle fibres. Little or no change in the activities of phosphagen, glycolytic or oxidative enzymes is observed subsequent to resistance training, contrasting with the adaptations observed following endurance training. Although the activities of key enzymes are not altered following resistance training, their concentration is reduced due to a dilution effect. Muscular hypertrophy results in a reduction in the number of mitochondria per unit of muscle. Despite this apparent disparity between endurance and resistance training, the vast majority of endurance athletes take part in at least some form of resistance training, and most believe it is effective in enhancing performance.

The different physiological responses between endurance and resistance training have prompted the question of their mutual compatibility within the same training programme. The evidence to date would suggest that taking part in strength and endurance training concomitantly interferes with the development of strength. For an in-depth examination of simultaneous strength and endurance training readers are directed to the work of Tanaka & Swensen (1998). The following section will, however, examine the influence of strength/resistance training upon endurance performance.

A wide variety of studies have investigated the use of strength training for endurance performance. To date, however, the results are equivocal, probably due to methodological disparities between studies. Tanaka et al (1993) investigated the influence of a land-based resistance-training programme in 24 highly trained swimmers over the course of a competitive season. The swimmers were split into two groups and matched for both stroke preference and ability. All athletes completed their swim training collectively; however, one group also engaged in an 8-week resistance-training programme. The resistance programme was designed specifically to develop the musculature involved with freestyle swimming using a model of progressive overload. Following completion of the 8 weeks of resistance training, the swimmers applied a 2-week taper before competing at their major competition. Strength testing before and after the 8-week programme revealed a 25–35% increase in absolute strength. Despite this improvement in absolute strength, swim performance was not increased. The authors concluded that the lack of transfer from land-based training to the pool might be due to a lack of specificity within the land-based training.

The influence of resistance training upon endurance performance has also been examined in cycling. A 12-week programme of combined upper and lower body resistance training has been shown to be effective in improving cycling time to exhaustion (Marcinik et al 1991). The use of time-to-exhaustion trials as a surrogate of endurance performance is questionable, however, as it does not replicate any competitive event and, as such, does not represent a true reflection of the physiological requirements of endurance performance. Additional cycling studies have demonstrated improved muscular strength of up to 30% and improved short-term cycling performance following the inclusion of resistance training programmes alongside typical endurance training. It should be noted, however, that these data largely pertain to previously sedentary groups of individuals. Thus, it is not clear whether these results can be extrapolated to the elite population. Data from the USA cycling federation examining an elite population indicates that higher ranked endurance cyclists tend to have higher anaerobic power outputs than their lower ranked cyclists. A compelling argument may therefore be to suggest that the improvements observed within the non-elite populations (improved strength, short-term cycling performance) may facilitate enhanced endurance performance. Such improvements may be rationalized when the stoichastic nature of competitive cycling is considered, when sprint efforts and hill climbing can often have a dramatic influence upon success.

Similar to cycling, competitive endurance running also includes periods of intense effort (sprint finish, hill climbs) that may be enhanced by improvements in muscular strength and anaerobic power. Studies to date examining endurance runners following the addition of resistance training to their programme have revealed an enhanced anaerobic capacity, an increased leg strength of 30–40% and improvements in short-term running performance. These adaptations will probably benefit the endurance runner through the ability to generate a greater force per stride – enabling the runner to exercise longer at each sub-maximal work rate by reducing the force contribution from each active muscle fibre and/or recruiting fewer fibres (Tanaka & Swensen 1998). It is also possible that strength/power training may result in a stiffer musculotendinous unit leading to an improved efficiency and decreased oxygen cost of running (this will be discussed in more detail later in the chapter).

Recent years have seen the development of additional supplemental strength/power training methods such as plyometrics. It is this form of power training that is increasingly advocated by strength and conditioning coaches to the elite endurance population. A recent paper from a Finish group (Paavolainen et al 1999) examined a number of athletic parameters, including 5-km running time, running economy, maximal 20-m speed, $\dot{V}O_2$max, and maximal running velocity before and after 9 weeks of 'explosive strength training' in 22 elite male cross-country runners. The athletes were split into a control group and an experimental group, with each respective group replacing 3% and 32% of their normal training volume with explosive training. The explosive training involved both basic sprint training and a variety of plyometric exercises. Significant improvements in 5-km running performance were observed in the experimental group following the 9-week training programme, which was not observed within the control group. Previously it may have been suggested that the observed improvements in performance were probably a function of an enhanced $\dot{V}O_2$max and/or lactate threshold (LT). Over the course of the study, however, no change in $\dot{V}O_2$max or LT was observed. Correlation data suggested that the improvement in 5-km running performance was a reflection of improved running economy and muscle power, defined as 'the ability of the neuromuscular system to produce power during maximal exercise when glycolytic and/or oxidative energy production are high and muscle contractility may be limited'. The authors went on to suggest that running economy was likely to be positively influenced by the explosive strength training via improved neuromuscular characteristics resulting in stiffer and more efficient musculature. Support for this theory is provided by additional data examining cross-country skiing. The efficacy of strength training in improving aerobic endurance performance as assessed on a highly sports-specific cross-country skiing ergometer was examined by Hoff et al (2002). Highly trained athletes were prescribed 8 weeks of resistance training (three times a week, three sets of six reps, a rest of 3–4 minutes between sets, at a workload of 85% of 1 RM), with much emphasis placed upon the maximal mobilization of force in the concentric movement, suggested by the authors to specifically target neuromuscular adaptation. Following the training programme, a number of positive outcomes were observed: strength as assessed by 1 RM, time to peak force, time to exhaustion and work economy were all improved.

As with the previous forms of training for endurance performance, the depth of empirical evidence examining the use of strength/power training in elite endurance athletes is sparse. Although early studies suggest that there may be physiological conflict in combining strength and endurance training within the same period of an athletes training cycle, recent studies examining explosive power training within an elite population provide compelling support for this type of training in endurance athletes.

## FLEXIBILITY

Flexibility has traditionally been an intrinsic component to training schedules for almost all athletes. Such universal acceptance is based largely on the belief that improved flexibility will improve performance and reduce the risk of injury. Recent investigation has begun to question the efficacy of flexibility in improving performance both in endurance and power events. The impact of flexibility upon power sports is covered in Chapter 6. The impact of flexibility and, more importantly, flexibility training, upon endurance performance is pertinent at this point.

A number of studies have examined the relationship between flexibility and running economy. From these studies it appears that flexibility is inversely related to running economy. Therefore, the less flexible an athlete is the lower the oxygen cost will be for a given running speed. It has been postulated that this relationship can be explained by an increase in musculoskeletal stiffness. Repetitive stretch–shortening cycles, as observed during prolonged exercise, result in a build-up of stored elastic energy. A stiffer musculotendinous system will enhance the return of this stored elastic energy, resulting in a lower overall energy cost to the activity, and hence lower oxygen cost. This apparent inverse relationship between flexibility and economy may result in a dilemma for coaches and athletes. Tradition suggests that stretching is an important component of any training programme, supposedly providing protection from injury. Yet, data drawn from these recent studies suggest that improving flexibility might negatively affect economy and therefore performance.

Further insight is provided by Nelson et al (2001) who highlight a number of issues associated with previous studies examining flexibility, and also question some of the firm beliefs held within the sporting fraternity regarding flexibility. The authors point out that correlation studies examining flexibility and running economy do not demonstrate cause and effect; further, there is a dearth of evidence regarding the relationship between risk of injury and an athlete's level of flexibility. Lastly, they questioned the premise that less flexible joints result in stiffer musculotendinous units.

The range of movement about a joint (flexibility) is not the same as musculotendinous stiffness. Improvements in flexibility may be gained via an improved tolerance to stretch rather than changes in the musculotendinous unit. Accordingly, it is possible to improve flexibility whilst retaining the 'stiffness' within the musculotendinous unit that is believed to be beneficial in terms of running economy. This contention is supported by the experimental work of Nelson et al (2001). Thirty-two physically active subjects were split into two groups. A control group (who maintained current activity levels) and an experimental group (who maintained current activity level, and added three 40-minute sessions of calf/thigh stretching a week) were examined over a 10-week period. Running economy was assessed prior to and following the 10-week period. Flexibility, assessed via a basic sit and reach test, significantly improved in the experimental group, concomitant to no change in running economy in either group. The authors note a number of limitations to their study, including a true assessment of musculotendinous stiffness and the use of the sit and reach test as an assessment of flexibility. Despite the limitations of the study the data set is none the less persuasive. Continuation, therefore, of stretching routines within an endurance athlete's preparation may not result in a reduction in running economy per se, rather athletes may wish to employ training methods that enhance the stiffness of the musculotendinous unit and therefore improve economy (such as resistance or plyometric work).

Further work is clearly needed before the issue of stretching and endurance performance is fully resolved, and requires a series of more in-depth investigations than are currently available. Such work needs to differentiate between flexibility and stiffness, and examine the interaction between programmes designed to enhance flexibility and musculotendinous stiffness. At present it appears that musculotendinous stiffness may be a far better determinant of running economy than flexibility.

Notwithstanding the fact that running economy does not appear to be impeded by improved flexibility, the lack of information regarding the benefits associated with stretching should also be reiterated. Presently much time is devoted to stretching routines in order to prevent injury, based largely upon a historical perspective rather than sound scientific evidence.

## WHAT PERCENTAGE OF TRAINING SHOULD BE DEVOTED TO EACH TYPE OF TRAINING?

The challenge faced by the coach or support scientist is to select the correct training method with the appropriate volume and timing (in terms of periodization), so as to optimize performance at key points within the athletes competitive season. Accordingly, the percentage of training that should be completed within each of the training zones (LSD, LT and HIT) is a source of much debate.

The distribution of training is largely dependent upon the athlete or group of athletes in question. Training status, physiological strengths and weaknesses coupled with the time point within the training macrocycle will all influence the percentage of training completed within each of the training zones. As such, it is not possible to provide a definitive answer to the above question. Despite this limitation, it is possible to broadly examine the typical division of training within elite endurance athletes over an entire training cycle and to draw some general recommendations from the available literature. It should be understood, however, that this information is purely a starting point. Coaches, athletes and support scientists should, via the process of a careful 'needs analysis', devise appropriate training programmes according to the individual needs of the athlete.

A limited number of studies have attempted to identify the characteristics of optimal endurance training programmes (Billat et al 2001, Steinacker et al 1998). Results from a South African study (Coetzer et al 1993) suggest that endurance runners with superior race performances train at a higher intensity than their slower counterparts. Slower runners spend 13% of their total training volume performing high-intensity training (defined as an intensity >80% $\dot{V}O_2$max) whereas faster runners spend 36% of the total training volume performing high-intensity exercise. This demonstrates a significantly greater proportion of training volume being completed within the LT and HIT training zones by the faster athletes.

The work of Billat et al (2001) attempted to quantify the training characteristics of elite marathon runners by comparing the characteristics of top-class versus high-level runners (all athletes within this study were of a very high standard). The differentiation of athletes, however, was based upon marathon personal bests; top-class males (2 hours 6 minutes 34 seconds to 2 hours 11 minutes 59 seconds), high-level males (2 hours 12 minutes to 2 hours 16 minutes), top-class females (2 hours 25 minutes to 2 hours 30 minutes) and high-level females (2 hours 31 minutes to 2 hours 38 minutes). Male top-class marathon runners complete a greater training volume than their high-level counterparts (206 km per week versus 168 km per week); further, the volume of high-intensity training (HIT) was also significantly greater for the top-class male runners. The top-class athletes completed 20.4 km per week at an intensity equal to or greater than the velocity associated with 10 km race pace, compared to the 17.8 km per week completed at the same intensity by the high-level athletes. Although the volume of training completed was significantly different between the top-class and high-level runners, the training load distribution was identical (18% of the total distance run was at a velocity greater than marathon running velocity, 4% at marathon running velocity and 78% at a running velocity less than their marathon running velocity). Differences between the training programmes of top-class and high-level female marathon runners were also evident within the study of Billat et al (2001). Top-class female marathon runners appear to engage in a greater number of high-intensity training sessions than their high-level counterparts (two sessions versus one session per week).

The division of training within elite rowers has also received some attention. Steinacker et al (1998) suggests that on-water training represents between 55 and 65% of total training volume, power-based training may represent between 16 and 20%, and general athletic training is in the range of 23 to 26% of total rowing training volume, dependent upon age. Although these data are somewhat informative, it is difficult to determine exactly how much time was spent in each of the three major training zones.

The limited data currently available regarding the appropriate division of endurance training programmes suggest that elite endurance athletes should perform the majority (70–80%) of training within the LSD training zone, with a smaller but still significant proportion (20–30%) of training being completed in the LT or HIT training zones. Undoubtedly, this suggested division of training is probably a little too simplistic. It does, however, provide a suitable starting point from which individual endurance training programmes may be developed.

## GENERAL SUMMARY

At the outset of this chapter, Figure 4.1 provided an overview of the determinants of endurance performance. Figure 4.4 provides an extension to the original schematic including greater detail with respect to each of the physiological determinants and the influence of the different training methodologies discussed in the present chapter, and as such provides a general summary to what has been discussed.

When examining the different types of training employed by endurance athletes, a considerable cross-over is apparent. Although specific training modalities are employed in an attempt to bring about specific physiological adaptations, it does not appear to be possible to specialize the training session to the extent of focusing on one specific determinant of performance (e.g. lactate threshold). LT training, for example, may increase mitochondrial size and density in a similar fashion to LSD training. Many of the individual training modalities discussed thus far stimulate physiological adaptations that beneficially affect a number of the underpinning determinants of endurance performance as highlighted in Figure 4.4.

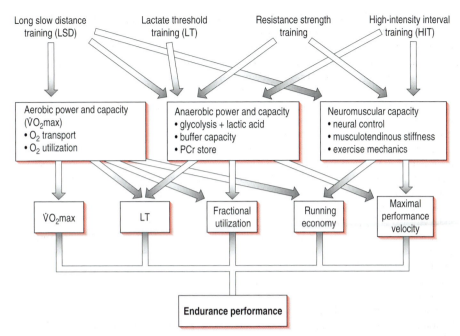

**Figure 4.4**  Hypothetical model of determinants of endurance performance in well-trained athletes as influenced by different training modalities. Based originally on a model provided by Paavolainen et al (1999).

In order for elite endurance athletes to achieve success at the highest level it is critical that they optimize all of the physiological determinants of performance. In order to do this they must employ the appropriate mixture of the different training stimuli within their training programme. Decisions regarding the appropriate periodization of the different training methods require careful consideration of each individual athlete's requirements at any given point within the training cycle. Thus, in order for a training programme to be truly effective, interdisciplinary assessment, discussion and review are required between the athlete, coach and support scientists on a regular basis.

## KEY POINTS

1. Endurance performance covers a wide variety of events ranging from competitive rowing (~6 minutes) through to marathon competitions (~2–3 hours), and beyond to some cycle stage races (~4 hours). The predominant source of ATP for endurance performance is via aerobic processes.
2. Endurance performance is underpinned by a number of physiological variables, all of which display varying degrees of trainability.
3. A well developed aerobic capacity ($\dot{V}O_2$max) is a prerequisite for endurance performance; however, other physiological parameters may be more important, especially in truly elite individuals.
4. Lactate threshold, economy, fractional utilization and maximum velocity/power are important factors in endurance performance.

5. Endurance training is broadly categorized into three distinct zones: long slow distance; moderate-duration, high-intensity training; short-duration, very-high-intensity training.

6. In addition to the basic training zones, a proportion of an endurance athlete's time will be devoted to strength training and flexibility.

## References

Acevedo EO, Goldfarb AH. (1989). Increased training intensity effects on plasma lactate, ventilatory threshold, and endurance. Medicine and Science in Sports and Exercise 21(5):563–568.

Bassett DR Jr, Howley ET 2000 Limiting factors for maximum oxygen uptake and determinants of endurance performance. Medicine Science Sports Exercise 32(1):70–84

Beaver WL, Wasserman K, Whip BJ 1985 Improved detection of lactate threshold during exercise using a log-log transformation. Journal of Applied Physiology 59(6):1936–1940

Billat VL, Demarle A, Slawinski J et al 2001 Physical and training characteristics of top-class marathon runners. Medicine and Science in Sports and Exercise 33(12):2089–2097

Bourdon P 2000 Blood lactate transition thresholds: Concepts and controversies. In: Gore C (ed.) Physiological tests for elite athletes. Human Kinetics, Champaign IL

Coyle EF 1995 Integration of the physiological factors determining endurance performance ability. Exercise and Sport Science Reviews 23:25–63

Coetzer P, Noakes TD, Sanders B et al 1993 Superior fatigue resistance of elite black South African distance runners. Journal of Applied Physiology 75(4):1822–1827

Convertino VA 1991 Blood volume: its adaptation to endurance training. Medicine and Science in Sports and Exercise 23(12):1338–1348.

Convertino VA, Brock PJ, Keil LC et al 1980 Exercise training-induced hypervolemia: role of plasma albumin, renin, and vasopressin. Journal of Applied of Physiology 48(4):665–669

Costill DL, Flynn MG, Kirwan JP et al 1988 Effects of repeated days of intensified training on muscle glycogen and swimming performance. Medicine and Science in Sports and Exercise 20(3):249–254

Evertsen F, Medbo JI, Bonen A 2001 Effect of training intensity on muscle lactate transporters and lactate threshold of cross-country skiers. Acta Physiologica Scandinavica 173(2):195–205

Franch J, Madsen K, Djurhuus MS, Pedersen PK 1998 Improved running economy following intensified training correlates with reduced ventilatory demands. Medicine and Science in Sports and Exercise 30(8):1250–1256

Gonzalez-Alonso J, Teller C, Andersen SL et al 1999 Influence of body temperature on the development of fatigue during prolonged exercise in the heat. Journal of Applied Physiology 86(3):1032–1039

Hoff J, Gran A, Helgerud J 2002 Maximal strength training improves aerobic endurance performance. Scandinavian Journal of Medicine and Science in Sports 12:288–295

Ingham SA, Whyte GP, Jones K, Nevill AM 2002 Determinants of 2000 m rowing ergometer performance in elite rowers. European Journal of Applied Physiology 88(3):243–246; Epub 2002 Oct 10

Ivy JL, Withers RT, Van Handel PJ et al 1980 Muscle respiratory capacity and fiber type as determinants of the lactate threshold. Journal of Applied Physiology 48(3): 523–527

Kinderman W, Simon G, Keul J 1979 The significance of the aerobic–anaerobic transition for the determination of work load intensities during endurance training. European Journal of Applied Physiology and Occupational Physiology 42(1):25–34

Laursen PB, Jenkins DG 2002 The scientific basis for high-intensity interval training: optimising training programmes and maximising performance in highly trained endurance athletes. Sports Medicine 32(1):53–73

Laursen PB, Shing CM, Peake JM et al 2002 Interval training program optimization in highly trained endurance cyclists. Medicine and Science in Sports and Exercise 34(11):1801–1807

Londeree BR 1997 Effect of training on lactate/ventilatory thresholds: a meta-analysis. Medicine and Science in Sports and Exercise 29(6):837–843

Marcinik EJ, Potts J, Schlabach G et al 1991 Effects of strength training on lactate threshold and endurance performance. Medicine and Science in Sports and Exercise 23:739–743

Nelson AG, Kokkonen J, Eldredge C et al 2001 Chronic stretching and running economy. Scandinavian Journal of Medicine and Science in Sports 11:260–265

Paavolainen L, Hakkinen K, Hamalainen I et al 1999 Explosive-strength training improves 5-km running time by improving running economy and muscle power. Journal of Applied Physiology 86(5):1527–1533

Pate RR, Branch JD 1992 Training for endurance sport. Medicine and Science in Sports and Exercise 24(9 suppl):S340–S343

Sjodin B, Jacobs I 1981 Onset of blood lactate accumulation and marathon running performance. International Journal of Sports Medicine 2(1):23–26

Sjodin B, Svedenhag J 1985 Applied physiology of marathon running. Sports Medicine 2(2):83–99

Steinacker JM, Lormes W, Lehmann M, Altenburg D 1998 Training of rowers before world championships. Medicine and Science in Sports and Exercise 30(7):1158–1163

Stepto NK, Hawley JA, Dennis SC, Hopkins WG 1999 Effects of different interval-training programs on cycling time-trial performance. Medicine and Science in Sports and Exercise 31(5):736–741

Tanaka H, Swensen T 1998 Impact of resistance training on endurance performance. A new form of cross-training? Sports Medicine 25(3):191–200

Tanaka H, Costill DL, Thomas R et al 1993 Dry-land resistance training for competitive swimming. Medicine and Science in Sports and Exercise 25:952–959

Tesch PA, Thorsson A, Kaiser P 1984 Muscle capillary supply and fiber type characteristics in weight and power lifters. Journal of Applied Physiology 56(1):35–38

Weston AR, Myburgh KH, Lindsay FH et al 1997 Skeletal muscle buffering capacity and endurance performance after high-intensity interval training by well-trained cyclists. European Journal of Applied Physiology and Occupational Physiology 75(1):7–13

## Further reading

Australian Sports Commission 2000 Physiological tests for elite athletes. Human Kinetics, Champaign IL

Docherty D, Sporer B 2000 A proposed model for examining the interference phenomenon between concurrent aerobic and strength training. Sports Medicine 30(6):385–394

Hawley JA, Myburgh KH, Noakes TD, Dennis SC 1997 Training techniques to improve fatigue resistance and enhance endurance performance. Journal of Sports Sciences 15:325–333

Hickson RC, Dvorak BA, Gorostiaga EM et al 1988 Potential for strength and endurance training to amplify endurance performance. Journal of Applied Physiology 65:2285–2290

Jones AM, Carter H 2000 The effect of endurance training on parameters of aerobic fitness. Sports Medicine 29(6):373–386

Kubukeli ZN, Noakes TD, Dennis SC 2002 Training techniques to improve endurance exercise performances. Sports Medicine 32(8):489–509

Chapter **5**

# The physiology of anaerobic endurance training

Ken A. van Someren

## CHAPTER CONTENTS

## LEARNING OBJECTIVES:

This chapter is intended to ensure that the reader:

1. Understands the physiological bases of anaerobic endurance.
2. Identifies the importance of anaerobic endurance to short-duration, high-intensity sports events.
3. Understands the scientific underpinning of training methods practised to develop anaerobic endurance.
4. Appreciates physiological adaptations to anaerobic endurance training.
5. Considers methods to evaluate anaerobic endurance.

## INTRODUCTION

High-intensity exercise requires the rapid re-synthesis of ATP to provide energy for muscular contraction. The demand for ATP and energy exceeds the rate at which oxygen delivery and consumption can support oxidative energy production. Consequently, a large part of the total energy demand is derived from anaerobic sources. While the oxidative pathway provides a relatively efficient but slow re-synthesis of ATP, the anaerobic pathways are relatively fast. There is, however, a limit to the energy yield from the anaerobic pathways during maximal exercise (for reasons discussed later in this chapter); this finite capacity for anaerobic energy production is the 'anaerobic capacity'. It is this capacity that determines an athlete's ability to sustain high-intensity exercise; because 'endurance' refers to the duration that work can be sustained, the term 'anaerobic endurance' is used to describe this ability and is often synonymous with 'anaerobic capacity'. Given that there is a finite capacity for anaerobic energy production, athletes must maximize this capacity through training and use it optimally during competition (i.e. effective pacing) to achieve optimal performance.

It is important to distinguish the term 'power', which is the rate at which energy is produced, from 'capacity', which is the total amount of energy produced. While it is anaerobic power that determines success in short-duration explosive events (e.g. javelin, shot-putt, high jump, see Ch. 6), it is anaerobic capacity that is important for many sprint and middle-distance events of between 10 seconds and approximately 4 minutes (e.g. 100–1500 m running, 50–400 m swimming, 200–1000 m canoeing and kayaking, 1000–4000 m track cycling). In these sprint and middle-distance events, athletes compete at exercise intensities exceeding their maximal rate of oxygen consumption ($\dot{V}O_2$max). In such events it is the ability to maintain a very high intensity, and therefore anaerobic endurance, that is crucial for success. In the middle-distance events athletes often require very high levels of both aerobic and anaerobic endurance and therefore coaches, scientists and athletes face an enormous challenge in the successful design of training programmes.

The term 'sprint' is normally used to describe the shortest event(s) within a sport. For example, flatwater canoeing and kayaking comprises sprint and marathon events; the sprint events are the 200 m, 500 m and 1000 m, which take approximately 40 seconds, 100 seconds and 220 seconds for men's single kayaks, respectively. 'Middle-distance' is a term often used to describe track running events of 800–1500 m and other sports events lasting a similar duration. Because there is a wide range of exercise durations that rely upon anaerobic endurance, for the purposes of this chapter, events lasting between 10 seconds and 4 minutes will be classified as short-duration, high-intensity exercise.

The measurement of anaerobic endurance or capacity is a problem that has confounded sports scientists for many years. In contrast to other physiological parameters such as aerobic power, which can be assessed by the direct measurement of oxygen consumption, no single gold standard technique for the measurement or calculation of anaerobic capacity exists today. Consequently, many scientists debate the relative merits of a number of measurement techniques to estimate anaerobic capacity, including the measurement of intramuscular substrate and enzyme content before and after exercise, the maximal accumulated oxygen deficit (MAOD), excess post-exercise oxygen consumption (EPOC), post-exercise blood lactate concentration, the Wingate anaerobic test, and sport-specific performance tests. Such lack of accepted and validated methods has hindered the progress of scientific research with respect to the importance of anaerobic capacity for short-duration, high-intensity sports. Consequently, the academic community has only been able to provide limited empirical evidence to the coach and athlete on which to base their training methods and evaluation techniques for anaerobic endurance. This presents a challenge for sports scientists in the future and means that at present much of the anaerobic endurance training techniques used by coaches and athletes are based upon anecdotal evidence and personal experience with only limited input from scientific data.

## PHYSIOLOGICAL BASES OF ANAEROBIC ENDURANCE

Energy for muscular contraction is derived from the hydrolysis of adenosine triphosphate (ATP). In order for exercise intensity to be maintained, ATP must be re-synthesized at the same rate at which it is used. If re-synthesis fails to keep pace with consumption, the athlete will be forced to reduce exercise intensity. ATP may be re-synthesized through a number of systems or pathways: (i) the hydrolysis of creatine phosphate (CP), (ii) anaerobic glycolysis, and (iii) the oxidation of carbohydrate, lipids and protein. A combination of these three pathways is used during exercise, with the relative contribution of each determined by the exercise intensity and duration. Table 5.1 provides empirical data quantifying the relative energetic demands of events of various durations. It is clear that as exercise duration decreases (and therefore intensity increases), the relative contribution of anaerobic energy increases; it is also evident that many of the 'middle-distance' events (e.g. 1500 m running, 400 m swimming, 4000 m cycling) have a significant anaerobic energy contribution.

Anaerobic endurance is determined by the capacities of the two anaerobic energy pathways: (1) the hydrolysis of intramuscular stores of ATP and CP (together known as high-energy phosphates or the ATP-CP system); (2) anaerobic glycolysis. Together, these pathways provide large energy contributions to short-duration, high-intensity exercise.

## ATP–CP PATHWAY

This pathway is often considered the immediate system that provides energy at the start of high-intensity exercise; it is however relatively short term in duration. The hydrolysis of intramuscular stores of the high-energy phosphates ATP and CP provide energy for muscular contraction during maximal exercise. The store of ATP in skeletal muscle is very small (5 mmol.kg$^{-1}$ of muscle) and can fuel exercise for just a couple of seconds. Rather than completely depleting this reserve of ATP, however, the CP system offers an immediate supply of energy for the rapid re-synthesis of ATP. The hydrolysis of CP by the enzyme creatine kinase (CK) provides energy and

**Table 5.1**  Percentage contribution of energy systems for short-duration, high-intensity maximal ergometry and sports events

| Event | ATP–CP (%) | Anaerobic glycolysis (%) | Oxidation (%) |
|---|---|---|---|
| **Cycle ergometry** | | | |
| 10 sec | 53 | 44 | 3 |
| 30 sec | 23 | 49 | 28 |
|  |  | 60* | 40 |
| 45 sec |  | 60* | 40 |
| 60 sec |  | 50* | 50 |
| 90 sec | 12 | 42 | 46 |
| 120 sec |  | 35* | 65 |
| **Running** | | | |
| 100 m |  | 90* | 10 |
| 200 m |  | 81* | 29 |
| 400 m |  | 62* | 38 |
| 800 m |  | 39* | 61 |
| 1500 m |  | 20* | 80 |
| **Cycling** | | | |
| 1000 m time trial | 10 | 40 | 50 |
| 4000 m pursuit | 1 | 14 | 85 |
| **Sprint kayaking** | | | |
| K1  200 m |  | 63* | 37 |
| K1  500 m |  | 38* | 62 |
| K1 1000 m |  | 18* | 82 |
| **Swimming** | | | |
| 50 m | 20 | 50 | 30 |
| 100 m | 19 | 26 | 55 |
| 200 m | 14 | 18 | 68 |
| 400 m | 6 | 10 | 83 |

(*represents combined percentage of ATP-CP and anaerobic glycolysis columns)

a free phosphate necessary for the phosphorylation of adenosine diphosphate (ADP) to ATP. Intramuscular stores of CP are approximately 15 mmol.kg$^{-1}$ of muscle and are rapidly depleted during maximal exercise. During a 30-second maximal sprint, CP is depleted by 55% in the first 10 seconds, a further 18% in the subsequent 10 seconds and a modest 10% in the final 10 seconds (Lakomy 2000). There is clear evidence from a number of scientific experiments that there is a concomitant decline in power output and ATP-CP depletion during short-duration maximal exercise. The rate at which CP is depleted is a function of exercise intensity, therefore it will be very rapidly depleted during all-out exercise of less than 30 seconds; however, it will be depleted at a somewhat lower rate during lower-intensity, longer-duration exercise (e.g. 1500 m running). Figure 5.1 illustrates the depletion of CP during a 10-minute bout of swimming; it is clear that the rate of depletion changes throughout the exercise bout. As exercise duration increases, anaerobic glycolysis contributes a major part of the total expended energy, although because this is a slower process than the ATP-CP system the same exercise intensity cannot be maintained.

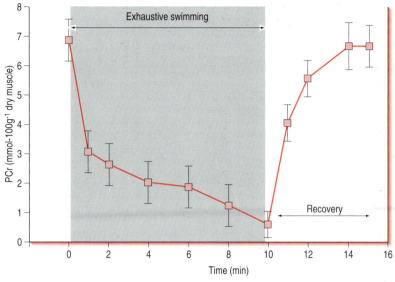

**Figure 5.1**   Creatine phosphate depletion and recovery following 10 minutes exercise. Reproduced with permission from Costill DL, Maglischo EW & Richardson AB (1992). *Swimming*. Blackwell Science, Oxford.

## ANAEROBIC GLYCOLYSIS

Glycolysis is an anaerobic process comprising 10 enzymatically controlled chemical reactions that catabolize muscle glycogen or glucose to provide energy for ATP re-synthesis. During high-intensity exercise it is almost entirely muscle glycogen rather than extracellular glucose that is metabolized. Although not quite as rapid as the ATP-CP system, glycolysis synthesises ATP at a faster rate than achieved through the oxidative pathway. This explains why a 100-m sprinter starts to slow down towards the end of a race and why a 400 m runner can maintain a high, albeit somewhat slower pace, for the duration of their race. Of course, the winner of a 400 m race is often the athlete who slows the least; the cause of this fatigue is for reasons other than the depletion of the ATP-CP system. Glycolysis results in the formation of pyruvate and it has long been accepted that when oxygen is available, such as during low-intensity exercise, pyruvate is converted to acetyl-CoA, which then enters the citric acid cycle (Krebs cycle) to allow the greater yields of ATP achieved through the oxidative pathway. During very high-intensity exercise where glycolysis occurs at a high rate, hydrogen ions ($H^+$) are produced faster than they can be removed via the oxidation of NADH in the electron transport chain. As a consequence of the accumulation of $H^+$, the pyruvate is converted to lactic acid under the control of the enzyme lactate dehydrogenase (LDH). This has been attributed to a lack of oxygen availability (hypoxia) within the mitochondria. It is likely, however, that oxygen availability is not the only cause of lactic acid production, the recruitment of fast-twitch motor units that preferentially work anaerobically is also responsible for the production of lactic acid. It is a different isoform of the enzyme lactate dehydrogenase (LDH) found in fast-twitch motor units that converts pyruvic acid to lactic acid. Although the production of lactic acid is associated with muscular fatigue (as discussed later), it does allow high rates of ATP re-synthesis, although the duration (or capacity) of this system is relatively short (2–3 minutes).

It is important to note that children typically demonstrate lower levels of anaerobic endurance than adults. This may in part be due to the slower rate of glycolysis observed in children, presumably a consequence of lower specific enzyme activity. This has implications for coaches and sports scientists involved with the coaching or evaluation of young athletes and should be considered in the design of training programmes.

## ENERGY CONTRIBUTIONS TO SHORT-DURATION, HIGH-INTENSITY EXERCISE

The ATP-CP system is the dominant energy pathway in short-duration, high-intensity sports of less than 10 seconds, for example 100 m sprinting and triple jump. In addition, the brief repetitive high-intensity bursts that characterize many field-sports and court games rely heavily upon this pathway. Longer-duration, high-intensity exercise (e.g. 10 seconds to 4 minutes) will place additional demands upon anaerobic glycolysis. A number of research studies have quantified the contribution of these systems and the oxidative energy system during maximal short-duration exercise. More dated literature tended to overestimate the anaerobic contribution to short-duration exercise; it is now evident that there is a significant aerobic component to even the shortest duration exercise. Table 5.1 illustrates the relative energy contributions to various durations of ergometry tests and sports events. Although there is some disparity between investigations in the same event (due primarily to methodological inconsistencies in the studies), it is clear that as the duration of the activity increases, the contribution of the three energy systems changes from predominantly anaerobic to predominantly aerobic; similarly the anaerobic contribution is in the main from the ATP-CP system in exercise lasting ≤10 seconds, and largely from the glycolytic system in longer-duration exercise (10 seconds to 4 minutes). While these generic data may be applied to any sports event, it is preferable and more accurate for scientists and coaches to source data specific to their sport and event.

It is also important to consider the importance of anaerobic energy production during the 'final sprint' in endurance events (e.g. 10 000 m running). Although this anaerobic energy yield may be very small in terms of percentage contribution of total energy, it may represent the difference between finishing inside or outside of the medals in competition. This is one of the reasons why even distance runners undertake some amount of anaerobic training.

Many of the field-sports (e.g. soccer, field-hockey, rugby) are characterized by repetitive changes of pace with sprinting superimposed upon relatively low-intensity activity. Time–motion analyses of field sports including soccer and field-hockey demonstrate that 90–95% of match time is spent standing, walking and jogging, and only 5% of the time spent undertaking, striding and sprinting (Bangsbo et al 1991, Spencer et al 2004). Although sprints rarely exceed a few seconds (≤ 5 seconds), they are typically interspersed with only short periods of recovery (15–90 seconds). It is this repetition of high-intensity activity that stresses the anaerobic endurance of players, particularly in respect of the capacity of the ATP-CP system and the ability to re-synthesize CP. Increases in blood lactate concentrations during the repetition of short-duration bouts of high-intensity exercise have been reported, reflecting the extent of metabolic acidosis and therefore the athlete's glycolytic capacity.

## CHARACTERISTICS OF SHORT-DURATION, HIGH-INTENSITY EVENT ATHLETES

There are a number of different sports that place high demands on an athlete's anaerobic capacity, which poses problems in characterizing the 'typical' physiological profile of such athletes. Athletes participating in short-duration, high-intensity sports, however, tend to exhibit relatively high distributions of fast-twitch (type IIa and IIx) muscle fibres, high levels of intramuscular ATP, CP and glycogen, high concentrations and activities of specific enzymes (e.g. creatine kinase (CK), phosphofructokinase (PFK), phosphorylase) and high post-exercise blood lactate concentrations. Consequent to these characteristics, the athletes competing in 'anaerobic' sports display superior measures of anaerobic capacity.

Identification of the energetic demands of sports events and the physiological characteristics of elite performers provides a comprehensive analysis of the physiological demands of a sport and therefore an understanding of the training required to improve performance. A sound understanding of both of these factors is imperative prior to the design of any specific training programme. Fortunately, there is much literature in these areas for most popular sports, although somewhat less for the minority sports. In addition, an individual's relative strengths and weaknesses must also be addressed to optimize the training programme.

## THE RELATIONSHIP OF ANAEROBIC ENDURANCE AND PERFORMANCE

By establishing the relationship between physiological attributes and athletic performance it is possible to identify the factors most closely related to success and indeed the percentage variance in performance explained by each attribute. Using these relationships it is possible to predict performance using multiple regression, thereby developing a structure of the physiological prerequisites for any sport. Inferences regarding the foci of physical training and physiological assessment may then be made. Of course, it must be remembered that a relationship does not demonstrate causation and it is, therefore, possible to misinterpret the relevance of some relationships. This is further confounded by the fact that many factors that are related to performance are also related to each other, particularly some of the indirect measures of anaerobic capacity.

There is extensive literature describing the relationships between physiological attributes and performance, although the majority of these data are confined to the popular sports and tend to focus on factors associated with cardiorespiratory fitness and endurance. In addition, there is a lack of data describing the relationship between physiological factors and performance in field sports due to the difficulties in defining and assessing performance in such sports.

The heterogeneity of the subjects used in the available research literature is also an important issue for the reader to consider. In many studies the samples are quite disparate in ability and therefore physiological status. This increases the likelihood of significant relationships between physiological parameters and performance; however, the relevance of such findings for scientists and coaches working with a homogenous group of highly-trained athletes may be limited.

## LIMITATIONS TO PERFORMANCE IN SHORT–DURATION, HIGH–INTENSITY SPORTS

The term fatigue is used to describe the general feeling of tiredness, but more specifically in relation to sports performance, it is the decline in muscular power output and thus performance. During short-duration, high-intensity exercise fatigue is caused by distinct physiological factors that are discussed below. These factors may also be considered as performance limitations and it is the improvement of these

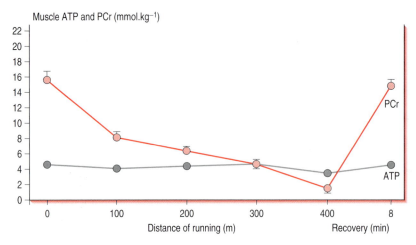

**Figure 5.2** Changes in muscle ATP and CP during running. Reproduced with permission from Hirvonen J, Nummela A, Rusko H, Rehunen S & Härkönen M (1992), Fatigue and changes of ATP, creation phosphate, and lactate during 400-m sprint, *Canadian Journal of Sport Science* 17:141–144.

factors that is the aim of any training programme designed for short-duration, high-intensity sports.

## Depletion of ATP–CP

As already discussed, intramuscular CP is depleted by 83% during 30 seconds of maximal exercise. In addition, 400 m running has been shown to result in an 89% depletion of CP and a 27% depletion of ATP (Fig. 5.2; Hirvonen et al 1992). The rate at which the high-energy phosphates are hydrolysed will determine the speed or power output an individual can attain, and the amount of CP stored within the muscle cell will determine the duration that very high-intensity exercise can be maintained. The depletion of CP has been consistently found to be associated with fatigue in short-duration, high-intensity exercise.

Many athletes have adopted dietary creatine supplementation to enhance intramuscular stores and therefore increase the capacity of the ATP-CP system. This subject has been a focus for much research over the last 10–15 years. Although confounded by many factors, there is sound evidence that creatine supplementation has an ergogenic effect in repeated sprint activities, suggesting that supplementation not only increases the intramuscular CP content but also accelerates the re-synthesis of CP between sprints.

## Re-synthesis of ATP–CP

It appears that power output during exercise is at least in part determined by the availability of CP. Therefore during intermittent sports, the ability to re-synthesize CP will affect an athlete's ability to perform subsequent bouts of high-intensity

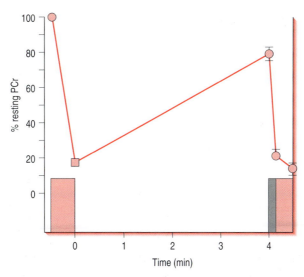

**Figure 5.3** CP depletion and re-synthesis during multiple sprint exercise. Reproduced with permission from Bogdanis GC, Williams C, Boobis LH & Lakomy HKA (1996), Contribution of phosphocreatine and aerobic metabolism to energy supply during repeated sprint exercise, *Journal of Applied Physiology* 80:876–884.

exercise. Not only is power output related to CP depletion during exercise, but also the recovery of power output following maximal high-intensity exercise is related to the re-synthesis of CP (Bogdanis et al 1995). Figure 5.3 illustrates CP depletion and repletion during repeated high-intensity exercise. Although there was considerable CP repletion during the 4-minute recovery period following a 30-second sprint, CP remained below resting values at the start of the second 30-second sprint, which was concomitant with an 18% reduction in power output. CP is re-synthesized at rest and at low to moderate exercise intensities via oxygen consumption; indeed an individual's rate of CP re-synthesis is related to their aerobic power ($\dot{V}O_2$max). Other factors that determine the rate of replenishment include creatine availability and the mode of recovery. It takes approximately 1–2 minutes for CP to be restored to 50% of pre-exercise levels and 3–4 minutes to be 90% restored. Due to the time required for CP repletion, intermittent sports will often be characterized by a decrease in exercise intensity throughout the training or competition bout, which is exacerbated by short-duration recovery periods. For this reason there is a concomitant decrease in the relative anaerobic contribution and an increase in the aerobic contribution as the exercise bout progresses.

## Metabolic acidosis

Since the early 20th Century lactic acid has been considered a primary cause of muscular fatigue during high-intensity exercise. Lactic acid rapidly dissociates to lactate and hydrogen ions ($H^+$). Because exercise physiologists often measure the concentration of lactate in blood to estimate anaerobic energy metabolism, many coaches, athletes and indeed students mistakenly believe that lactate is the cause of fatigue. Rather, it is the accumulation of $H^+$ that causes metabolic acidosis.

During high-intensity exercise when $H^+$ accumulates in the cytosol, intracellular proteins provide buffering of some of the excess acidity; in addition, hydrogen ions effluxing from the cell are buffered by extracellular bicarbonate. The ingestion of exogenous buffering agents (e.g. sodium bicarbonate and sodium citrate) to enhance this buffering capacity has been practised by athletes and widely researched by scientists over the last 20 years. Although results are equivocal, there is evidence that this practice can increase the body's buffering capacity and improve anaerobic performance. Any such buffering is not, however, capable of completely preventing acidosis and the decline in intracellular pH, which drops from normal resting levels of 7.1 to $\leq 6.5$, and possibly lower within individual fast-twitch fibres. The reduction in pH disturbs the homeostasis of the muscle cell and inhibits key glycolytic enzymes, particularly phosphofructokinase and phophorylase, thereby slowing glycolytic energy production. Acidosis also displaces calcium ($Ca^{2+}$) from the sarcoplasmic reticulum within the muscle cell and impairs its affinity for binding to the intramuscular protein troponin. This prevents troponin from regulating the exposure of the active binding sites on the actin filament and thus the cycling of cross-bridges between the actin and myosin filaments. This in turn reduces muscle tension and the force of contraction, which will manifest as a reduction in exercise intensity. The reduction in pH caused by high-intensity exercise may persist for several minutes following exercise, as shown in Figure 5.4. Metabolic acidosis has also been suggested to exert an osmotic pressure that could cause muscle swelling and blood flow restriction following high-intensity exercise (Sahlin 1986).

Recent evidence suggests that the production of lactic acid and metabolic acidosis may not be as important a cause of physiological fatigue as previously accepted. Much of the previous research that has shaped popular understanding of the role of acidosis in fatigue was either based on the observation of relationships between

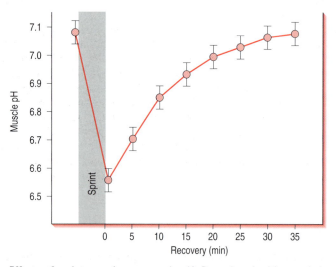

**Figure 5.4** Effects of sprint exercise on muscle pH. Reproduced with permission from Costill DL, Maglischo EW & Richardson AB (1992) *Swimming.* Blackwell Science. Oxford.

intramuscular pH and fatigue or was undertaken on in-vitro muscle preparations at non-physiological temperatures. More recent work that has been undertaken at normal muscle temperatures suggests that acidosis is not the cause of fatigue; rather it is one of many associated symptoms (e.g. Westerblad et al 1997). Support for this argument is that recovery of power output following maximal exercise occurs before muscle pH is restored; in fact it is closely related to the re-synthesis of CP (Bogdanis et al 1996). More recent evidence indicates that rather than a cause of muscle fatigue, acidosis may in fact protect the muscle against fatigue that is in fact caused by other mechanisms (Nielsen et al 2001).

Another suggested cause of fatigue is an increase in intramuscular inorganic phosphate (Pi) during intense exercise, which may interfere with the release of $Ca^{2+}$ by the sarcoplasmic reticulum (Fryer et al 1995), which in turn would inhibit cross-bridge cycling. However, much of the evidence for the role of Pi in muscle fatigue is again derived from experiments carried out at temperatures below those of exercising skeletal muscle.

It is clear that further research is necessary to clarify the mechanisms of fatigue during short-duration, high-intensity exercise. Whatever the exact mechanisms of fatigue, a reduction in anaerobic energy metabolism will result in a greater contribution of aerobic energy as both high-intensity constant load exercise and intermittent exercise progress, concomitant with a decrease in exercise intensity.

## Glycogen depletion

Although high-intensity exercise demands high rates of anaerobic glycolysis (~35–40 times higher than during low-intensity, long-duration exercise) and therefore depletes the body's carbohydrate stores fairly quickly, it is unlikely that glycogen availability will limit high-intensity anaerobic exercise due to the fact that metabolic acidosis and/or other associated mechanisms of fatigue will normally precede such depletion. For instance, the body's glycogen and glucose stores are capable of fuelling ATP re-synthesis for up to an hour, or longer in well-trained individuals, at lower exercise intensities at which metabolic acidosis and associated mechanisms are not the primary cause of fatigue.

It is possible, however, that for those sports consisting of repetitive sprints or high-intensity bursts, carbohydrate availability may become a limiting factor towards the end of the training or competition bout. For example, soccer is an intermittent sport with an average exercise intensity of 75% $\dot{V}O_2$max for outfield players (van Gool et al 1988). Repetitive demands on anaerobic energy metabolism during intermittent sprinting, in addition to the ongoing oxidation of carbohydrate, can significantly deplete muscle glycogen stores throughout a game. Even greater depletion is experienced in fast-twitch fibres, thereby greatly reducing the muscle's ability to perform glycolysis and generate force. Indeed, time–motion analysis has demonstrated that players cover significantly less distance and achieve lower average exercise intensities in the second half of matches, presumably in part due to glycogen depletion.

## Neuromuscular

The contraction of muscle fibres requires a complex series of neuromuscular mechanisms. This includes innervation of the motor nerve, propagation of the electro-chemical nerve impulse along the nerve, neurotransmission across the motor end-plate and propagation of the impulse across the sarcolemma and through the T tubules. It is possible that fatigue is in part caused by failure of one or more of these mechanisms. There is evidence that the accumulation of potassium ($K^+$) within muscle fibres during contraction can stimulate an associated reflex inhibition (Garland & McComas 1990) and inhibit action potential propagation across the sarcolemma and through the T tubules. Further evidence is provided by the fact that the recovery of muscular force exhibits a similar temporal pattern to the return of $K^+$ to normal levels following exhaustive exercise.

## Neural

While many coaches and athletes may argue that mental toughness is key to top-level sports performance, it is apparent that fatigue in high-intensity exercise is a physiological rather than purely psychological state. Recently, however, the role of the central nervous system (CNS) has been highlighted in the perception of fatigue and the ability to sustain physical effort. There is now some convincing evidence that local physiological mechanisms may trigger a down-regulation of CNS activity and therefore muscle recruitment, thereby causing a decrease in power production. In addition, the cytokine response to exercise (cytokines are proteins that mediate the immune response) appears to have an effect upon the CNS and thus the sensation of fatigue.

Having identified the physiological demands and limitations to performance in a sports event the sports scientist and coach may prescribe a training programme with scientific underpinning. Specific training that targets the necessary physiological adaptations is required to reduce an individual's performance limitations and thus enhance athletic performance. The remainder of this chapter will discus the training methods for the improvement of anaerobic endurance and provides examples of specific training techniques used by athletes in short-duration, high-intensity sports.

## TRAINING METHODS

The aim of any physical training programme is to stress the physiological systems of the body in order to bring about adaptation that in turn improves performance. An athlete's capacity for adaptation and their response to training is in part determined by their genotype (genetic make-up) and phenotype (physical characteristics resulting from the genotype); however, with appropriate training prescription allowing, an athlete will be able to fulfil their potential. With the appropriate training, physiological adaptation and improvements in performance will take place. Understanding the demands of the athlete's event and the importance of anaerobic endurance to their sport is crucial in developing an appropriate training strategy.

One of the most challenging tasks for the sport and exercise physiologist is to interpret scientific knowledge and assist in the prescription of effective physical training programmes for athletes. The understanding of the physiological demands of a specific sporting event and the identification of the physical characteristics of successful athletes provides relevant information to facilitate this. The description of the physiological profiles of elite performers has been widely reported in a number of sports, which has allowed for the identification of key physiological variables related to successful performance in these events. Subsequently, an understanding of these physiological performance-influencing factors will aid the sports scientist and coach in the prescription of appropriate physical training regimes.

While there has been considerable research investigating the physiological adaptations to specific training programmes, most of the literature in this area has focused on endurance performance. Typically, it has been the effects of endurance training on markers of endurance capacity, such as the anaerobic threshold and maximal oxygen consumption which have been investigated. Conversely, there is a relative paucity of literature reporting the physiological adaptations to specific training for short-duration, high-intensity sports events. The fact that some authorities have suggested that most of the existing knowledge regarding the training practices of today's elite athletes has come from the field-based observations of successful coaches, rather than from a scientific basis provided by exercise physiologists, is perhaps in part a consequence of this.

Many of the adaptations that underpin anaerobic endurance are peripheral and therefore specific to the muscle and will occur only during high-intensity exercise (i.e. > 90% $\dot{V}O_2$max) when the fast-twitch (type II) motor units are recruited. Lower-intensity training will recruit predominantly slow-twitch (type I) motor units and have little effect on anaerobic endurance or capacity. This is not to say that lower-intensity aerobic training is not necessary for athletes in short-duration, high-intensity sports; indeed, a well-developed aerobic fitness is necessary in order to perform the volume of high-intensity training needed to develop anaerobic endurance. Further, a well developed aerobic capacity is a pre-requisite for many team game athletes. For this reason many athletes in sports with only modest aerobic energy demands will perform a considerable amount of aerobic endurance training, particularly in the off-season. This has implications for the periodization of training and will be discussed later.

The primary characteristic of anaerobic endurance training is the high-intensity at which it is performed. At perimaximal ($\sim\dot{V}O_2$max) and supramaximal ($>\dot{V}O_2$max) exercise intensities the anaerobic energy systems will be heavily taxed. The aim of anaerobic endurance training is to maximally stress these systems and thereby elicit the required adaptations. As a consequence of the intensity of training and the resultant fatigue, exercise bouts will be of short-duration, therefore training is normally divided into repeated bouts or intervals of short duration. This form of training is termed 'high-intensity training'. This should not be confused with 'interval training' which comprises the repetition of longer exercise bouts to develop aerobic endurance capacity. Interval training was brought to popular attention in the 1930s by Rudolf Harbig, the German 800 m world record holder; the repetition of intervals allows the athlete to undertake a greater volume of training at the appropriate intensity in any one training session. In contrast, high-intensity training involves the repetition of short bouts of exercise at supramaximal intensities to elicit adaptations in anaerobic capacity or anaerobic endurance. In the 1980s the importance of high-intensity training for middle-distance running was illustrated by the training methods employed by Sebastian Coe (1984 Olympic medallist in 800 m and 1500 m), and his father and coach, Peter. Coe's training adopted a greater amount of high-intensity training than had previously been considered appropriate for middle-distance running. Coe's success turned coaching and scientific attention to the role of high-intensity training and the importance of anaerobic capacity for middle-distance events.

The nature of some sports in which training may be undertaken on varying terrain, for example running and cycling, allows the use of 'hill sprints' to be used to increase the training intensity. In other sports where the terrain remains constant (e.g. swimming, rowing, kayaking), however, coaches and athletes must employ structured training sessions to manipulate the training intensity and duration, as well as the recovery duration. Factors that must be considered in the design of the training session include:

1. The required adaptations – these will be specific to the athlete's event; it may be to improve the capacity of the ATP-CP system in the shorter-duration events (e.g. 100 m running) or the capacity of the glycolytic system in the longer duration events. This factor must be decided upon prior to consideration of any of the following factors.

2. Repetition intensity – gross recruitment of the fast-twitch motor units requires training intensities of > 90% $\dot{V}O_2$max; at higher intensities the relative energy contribution from the anaerobic sources will be greater, thereby focusing the training session on the required adaptations. Many athletes make the mistake of trying to complete repetitions that are too long and/or too many in number. While they may believe that 'more is better', this is simply not the case. By attempting to undertake excessive volume, training intensity will be compromised. Given that anaerobic adaptations require high-intensity training, any repetitions that fail to meet the required intensity will also fail to have the desired effect.

3. Repetition duration – this will be largely determined by the training intensity and consequent physiological fatigue. Very high-intensity bouts designed to stress the ATP-CP energy system will be limited to a short duration ($\leq 15$ seconds) by CP depletion. On the other hand, repetitions that stress the glycolytic energy system may be longer with acidosis and other associated mechanisms causing fatigue over a longer period (e.g. up to 3 minutes).

4. Recovery duration – this will determine the intensity and number of subsequent repetitions that may be achieved. The duration will also depend upon the aim of the training session. Recovery of the various mechanisms of fatigue display different temporal patterns, for example, while cellular CP is re-synthesized relatively quickly, metabolic acidosis takes somewhat longer to recover to homeostasis. Therefore, if the aim of the session is to tax the ATP-CP system then only relatively short recovery periods will be needed and will be determined by the duration of the exercise interval. If, however, the restoration of normal pH levels is required then longer duration recovery will be required between exercise repetitions. Again, muscle acidity should not be confused with blood lactate concentrations. Blood lactate is merely an indirect marker of metabolic acidosis and can demonstrate a quite different rate of return to resting levels than that of cellular pH.

5. Number of repetitions and sets performed – this is the factor that can be manipulated to control the volume of each training session. The training intensity together with the duration of the recovery periods will largely determine the volume of training that an athlete can complete.

6. Recovery period between training sessions – while the purpose of recovery periods between repetitions is to allow the re-synthesis of energy substrates and restoration of cellular homeostasis, the rationale for recovery between training sessions is to provide for the complete recovery of the whole organism and adaptation to the imposed demands. At best, failure to incorporate sufficient recovery in the training programme will prevent physiological adaptation and improvements in performance; at worst, full recovery will not be achieved. This is known as 'over-reaching' (see Ch. 1); long-term over-reaching will compromise physiological adaptation and may result in overtraining, or as it is now referred to in the literature, the 'unexplained under-performance syndrome' (UUPS) (see Ch. 9).

This condition is characterized by a reduction in athletic performance in the absence of any clinically diagnosed illness. Many athletes who have experienced this condition have suffered long-term fatigue with the inability to continue their training and athletic careers.

## TYPES OF ANAEROBIC ENDURANCE TRAINING

The demands of an athlete's event and therefore the targeted adaptations will shape the type of training session performed. For example, performance in the shorter duration events (≤ 20 seconds) is greatly influenced by both the amount of cellular CP stored within skeletal muscle and the rate at which it can be degraded to re-synthesize ATP. Therefore a 100 m track athlete wanting to improve their average speed would need to perform repetitions of 10–15 seconds with recovery periods of adequate duration to allow almost complete CP re-synthesis. Athletes competing in longer events (e.g. 20 seconds to 4 minutes) will strive to increase their ability to tolerate high levels of metabolic acidosis. This can be attained by performing training repetitions of between 10 and 120 seconds, during which cellular pH will fall and very high levels of blood lactate will be generated (e.g. >12 mmol.L$^{-1}$). For this reason, this type of longer-duration anaerobic endurance training is often referred to as 'lactate tolerance' training. This chapter will adopt the terms 'short-term anaerobic endurance' and 'long-term anaerobic endurance' to classify training that targets the ATP-CP capacity and the glycolytic capacity, respectively.

For those athletes whose race distance imposes high demands on anaerobic energy production and the capacity to produce such energy, race-pace training presents an effective way of achieving the goals of anaerobic endurance training. This type of training has the additional benefits of practising and developing specific coordination and muscle fibre recruitment, and pace judgement. It is likely, however, that this type of training will be more effective when split into repetitions, thereby allowing a greater volume of high-intensity training to be completed during the session.

Many endurance athletes control training intensity by monitoring their heart rate. Heart rate monitors today are very accurate and affordable; however they are of limited use during high-intensity training. Because such training is supramaximal and of short-duration, heart rate is not a sensitive indicator of exercise intensity. Instead it is more appropriate to control intensity either by speed or power output, or simply by maximal effort.

## Short–term anaerobic endurance training

The repetition of short-duration exercise bouts (≤ 15 seconds) will develop the capacity for intramuscular CP storage and the rate of ATP re-synthesis, thus resulting in a greater power output as well as an ability to sustain this power for longer. While previous research has clearly demonstrated that repetitive sprint exercise of short duration bouts results in considerable metabolic acidosis and blood lactate accumulation, this can be reduced if recovery periods allow for the restoration of cellular CP. As previously discussed, CP is re-synthesized relatively quickly (90% in 3–4 minutes), therefore such training sessions may employ work:rest duration ratios in the order of 1:10, thereby allowing the repetition of maximal short-duration exercise bouts. Research has consistently shown that CP is re-synthesized at a higher rate during low-intensity exercise than at rest, therefore rest intervals should be active rather than passive. Short-term anaerobic endurance training increases the capacity of the ATP-CP energy pathway and enhances muscular power.

## Long-term anaerobic endurance training

Maximal exercise of 1–3 minutes duration will place very high demands on the anaerobic glycolytic system and, as a consequence, on the intra- and extra-muscular buffering capacities. Long recovery intervals between repetitions allow for the restoration of cellular homeostasis, including return of pH towards resting levels and the removal and oxidation of lactate. A work:rest duration ratio in the region of 1:4 should be used for such training.

An alternative form of anaerobic endurance training that is commonly used by athletes in the longer-duration, high-intensity events (i.e. 30–180 seconds) is the repetition of short-duration (20–120 seconds), maximal exercise bouts interspersed with short-duration rest periods (work:rest duration ratios of 1:1). This is termed 'lactate tolerance training', an example of which is repetitions of 30-second work periods separated by 30 seconds of rest; four to six repetitions may comprise a set, after which a longer rest period allows restoration of cellular homeostasis. A total of four to six sets might be completed in a training session. Such training also results in very high levels of metabolic acidosis but rather than allowing full recovery between each repetition, the athlete performs further repetitions (within the set) while the muscle is in a fatigued state. There is a paucity of research investigating the acute and chronic physiological responses to this type of training; however, it is widely used by coaches and athletes. It is interesting to note that there is recent evidence that such training methods with similar work and rest durations may be one of the most effective methods to develop $\dot{V}O_2max$ (Billat et al 2000), although repetitions are normally performed at 100% $\dot{V}O_2max$ rather than at supramaximal intensities, and a greater number of repetitions are completed within a given training session.

## Resistance training

Gym-based training may also be used to develop anaerobic endurance. By manipulating the intensity, the number of repetitions and sets, and the duration of rest periods (as previously discussed in this chapter), training may be designed to target specific physiological adaptations to enhance the ability to sustain force production (sometimes referred to as 'strength endurance'). It must be remembered, however, that the physiological adaptations that underpin anaerobic endurance are specific to the trained muscle. Great care must therefore be taken to ensure that the resistance training exercises target the relevant muscle in the same way in which it is recruited during the sports performance (see Ch. 6).

## THE IMPORTANCE OF A WARM-DOWN

While many athletes undertake a warm-down after intense training there is a surprising lack of scientific evidence for this practice. The proposed benefits of warming-down following high-intensity training include a more rapid removal of lactate from the blood and conversion to glucose within the liver, an accelerated removal of other metabolic by-products from the muscle, prevention of blood pooling and the avoidance of the potentially negative effects of increased circulating catecholamines on cardiac function. It is possible that the rate of recovery following training is increased as a consequence of performing a warm-down; however, as yet there is a lack of supporting evidence.

# EXAMPLES OF SPORT-SPECIFIC TRAINING SESSIONS

## Running

Running provides the flexibility of using the terrain to manipulate training intensity; the use of hill sprints is a common training method for middle-distance runners. Hill sprints are effective in increasing the intensity and stress on the muscular system and may therefore be incorporated as part of anaerobic endurance training; many middle-distance runners use hill sprints as an alternative to gym-based resistance training to improve strength. A note of caution, however, is that hill running involves the recruitment of slightly different motor units to that of running on the flat; given that improvements in anaerobic capacity reside within the muscle, this may therefore have limited benefit for flat terrain running. Despite this, there is a consensus of opinion that hill-running can greatly improve anaerobic endurance and strength of runners.

### *Typical sessions*

### Short-term anaerobic endurance training
- 10 repetitions of 100 m, with 3-minute rest intervals

### Long-term anaerobic endurance training
- 6 repetitions of 500 m, with 3-minute rest intervals
- 8 repetitions of hill sprints of approx. 45 seconds, with 4-minute rest intervals
- 3 sets of 4 repetitions of 200 m intervals at 400 m pace, 200 m steady; rest intervals of 6–8 minutes between sets

## Cycling

Cyclists, like runners, may take advantage of hills to perform their high-intensity training. Alternatively, a structured session on flat terrain or a track may be performed.

### *Typical sessions*

### Short-term anaerobic endurance training
- Maximal sprints of 10 seconds, with complete recovery

### Long-term anaerobic endurance training
- 8 repetitions of 1000–2000 m, with rest intervals of 5–10 minutes
- 12 repetitions of 30 seconds, with rest intervals of 4–5 minutes

## Swimming

Swimming is a sport in which the environment is constant. This has the advantage of allowing for day-to-day comparison of training performance. The use of hand paddles may also be effective in increasing the load on the upper body musculature and therefore promoting adaptation.

### *Typical sessions*

### Short-term anaerobic endurance training
- Maximal sprints of ≤25 m with complete recovery

### Long-term anaerobic endurance training

- 3 sets of 6–10 repetitions of 50 m, with rest intervals of 10–30 seconds; rest intervals of 3–5 minutes between sets
- 2 sets of 200 m, 150 m, 100 m, 50 m, with equal-duration rest intervals; rest intervals of 5 minutes between sets

## Canoeing and kayaking

Structured training sessions may be used to develop anaerobic endurance, either on the water, or through dry-land ergometer training. Although modern ergometers provide accurate replication of the on-water action, athletes are best advised to carry out their high-intensity training on the water (due to the specificity of the training adaptations). Canoeists and kayakers often increase the resistance on the boat through the water by attaching ropes around the hull; this increases the drag and therefore the intensity of effort required.

### Typical sessions

### Short-term anaerobic endurance training

- 15 repetitions of 10 seconds, with 2-minute rest intervals; rolling starts

### Long-term anaerobic endurance training

- 6 sets of 6 repetitions of 30 seconds, with 30-second rest intervals; rest intervals of 5–7 minutes between sets
- 8 repetitions of 2 minutes, with 6-minute rest intervals

## Field sports and court games

Field sports and court games players can make use of the pitch or court to structure their anaerobic endurance training. By performing repeated shuttle sprints not only can players stress the appropriate physiological capacities but they can also develop acceleration and agility.

### Typical sessions

### Short-term anaerobic endurance training

- 3 sets of 10 repetitions of width of pitch, with 1-minute rest intervals; 4-minute rest intervals between sets

### Long-term anaerobic endurance training

- 10 repetitions of 60 seconds, with 2-minute rest intervals
- Repetitions of shuttle runs (5–15 seconds) up and down length of pitch, with equal rest intervals; rest intervals of 4–6 minutes between sets

Endurance athletes will often perform what they refer to as 'speed training'. Of course they have little need for all-out speed and this training is in fact 'anaerobic endurance' and quite similar to some of the training methods described above. Endurance athletes will often perform high-intensity training twice a week with bouts as short as 90 seconds with complete recovery (4–7 minutes) in the final few weeks prior to major competition. It is clear that such a training plan will be insufficient to maximize anaerobic endurance for most sprint and middle-distance athletes; however, it does provide the endurance athlete with their equivalent of speed work.

## PLANNING OF ANAEROBIC ENDURANCE TRAINING DURING THE YEAR

When anaerobic endurance training should commence in the periodized year is a question that has largely gone unanswered in the scientific community. Some authorities recommend that anaerobic endurance training should take place for a period of 4–8 weeks prior to the start of the taper for major competition. It must be stressed that these guidelines have largely been derived from endurance-based sports in which athletes perform only a relatively small amount of anaerobic training superimposed upon an extensive base of aerobic conditioning. Clearly the training principle of specificity dictates that the amount and duration of anaerobic endurance development will differ according to the sports event and the individual. What is more generally accepted, however, is that anaerobic endurance training, due to the high-intensity at which it is performed, places a high stress on the physiological capacities of the athlete; consequently the prescription of appropriate rest and recovery is paramount.

For most short-duration, high-intensity sports, the latter part of the preparatory phase (specific preparatory sub-phase) or the early part of the competitive phase (pre-competitive sub-phase) is the time that most of the training for anaerobic capacity should take place. During this time the total volume of the training plan will be reduced as intensity is increased. Anaerobic endurance training may be spread throughout these sub-phases but will normally be concentrated within alternate macro- or microcycles (see Ch. 1). Whatever the duration of the event, the anaerobic endurance training will commence with longer duration, lower intensity intervals, moving to shorter duration and higher intensity intervals as the competitive phase progresses. While there is no consensus on the amount of anaerobic endurance training that should be performed during this phase of training, a guideline of 50% is recommended, with the other 50% being made up of endurance maintenance, and strength and power training.

Well-developed aerobic fitness decreases the recovery time between high-intensity exercise bouts, which in turn will prepare the athlete for the necessary volume of anaerobic training. Aerobic fitness must therefore be incorporated and targeted in the preparatory phases of training. Indeed, for the many sports that require high levels of both aerobic and anaerobic endurance (e.g. middle-distance running, 50–400 m swimming, 500 m and 1000 m canoeing and kayaking, 4000 m track cycling) this will be particularly relevant. There is, however, some evidence both in human and in-vitro equine muscle that high-intensity training reduces the aerobic capacity of muscle (see Ch. 3). This highlights the importance for those middle-distance athletes whose events demand high levels of both aerobic and anaerobic endurance of not neglecting aerobic conditioning at any time of the training year.

High-intensity anaerobic training imposes a high stress upon the organism and as such requires considerable recovery. The recovery period required for the optimization of adaptation and prevention of chronic overreaching will depend upon the individual. Genetic endowment will have a large influence on an individual's rate of recovery from training. Young athletes (<18 years) and older athletes (>25 years) will require longer to recover and adapt, as will less experienced athletes.

Hormonal differences between males and females usually necessitate longer recovery periods for female athletes.

## PLANNING OF DAY-TO-DAY ANAEROBIC ENDURANCE TRAINING

High-intensity training results in a number of causes and symptoms of fatigue, including ATP-CP depletion, metabolic acidosis, glycogen depletion and CNS disturbances. High-intensity training also predisposes athletes to 'high-frequency fatigue', which manifests as impaired electrochemical function and excitation-contraction coupling within the muscle cell. In addition, such high-intensity training may cause microtrauma and damage to skeletal muscle fibres, particularly if the training is unaccustomed, as it may be at the start of the training phase in which anaerobic endurance is developed. All of these factors require recovery before further anaerobic training can be effectively completed. For this reason athletes are advised to alternate types of training sessions and structure their training so that high overload sessions and low to moderate overload sessions are undertaken on alternate days. While some of these symptoms and causes of fatigue recover fairly quickly, depleted glycogen can take up to 48 hours to be restored. Skeletal muscle damage takes somewhat longer to recover; however, skeletal muscle demonstrates a very high capacity to adapt to unaccustomed exercise so as to reduce or prevent further damage when that same exercise is repeated.

There are many ways that the training type and load can be cycled throughout a week or microcycle, which makes the provision of exact guidelines difficult. The prescription of training must take account of the other elements of physical training that are also being targeted within that period of training. This will dictate the amount of recovery required between training sessions and therefore the volume of training that can be achieved. It is not uncommon for a single training session to target a number of different physiological capacities and adaptations, for example: base endurance and sprint training. While the alternating of types of training within a session is one way in which training may be cycled it does limit the volume of any one type of training that can be performed within a single training bout. In addition, the fatigue induced by one type of training may well limit the ability to perform another. Athletes are therefore best advised to focus on one component of fitness in any single training session and to structure the session to target specific adaptations accordingly.

## EXAMPLES OF TRAINING SCHEDULES

Tables 5.2 and 5.3 provide examples of training programmes during the pre-competitive and competitive phases of the periodized year. A training programme for an elite 400 m runner devised by athletics coach Bruce Tulloh is shown in Table 5.2; Table 5.3 details the training carried out by Sebastian Coe in preparation for the 1984 Los Angeles Olympics in which he won gold in the 1500 m and silver in the 800 m. Both programmes illustrate how anaerobic endurance training may be structured within the overall training plan.

The presentation of training schedules is in some ways in stark conflict with the primary purpose of this chapter, which is to discuss the *physiology* of training for anaerobic endurance. Unfortunately these schedules, and indeed any others, are not the direct result of scientific investigation alone but rather a result of the interpretation and synthesis of scientific training principles, empirical research findings and a wealth of anecdotal evidence accumulated by coaches. While these training

**Table 5.2**    Training programme for an elite 400 m runner

| (a) Pre-competition phase | | |
|---|---|---|
| | Session 1<br>(07:00 hours) | Session 2<br>(12:00 hours approx.) | Session 3 (18:00 hours approx.) |
| Day 1 | 2 mile run at<br>6 min/mile | 1 × 500 m<br>(50 s/400 m).<br>10 min rest.<br>6 × 60 m bounding;<br>10 × 60 m hopping.<br>1 mile slow run. | 4 × 60 sec hard effort through<br>sand or uphill; 3 min rest.<br>4 × 30 sec hard effort through<br>sand or uphill; 2 min rest. |
| Day 2 | as above | 3 × 5 × 40 m sprint<br>drills.<br>1 mile slow run. | 4 × differential 400 m with<br>first 200 m in 28–29 sec<br>then accelerating.<br>1–2 mile warm-down. |
| Day 3 | as above | 3 mile brisk run at<br>6 min/mile. | 6 × 400 m (60–62 sec);<br>2 min jog recovery.<br>1–2 mile warm-down. |
| Day 4 | as above | 30 min weight-training.<br>6 × 60 m bounding;<br>10 × 60 m hopping.<br>1–3 mile slow run. | 100 m – 200 m – 100 m –<br>250 m – 150 m – 300 m –<br>200 m – 200 m<br>(11–12 sec/100 m, with rolling<br>starts); 2 min recovery.<br>1 mile warm-down. |
| Day 5 | as above | 3 × 5 × 40 m sprint<br>drills.<br>1 mile slow run. | REST |
| Day 6 | REST | Warm-up only. | 3–4 × 300 m; 10 min recovery<br>(with blood lactate tests).<br>2–3 mile warm-down. |
| Day 7 | REST | 30 min weight-training. | 6 × 150 m sprint – coast – sprint.<br>Warm-down. |

Session 1: daily warm-up
5 min jogging
10 min loosening and stretching

Sessions 2 and 3: daily warm-up
5 min jogging
10 min loosening and stretching
5 min abdominal and back-strengthening exercises
10 min jogging and striding

| (b) Competition phase | |
|---|---|
| | Session 1<br>(07:00 hours) | Session 2 (12:00 hours approx.) |
| Day 1 | 1–2 mile run slow | 200 m – 300 m – 300 m – 200 m (race speed);<br>8–10 min recovery.<br>2 mile slow jog. |

*Continued*

Table 5.2    Training programme for an elite 400 m runner—Cont'd

| | (b) Competition phase | |
|---|---|---|
| | Session 1 (07:00 hours) | Session 2 (12:00 hours approx.) |
| Day 2 | 1–2 mile slow run | 3 × 150 m; 3 × 100 m (sub-11 sec/100 m, rolling start); 5 min recovery. 2 mile warm-down. |
| Day 3 | as above | 6 × 120 m fast relaxed running. 1 mile warm-down. |
| Day 4 | as above | 3 × differential 400 m with first 200 m in 25–26 sec then maximum effort to finish; 12 min recovery. 2 mile slow jog. |
| Day 5 | as above | Warm-up only |
| Day 6 | as above | 200 m – 300 m – 300 m – 200 m (race speed); 8–10 min recovery. 2 mile warm-down. |
| Day 7 | as above | 5–6 × 150 m tactical running, changing pace every 50 m. |
| Day 8 | as above | Warm-up only |
| Day 9 | as above but omit strengthening exercises | Warm-up only, omit strengthening exercises |
| Day 10 | as above but omit strengthening exercises | RACE, omit strengthening exercises in warm-up |

Session 1: daily warm-up
5 min jogging
10 min abdominal and back-strengthening exercises 10 min loosening and stretching
10 min either leg strength exercises or sprint drills

Session 2: daily warm-up
5 min jogging
10 min loosening exercises
10–15 min jogging and striding

Reproduced from Newsholme EA, Leech T, Duester G 1994 *Keep on running: the science of training and performance*, with permission from Wiley, Chichester.

schedules have not been tested in a research context, they have produced impressive results for high-level athletes. It is refreshing that sports scientists are able to learn so much from coaches and athletes in competitive sports. Hopefully our learning will stimulate further applied scientific research to better understand the acute and chronic responses to physical training, particularly in the case of anaerobic endurance training, which at present is perhaps the least researched component of physiological fitness.

While these schedules provide guidelines for training, it is important to remember the training principle of individualization. This states that training must take account of the individual characteristics of the athlete, as previously discussed in this chapter. The sports scientist and coach must therefore evaluate the

**Table 5.3**   Training programme of Sebastian Coe, July 16–22 1984, leading up to the Los Angeles Olympics

|        | Session 1 | Session 2 |
|--------|-----------|-----------|
| Day 1 | 6 mile recovery run | |
| Day 2 | Tempo run: 6 × 800 m in 2 minutes with 3 minute recovery; 2 lap cool-down at 90 sec lap the easy jogging | 4 miles easy |
| Day 3 | 5 miles easy | 10 × 100 m steady accelerations to 60 m, maximum speed to 80 m, then float to 100 m; walk back to start recovery |
| Day 4 | 6 × 300 m at 41 sec with 3 minute recovery | 4 miles easy |
| Day 5 | 20 × 200 m in 27–28 sec | 5 miles easy |
| Day 6 | 11 sprints progressing in distance from 100 m to 200 m in 10 m increments, increasing from 14 to 35 sec, with jog-back recovery | |
| Day 7 | 6–7 miles endurance run including mixed accelerations | |

Reproduced from Sandrock M 1996 *Running with the legends. training and racing insights from 21 great runners*, with permission from Human Kinetics, Champaign IL.

individual's unique capacity and response to training before effective training can be prescribed.

## ADAPTATION TO ANAEROBIC ENDURANCE TRAINING

All of the limitations to anaerobic endurance discussed earlier in this chapter may be addressed and improved through specific training. In contrast to the adaptations to aerobic endurance training that occur at both central and peripheral sites, adaptations in anaerobic capacity occur peripherally and predominantly within the muscle cell. Unfortunately there have been relatively few well-controlled scientific investigations examining the physiological adaptations to high-intensity training; however Table 5.4 provides a summary of the key findings of a selection of training intervention studies that have addressed this question.

The primary adaptations that improve the capacity of the ATP-CP system, and therefore short-term anaerobic endurance, are increased:

- intramuscular ATP and CP stores;
- intramuscular free creatine stores;
- concentration and activity of specific enzymes (creatine kinase, myokinase).

The primary adaptations that improve the capacity of the glycolytic system, and therefore long-term anaerobic endurance, are increased:

- glycolytic enzymes (e.g. PFK, phosphorylase);
- intracellular and extracellular buffering capacity.

These and other adaptations to high-intensity training are discussed below.

Table 5.4  A summary of the findings of high-intensity training studies

| Duration | Training activity | Adaptations | No change | Reference |
|---|---|---|---|---|
| 6 weeks | Intermittent hill-running | 17% ↑ high-intensity treadmill test<br>14% ↑ peak blood lactate<br>15% ↑ high-energy phosphates | $\dot{V}O_2$max<br>anaerobic power<br>fibre composition | Houston & Thomson (1977) |
| 8 weeks | Sprint training | 20% ↑ peak muscle lactate<br>no change in intramuscular pH *<br>46% ↑ PFK activity | | Sharp et al. (1986) |
| 6 weeks | Cycle ergometry sprints, 2–3 times weekly<br>either: 2 × 15 sec & 2 × 30 sec in week 1 progressing to 6 × 15 sec & 6 × 30 sec | ↑ peak blood lactate<br>↑ % IIa muscle fibres<br>↑ PFK activity<br>↓ Mb | Wingate performance | Jacobs et al. (1987) |
| 6 weeks | Treadmill running, 3 times weekly<br>either: 3 × 2 min, 8 min rests<br>or: 8 × 20 sec, approx. 5 min rests | 10% ↑ MAOD in both groups | peak blood lactate | Medbo & Burgers (1990) |
| 3 weeks | Cycle ergometry all-out sprints<br>10 × 6 sec sprint, 24 sec rests<br>10 sessions in total | ↑ mean power in 2 out of 10 sprints<br>↑ peak power in 3 out of 10 sprints<br>↑ peak blood lactate<br>no change in post-ex. blood pH * | $\dot{V}O_2$max<br>plasma volume<br>blood glucose | Jenkins et al. (1994) |
| 8 weeks | Treadmill running, 3–4 times each week<br>2 × maximal 30 sec, 10 min rest<br>6–10 × maximal 6 sec, 54 sec rests<br>2–5 × 2 min at 110% $\dot{V}O_2$max, 5 min rests | 12% ↑ peak power in 30 sec sprint test<br>6% ↑ mean power in 30 sec sprint test<br>↑ post-ex. muscle lactate<br>↓ post-ex. blood pH | in-vitro muscle buffering capacity<br>metabolic responses to 2 min test at 110% $\dot{V}O_2$max | Nevill et al. (1989) |

* No change in muscle/blood pH following exhaustive exercise is indicative of increased buffering capacity.

## ATP–CP CAPACITY

Short-term anaerobic endurance training (repetitions of ≤15 seconds) increases resting intramuscular concentrations of ATP and CP. An increase in the amount of free creatine, used in the re-synthesis of CP, is also observed following training. While the promotion of substrate storage will increase the duration over which this pathway may contribute energy, the rates of ATP and CP depletion during maximal exercise appear to be similar for trained and untrained subjects. Strength training has been shown to increase creatine kinase and myokinase concentrations in fast-twitch muscle fibres, although surprisingly there is little evidence of such adaptations in response to other forms of high-intensity training.

## GLYCOLYTIC CAPACITY

Long-term anaerobic endurance training has been shown to increase the rate of glycogen metabolism during high-intensity exercise and to increase post-exercise levels of muscle acidity and blood lactate, indicating either a higher rate or amount of anaerobic glycolysis. Indeed, post-exercise blood lactate has been shown to correlate with performance in short-duration, high-intensity events. Consequently, sports scientists often use post-exercise blood lactate concentration as an indication of anaerobic contribution during exercise. Concentrations in the blood usually peak a few minutes after the cessation of maximal exercise and the highest concentrations are seen in maximal exercise of 2–3 minutes duration. This increase in anaerobic glycolysis may be due to increases in specific enzyme activity and/or an enhanced buffering capacity to cope with the metabolic acidosis. Increases in glycolytic enzymes enhance the rate of ATP re-synthesis via glycolysis, thereby increasing exercise intensity that can be achieved during short-duration exercise. Care must be taken not to confuse blood lactate concentrations with muscle and blood acidity (pH). Sharp et al (1986) and Jenkins et al (1994) have shown that training-induced increases in buffering capacity result in increases in blood lactate with no change in muscle or blood pH (Table 5.4). This is due to an increased buffering capacity that 'mops up' the hydrogen ions produced by the rapid dissociation of lactic acid; as a consequence, the rate of glycolysis and therefore exercise intensity are maintained, thus elevating lactate concentrations. The performance gains resulting from an increase in buffering capacity are also demonstrated by the administration of exogenous buffers (e.g. sodium bicarbonate, sodium citrate), that have been shown to increase blood alkalinity prior to exercise and enhance anaerobic exercise performance. Ingestion of these buffers is not, however, widespread among athletes due partly to the fact that they can often cause gastrointestinal disturbance.

## OTHER ADAPTATIONS

### Performance

Performance tests are often used in sports science laboratories to provide a sport-specific estimation of anaerobic capacity in a controlled environment. These tests may be used to evaluate the efficacy of anaerobic training in increasing anaerobic endurance. Perhaps due to the lack of specificity of some methods used to identify anaerobic capacity, however, some research has demonstrated adaptations in a number of physiological measures in the absence of a concomitant improvement in laboratory performance tests. For example, Jacobs et al (1987) found that 6 weeks of training results in a number of adaptations with no concomitant improvement in Wingate cycle test performance (see Table 5.4). This suggests that either cellular adaptations do not necessarily result in performance gains or that the Wingate test is not a sensitive measure of anaerobic capacity.

## Muscle fibre composition

The question of whether an individual's muscle fibre composition is genetically determined or a result of long-term athletic training has been debated for many years. The first study showing that athletes from different sports were characterized by different distributions of fibre type was published in 1972 (Gollnick et al 1972). Subsequent work by the same group also demonstrated that endurance training could increase the percentage of slow-twitch fibres by up to 36% (Gollnick et al 1973). This was supported by Tesch & Karlsson (1985) who reported that long-distance runners exhibit a 67% and 49% slow-twitch fibre composition in the vastus lateralis and medial deltoid, respectively; in contrast, marathon kayakers demonstrated an opposite profile of 71% and 41% slow-twitch fibres in the medial deltoid and vastus lateralis, respectively. Differences in fibre composition between trained and untrained individuals, and indeed between trained and untrained muscles within individuals, are evidence that long-term training and not heredity alone determine muscle fibre characteristics. The transition towards a predominance of fast-twitch fibres as a result of high-intensity training is less well-documented. It is possible, however, that muscle plasticity would also allow some adaptation in athletes in short-duration, high-intensity events. Selective muscle fibre hypertrophy is also evident with training. Gollnick et al (1972) noted considerable hypertrophy of slow-twitch muscle fibres in endurance athletes, while Clarkson et al (1982) revealed that although there was no difference in the percentage fibre composition of the biceps brachii and vastus lateralis in sprint kayakers, the fast-twitch fibres in the biceps brachii exhibited hypertrophy and an increase in the percentage of total muscle area (as opposed to number) compared to the vastus lateralis. Therefore, both muscle fibre composition and selective fibre hypertrophy are a consequence of specific physical training. Contemporary understanding of skeletal muscle indicates that the categorization of fibres into three discrete types is probably overly simplistic; rather, there is a continuum of fibre types based on a number of biochemical characteristics, all of which exhibit adaptation to exercise training.

## Neural

It has been suggested that anaerobic endurance training may result in an increase in an athlete's mental toughness or pain tolerance. While it is possible that this occurs it is likely to only be responsible for improved performance in previously untrained individuals. It is, however, likely that the high intensities characteristic of anaerobic training will demand high levels of neural input and coordination. Short-term anaerobic endurance training in which maximal speeds/power outputs are attained will result in a greater number and synchronicity of motor unit recruitment, thereby increasing muscle force generating capacity. Such neural adaptations occur relatively quickly in response to training. This is clearly demonstrated by the initial response to resistance training exercise in which strength gains are observed without any concomitant muscle hypertrophy.

## Aerobic

Training for anaerobic endurance must be performed at high intensities to elicit the required training adaptations. As previously highlighted, however, the aerobic contribution to short-duration, high-intensity exercise can be considerable, particularly over the course of a complete training session. Further, recent research has highlighted that an effective way of improving aerobic power ($\dot{V}O_2$max) is by performing repetitions of short-duration, high-intensity exercise interspersed with active recovery periods, e.g. 30-second bouts at 100% $\dot{V}O_2$max with 30-second recovery periods at 50% $\dot{V}O_2$max (Billat et al 2000). It is therefore probable that training for anaerobic endurance will have some effect on $\dot{V}O_2$max, a fact that may be particularly important for athletes participating in middle-distance events in which there is a large anaerobic and aerobic energy contribution, and in which performance has been correlated with both aerobic and anaerobic endurance.

## ASSESSMENT OF ANAEROBIC ENDURANCE

It is important to monitor training progression in all components of physical fitness. This will allow the evaluation of training and the modification of training if necessary. The monitoring or assessment of anaerobic endurance can be undertaken in either a laboratory of field environment. While field tests may lack some of the control and reliability of laboratory tests, they often provide a greater degree of sport-specificity. In contrast to the testing of aerobic power (i.e. maximal oxygen consumption) there is no one method capable of quantifying anaerobic energy yield. There are two approaches to measuring anaerobic capacity. Firstly, to estimate anaerobic energy yield during exercise. Secondly, to simply measure the work performed during a short-duration performance test. Some commonly used tests for the assessment of anaerobic endurance are briefly outlined here.

## ESTIMATION OF ANAEROBIC ENERGY YIELD

### Maximal accumulated oxygen deficit (MAOD)

Proposed in 1988 by Medbo et al, the maximal accumulated oxygen deficit provides a method for estimating the anaerobic energy contribution during supramaximal exercise. This procedure requires the calculation of the individual's submaximal oxygen consumption–power relationship, which can be attained from an incremental submaximal exercise test. This relationship is then applied to the power output achieved during a supramaximal test to estimate the oxygen cost of the exercise. The difference between this estimated oxygen cost and the total oxygen consumed is termed the oxygen deficit. During exhaustive supramaximal exercise of 2–3 minutes duration, in which the anaerobic capacity is fully utilized, this deficit represents the maximal accumulated oxygen deficit. Although this procedure relies on a number of assumptions that have been disputed in recent literature, it is perhaps one of the most robust ways of estimating anaerobic energy yield.

### Excess post–exercise oxygen consumption (EPOC)

Following supramaximal exercise, oxygen consumption remains elevated above resting levels for a period of time. It has been proposed that this represents the repayment of an 'oxygen debt' incurred during an exercise bout. It is suggested that the elevated oxygen consumption was required to replenish the depleted ATP and CP stores and to oxidize the lactate produced. More recently the term EPOC has replaced 'oxygen debt' because the excess oxygen consumption is now known to be influenced by endocrinal and thermal factors. The use of EPOC to estimate anaerobic energy yield has largely been replaced by the MAOD procedure.

## Quantification of intramuscular substrate and enzyme activity

The use of muscle needle biopsy provides researchers with an invasive method of determining cellular changes in response to exercise and to chronic training. This procedure may be used to identify depletion rates of ATP, CP and glycogen together with enzyme activities and intramuscular pH. While research has used this technique to elucidate cellular responses to high-intensity exercise and training, in practice it is clearly not a suitable method for the routine assessment of athletes (see Ch. 6).

## Post-exercise blood lactate concentration

Blood lactate measurements taken after an exercise bout are often used to monitor the contribution of anaerobic glycolysis to exercise. While this method attempts to estimate anaerobic energy yield via the measurement of a glycolytic by-product, it should be noted that blood concentration is a relatively poor indicator of muscle lactic acid production. The concentration of lactate in blood reflects a balance between production and clearance. It is therefore affected by differences in lactate clearance rates as well by the extent of glycolysis. A number of studies have, however, interpreted an increase in post-exercise blood lactate concomitant with no change in muscle or blood pH as an indication of enhanced buffering capacity. While this is a reasonable assumption it is difficult to quantify the magnitude of adaptation in this way.

## PERFORMANCE TESTS

Sports scientists use a variety of performance tests to measure short-duration, high-intensity power output, and thus estimate anaerobic capacity. The most well-known of these, the Wingate anaerobic test, is an all-out 30-second cycle ergometry test. Measures of peak power output, total work done and the rate of fatigue (fatigue index) are recorded. Work done in the first 10 seconds of the test can be used as an indirect estimate of the capacity of the ATP-CP system, and the 30-second work output an estimate of total anaerobic capacity. Despite much debate as to the validity and sensitivity of the Wingate test it remains a popular method of physiological assessment. The Wingate test has since been modified for use in a variety of exercise modalities and durations.

Other performance tests include Cunningham & Faulkner treadmill test. This is a supramaximal running test performed at a constant speed of 12.8 km.h$^{-1}$ and gradient of 20%. Time to exhaustion is recorded and used as an index of anaerobic endurance. More recently the test has been modified to a speed of 16 km.h$^{-1}$ so as to elicit fatigue in less time and therefore reduce the aerobic energy contribution to the exercise.

Multiple sprint tests are commonly used in the assessment of field sports players (e.g. soccer, hockey, rugby). These tests comprise a series of repeated sprints over a specified distance, separated by timed recovery periods; the recording of the fastest time and the fatigue index provides an indirect estimation of anaerobic endurance.

Variations of such tests include the Bangsbo test (Bangsbo 1994), which consists of seven repeated sprints over a 34 m course that includes a change of direction, and which are separated by 25 seconds active recovery.

The major limitation of such performance tests is that they fail to take account of aerobic energy contribution which, as shown in Table 5.1, can account for up to 40% of total energy during exhaustive 30-second cycle ergometry. For this reason performance tests often lack validity and may be insensitive to specific training-induced adaptations in anaerobic endurance.

## CONCLUSIONS

Sports events of between 10 seconds and 4 minutes demand a considerable anaerobic energy contribution; for many of these events anaerobic endurance may present a limitation to performance. Similar characteristics also apply to high-intensity intermittent sports (e.g. field and court sports). With appropriate training an athlete can increase their average power production over a short to medium-duration through physiological adaptation to promote the capacity for anaerobic energy metabolism. The prescription of effective training requires an understanding of the principles of training together with an appreciation of the empirical evidence demonstrating the physiological adaptations to training. It should be noted, however, that training is not a solely scientific practice; rather it is informed by the practical experience of coaches and athletes. Indeed, many training methods used by coaches and athletes today are not yet supported by scientific evidence.

The physiological assessment of athletes can be used to identify factors related to performance and to monitor specific adaptation, which provides further evidence for the prescription of training. It is clear that at present high-intensity exercise and training are relatively under-researched areas of exercise physiology. Further applied research in this area is needed to elucidate the physiology of training for anaerobic endurance.

## KEY POINTS

1. Sports events of between 10 seconds and 4 minutes duration rely upon a significant energy contribution from the anaerobic energy pathways.
2. Performance in such events is limited, at least in part, by anaerobic capacity, which in turn is determined by a range of physiological factors.
3. An understanding of the physiological bases of anaerobic endurance and the principles of training provide the scientific underpinning for the prescription of anaerobic endurance training.
4. There is limited empirical evidence regarding adaptation to high-intensity training and therefore further research is required to support training methods to enhance anaerobic endurance.

## References

Bangsbo J 1994 Fitness training for football: a scientific approach. HO & Storm, Copenhagen.

Bangsbo J, Norregaard L, Thorso F 1991 Activity profile of competition soccer. Canadian Journal of Sport Science 16:110–116

Billat V, Slawinski J, Bocquet V et al 2000 Intermittent runs at $\dot{V}O_2$max enables subjects to remain at $\dot{V}O_2$max for a longer time than intense but sub maximal runs. European Journal of Applied Physiology 81:188–196

Bogdanis GC, Nevill ME, Boobis LH et al 1995 Recovery of power output and muscle metabolities following 30 sec of maximal sprint cycling in man. Journal of Physiology 482:467–480

Bogdanis GC, Williams C, Boobis LH, Lakomy HKA 1996 Contribution of phosphocreatine and aerobic metabolism to energy supply during repeated sprint exercise. Journal of Applied Physiology 80:876–884

Clarkson PM, Kroll W, Melchionda AM 1982 Isokinetic strength, endurance, and fiber type composition in elite American paddlers. European Journal of Applied Physiology 48:67–76

Fryer MW, Owen VJ, Lamb GD, Stephenson DG 1995 Effects of creatine phosphate and Pi on $Ca^{2+}$ movements and tension development in rat skinned skeletal muscle fibers. Journal of Physiology 482:123–140

Garland SJ, McComas AJ 1990 Reflex inhibition of human soleus muscle during fatigue. Journal of Physiology 429:17–27

Gollnick PD, Armstrong RB, Saubert CW et al 1972 Enzyme activity and fiber composition in skeletal muscle of trained and untrained men. Journal of Applied Physiology 33:312–319.

Gollnick PD, Armstrong RB, Saltin B et al 1973 Effect of training on enzyme activity and fiber composition of human skeletal muscle. Journal of Applied Physiology 34:107–111

Hawley JA (ed.) 2000 Running. Blackwell Science, Oxford

Hirvonen J, Nummela A, Rusko H et al 1992 Fatigue and changes of ATP, creation phosphate, and lactate during 400-m sprint. Canadian Journal of Sport Science 17:141–144

Houston ME, Thomson JA 1977 The response of endurance-adapted adults to intense anaerobic training. European Journal of Applied Physiology and Occupational Physiology 36:207–213

Jacobs I, Esbjörnsson M, Sylvén C et al 1987 Sprint training effects on muscle myoglobin, enzymes, fiber types, and blood lactate. Medicine and Science in Sports and Exercise 19:368–374

Jenkins DG, Brooks S, Williams C 1994 Improvements in multiple sprint ability with three weeks of training. New Zealand Journal of Sports Medicine 22:2–5

Lakomy HKA 2000 Physiology and biochemistry of sprinting. In: Hawley JA (ed.) Running. Blackwell Science, Oxford

Medbo JI, Burgers S 1990 Effect of training on the anaerobic capacity. Medicine and Science in Sports and Exercise 22:501–507

Medbo JI, Mohn A, Tabata I et al 1988 Anaerobic capacity determined by the maximal accumulated oxygen deficit. Journal of Applied Physiology 64:50–60

Nevill ME, Boobis LH, Brooks S, Williams C 1989 Effect of training on muscle metabolism during treadmill sprinting. Journal of Applied Physiology 67:2376–2382

Nielsen OB, de Paoli F, Overgaard K 2001 Protective effects of lactic acid on force production in rat skeletal muscle. Journal of Physiology 536:161–166

Sahlin K 1986 Muscle fatigue and lactic acid accumulation. Acta Physiologica Scandinavica 128:83–91

Sharp RL, Costill DL, Fink WJ, Kings DS 1986 Effects of eight weeks of bicycle ergometer sprint training on human muscle buffer capacity. International Journal of Sports Medicine 7:13–17

Spencer M, Lawrence S, Rechichi C et al 2004 Time motion analysis of elite hockey, with special reference to repeated-sprint activity. Journal of Sports Science 22:843–850

Tesch PA, Karlsson J 1985 Muscle fiber types and size in trained and untrained muscles of elite athletes. Journal of Applied Physiology 59:1716–1720 van Gool D, van Gerven D, Boutmans J 1988 The physiological load imposed on soccer players during real match-play. In: Reilly T et al (eds) Science and football. E. and F.N. Spon, London

Westerblad H, Bruton JD, Lannergren J 1997 The effect of intracellular pH on contractile function of intact, single fibers of mouse declines with temperature. Journal of Physiology 500:193–204

## Further reading

Bogdanis GC, Williams C, Boobis LH, Lakomy HKA 1996 Contribution of phosphocreatine and aerobic metabolism to energy supply during repeated sprint exercise. Journal of Applied Physiology 80:876–884

Bompa T 1999 Periodization. Theory and methodology of training. Human Kinetics, Champaign IL

Green S 1995 Measurement of anaerobic work capacity in humans. Sports Medicine 19:32–42

Medbo JI, Tabata I 1989 Relative importance of aerobic and anaerobic energy release during short-lasting exhausting bicycle exercise. Journal of Applied Physiology 67:1881–1886

Spencer MR, Gastin PB 2001 Energy system contribution during 200- to 1500-m running in highly trained athletes. Medicine and Science in Sports and Exercise 33:157–162

## Chapter **6**

# The physiology of sprint and power training

Colin Boreham

## LEARNING OBJECTIVES:

This chapter is intended to ensure that the reader:

1. Recognizes the main determinants of human speed and power, namely muscle strength, muscle fibre – type proportions, and muscle and tendon elasticity.
2. Appreciates how specific forms of resistance training and plyometric training can lead to adaptations in these properties that are beneficial to speed and power.
3. Appreciates how athletes and coaches might optimize these adaptations by mixing various training options.

## INTRODUCTION

With few exceptions (target activities such as darts, snooker, bowls and shooting being notable among them), human power production is central to performance in competitive sport. Power (P) can be defined as work done (force [f] × distance [d]) divided by velocity (v); [P = (f.d)/v]. As distance is usually fixed in sporting contexts (e.g. the height the barbell must be raised; the distance a sprinter must run; the circumference of a pedal revolution, etc.) this definition of power can be simplified for practical purposes to P = f/v. As both movement force and movement velocity are largely dependent upon the quantity and quality, respectively, of muscle tissue, these topics will form a major portion of subsequent discussion in this chapter. For the time being, it is clear that both strength and speed are essential components of power production, their relative contribution being determined by the specific requirements of the sport. Huge amounts of human power can be generated in both speed-dominated events (e.g. 100 m sprinting generates about 1500–2000 W) and strength-dominated events (e.g. Olympic weightlifting up to 4000–5000 W), although it has been shown that optimum power production occurs at about 40–60% of maximal voluntary contraction (MVC; Izquierdo et al 2002). Although optimal power production is an important consideration for activities of varying duration, involving energy sources from aerobic (1 minute or greater) to anaerobic alactic (under 10 seconds), the former (aerobic) types of activity are covered elsewhere in this text (see Chapters 4 and 5). Accordingly, the current chapter will concentrate on those activities which involve high levels of force development and mechanical and metabolic power production, relying primarily on high-energy phosphates or anaerobic glycolysis to generate the necessary adenosine triphosphate (ATP). Such activities may be repetitive in nature, lasting for several seconds, as in sprinting, or, commonly in sport, single explosive muscular actions lasting less than 300 milliseconds. In the case of the latter, large forces (up to 4000 N in both legs) need to be produced in less than one-third of a second; thus, power production will be dominated by maximal absolute strength and the time it takes to reach maximal force (so-called force–time characteristics).

Although skeletal muscle is of obvious importance in the generation of short-term power, it is necessary to stress at this stage that muscles and their tendons act as the functional unit to augment and transmit power production to the limbs. Indeed, most movement involves both an eccentric (muscle- and tendon-lengthening) phase closely followed by a concentric (shortening) phase, commonly termed the 'stretch-shortening cycle' (SSC). The stretching of tendon and other elastic structures in the muscle during the early phase of the SSC stores a considerable amount of energy which is subsequently used to boost contractible force production during the concentric phase. Due to the high coefficient of restitution of tendon, up to 90% of the stored elastic energy can be re-used in this way, producing a 'catapult' action which can boost subsequent power production considerably, perhaps over 50% of the total power in jumping (Huijing 1992). Furthermore, such elastic energy is essentially 'free' in the metabolic sense, making the enhancement of this elastic component through training an important consideration both for power production and for the metabolic efficiency of movement. Subsequent sections will deal at length with aspects of the stretch-shortening cycle and the training of elastic recoil by, for example, plyometric training. The effects of various training regimes on muscle tissue and consequences for power production will also be covered in depth in the following chapter. Muscle tissue is known to be highly adaptable to environmental stresses, including habitual training, and several recent studies have highlighted the role that specific types of resistance training can play in enhancing power production for sport.

To return to our simplified definition of power ($P = f/v$), it is clear that an understanding of the training of human muscle power and speed can only be attained through an examination of the main physiological factors influencing both force and velocity of contraction, and how they may be modified by specific training regimes.

## FACTORS AFFECTING POWER AND SPEED

### (i) Strength

Strength can be defined as the ability to produce force. Force may be generated isometrically (as observed by the opposing forwards in a rugby scrum) or dynamically, the latter being more common in sporting contexts. Although anecdotally, strength and speed/power were often regarded as mutually exclusive (as in 'too much strength training slows you down'), this view is now accepted as outmoded and misinformed. As has already been shown, force is an integral component of power production and, as maximal muscle force is relatively easily trained (compared with muscle speed), most power-based athletes spend an inordinate amount of time pursuing this goal. Furthermore, Newton's second law (F = ma) demonstrates that acceleration (a critical component in most sports) depends proportionately on the ability of the musculature to produce force. Although muscle strength and its training are covered comprehensively elsewhere in this volume (see Ch. 7), certain aspects with specific relevance to power and speed require emphasizing at this point. We will start with some intrinsic properties of skeletal muscle governing force development, and their modification with training.

## (ii) Length–tension relationship

Although individual muscle sarcomeres can range in length from approximately 1.2 μm (fully contracted) to 3.6 μm (fully relaxed), the amount of tension (force) that can be generated by the cross-bridges at these extremes is not optimal. At the fully contracted, shortened state, the actin filaments overlap and interfere with cross-bridge attachment, while in the lengthened (relaxed) state, there is insufficient overlap between actin and myosin filaments, thus reducing the proportion of cross-bridges which can attach and generate force. In fact, optimal conditions for cross-bridge attachment occur when the sarcomeres are about 2.2 μm in length, or about 60% of resting length. In this position, the maximal number of myosin cross-bridges can attach to the active sites on the actin molecules, and as this happens simultaneously in all sarcomeres throughout the contracting muscle, whole muscle force production is maximized. This physiological relationship between muscle length and force output has major implications for power production in sport, most obviously in activities which require high force production. In the sprint start position, for example, the sprinter unwittingly 'sets up' his or her sarcomeres for optimal force production in the initial push off the blocks; the volleyball player squats to the correct position (approximately one-third squat) to achieve maximum force in the subsequent jump, and so on. As far as is known, training has no effect on the length–tension relationship.

## (iii) Force–velocity relationship

The force–velocity relationship was first described in the 1930s and refers to the reciprocal association between muscle contractile force and contractile velocity, i.e. the greater the force required, the slower the speed of contraction (see Fig. 6.1). This phenomenon has been experienced by anyone who has lifted a series of progressively heavier weights in the weight training room. As the weight (resistance) increases, so does the force produced by the muscle, but at the expense of contractile speed (velocity). Thus, at one extreme, an unloaded barbell can be moved at cosiderable speed relatively easily, while a maximal lift can be lifted only once with a reduced velocity. It is apparent that any change in the force–velocity curve – specifically a shift upwards and to the right (see dotted line) – will have important repercussions for power production, and, therefore, sporting performance. Not surprisingly, there has been much illuminating research on the effects of specific strength and power training practices on the force–velocity relationship, much of it

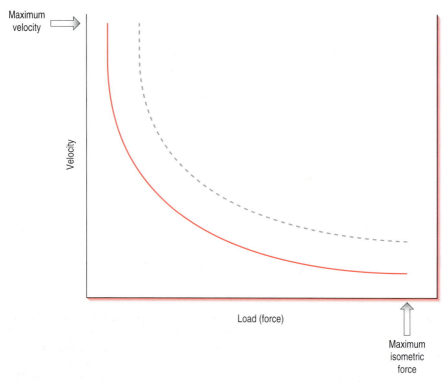

**Figure 6.1** The force–velocity curve. The solid line represents the classic inverse relationship between the force a muscle exerts and its speed of contraction. The dotted line represents the shift upwards and to the right which characterizes adaptation to strength and power training.

by Keijo Häkkinen and colleagues in Jyväsklyä, Finland. Details of this work are available elsewhere (Häkkinen 2002). In brief, such research shows that different types of resistance training can result in specific alterations to the shape of the force–velocity curve. Heavy resistance training (80–100% of 1 repetition maximum (RM)) results in a shift to the right predominantly at the 'force' end of the curve (as in Fig. 6.2A), while lighter resistances (30–60% 1RM) lifted explosively tend to shift the 'velocity' end of the curve to the right (Fig. 2B). Furthermore, such training variations may also initiate change in the 'force–time' curves, as seen in Figure 6.3. These latter results show that while absolute increases in force may be greater following a period of heavy resistance training (Fig. 6.3A), these increases only manifest themselves in contractions lasting longer than about 150 milliseconds. Explosive strength training, on the other hand (Fig. 6.3B), appears to shift the force–time curve to the right along its entire length (albeit to a lesser absolute extent). Thus, force production in very rapid contractions (lasting less than 150 milliseconds) is also enhanced.

The implications of such findings for speed and power training are twofold. Firstly, all sports and activities that rely on power and speed should endeavour to shift the force–veloicty and force–time curves of the relevant musculature to the right. Secondly, this is best achieved by a combination of different types of resistance training, such that heavy, slow lifting is mixed with lighter, more explosive

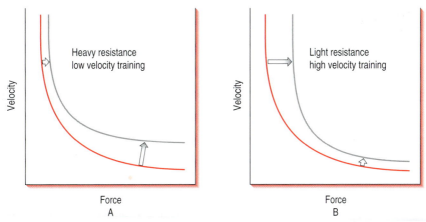

**Figure 6.2** If the training programme concentrates on heavy strength exercises, the shift in the force–velocity curve will tend to concentrate at the 'force' end of the curve (A). If the training is more explosive in nature, using lighter resistances, the shift will tend to concentrate at the 'velocity' end of the curve (B).

actions. This should result in an optimal shift along the whole length of the force–velocity and force–time curves such that power production is enhanced at all speeds of movement. Taking sprinting as an example, it is clear that the start involves relatively high muscular forces applied over a relatively long contact time (approximately 300 milliseconds). By 50 metres, however, relatively small forces are applied for much shorter durations (foot contact is about 100 milliseconds at top sprinting speed). Training studies carried out to date have reported results generally in favour of lighter, more explosive resistance training to enhance sprinting and jumping power (Delecluse et al 1995, Newton et al 1999, Wilson et al 1993). Blazevitch & Jenkins

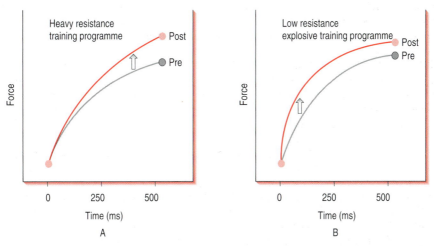

**Figure 6.3** Typical force–time curves for isometric leg contractions pre- and post-training with heavy resistances (A) or lighter, explosive weights (B).

(2002), however, found no differences in the high versus low velocity training approach, while Aargaard et al (2002) reported a 15% increase in the rate of force development following 14 weeks of heavy resistance training. Furthermore, it should be remembered that so-called 'explosive' resistance training is prescribed on the basis of a percentage of maximum strength (1 RM). This prescription is normally between 30 and 60% of 1 RM, corresponding to the resistance which enables maximal power output for the upper body (30–45% 1 RM) and lower body (45–60% 1 RM) (Izquierdo et al 2002). Thus, the quality of explosive resistance training is directly related to maximal strength levels, enabling the stronger athlete to both train and perform at higher absolute power outputs. Resistance training, in any given training cycle, should therefore probably start by enhancing the base of maximal strength. Thereafter (possibly following 6–8 weeks of heavy resistances), lighter, more dynamic exercises should be progressively incorporated so that power output is enhanced throughout the range of contraction velocities. There is some experimental evidence to corroborate the effectiveness of such mixed light and heavy resistance training (Harris et al 1996).

## STRENGTH AND THE ABILITY TO SUSTAIN POWER OUTPUT

While strength training is generally associated with a reduction in aerobic power output (Tesch & Alkner 2003), there are good theoretical and experimental grounds to support the view that enhanced strength improves power output in sustained high-intensity exercise lasting as long as 40 or 50 seconds (also known as 'speed endurance'). The theoretical case is illustrated in Figure 6.4. 'X' represents the proportion of pre-training maximal strength required to carry out a repetitive task (say press ups). For argument's sake, we will say that X = 50% of 1 RM for the muscle group in question. If this individual undertakes an intensive strength-training programme and doubles his/her strength, X becomes only 25% of 1 RM. Consequently,

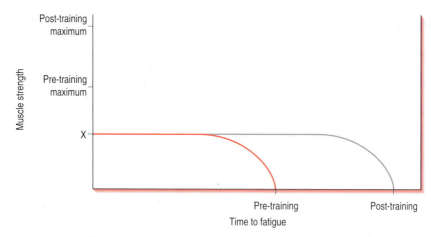

**Figure 6.4**  The effect of strength training on local muscular endurance. Before strength training, X represents a given resistance (in this case, about 50% of maximal strength). After strength training, maximal strength is almost doubled, so that X is now 25% of maximal strength. The resulting improvement in the ability to move X repeatedly to fatigue is shown on the Y axis.

in theory at least, the number of press-ups completed, or the time to fatigue, should double also. Limited experimental data support this association between short-term power output (speed endurance) and maximal strength (Costill et al 1980, Robinson et al 1995). The correlate of this relationship is that a task performed at the same absolute load (e.g. bench pressing 10 repetitions at 50 kg) after a period of training becomes less fatiguing. This is thought to be due to the stronger muscles requiring less neural activation, as shown by electromyographical (EMG) experiments (Sale 2003).

## OPTIMIZING THE POWER: WEIGHT RATIO

Muscle strength, as we have just seen, has a direct bearing on human speed and power output. As muscle strength is proportional to muscle size (about 3–4 kg per $cm^2$ of cross-sectional area) it might be supposed that increasing muscle size (hypertrophy) might be the principal goal of the athlete or coach interested in enhancing power. This probably is true of sports such as weight lifting or rowing, which are non-ambulatory (i.e. either the body does not need to transport itself great distances horizontally or vertically, or, the body mass is supported). The majority of sports, however, do incorporate ambulatory running and jumping activity, and for these sports it is imperative to maximize the improvements in muscle strength while minimizing increases in muscle mass. This is because, while muscle strength is a squared function (proportional to $cm^2$ of muscle cross-sectional area, as mentioned above), muscle mass is a cubed function, proportional to $cm^3$ of muscle tissue. Thus, as muscle size increases, strength increases at an exponentially slower rate than muscle mass. Recent findings relating to the 'time course' of training-induced changes in muscle strength provide guidance as to how the athlete might avoid the pitfalls of accumulating too much bulk in the pursuit of greater strength and power.

It is now accepted that the major proportion of strength gains in the initial stages (4–6 weeks) of a strength-training programme are due to adaptations in the facilitatory and/or inhibitory neural pathways controlling muscle contraction, rather than muscle hypertrophy. This lack of hypertrophy, however, may be more apparent than real. Indeed, individual muscle fibres may increase their cross-sectional area by 5–8% in the first month of strength training, but much of this increase may be 'absorbed' by inter- and intra-fibre space, resulting in no measurable changes in gross appearance (Sale 2003). Neural adaptations to strength training have been reviewed extensively elsewhere (Robinson et al 1995), but can be summarized as: (i) increased activation of the agonists, and/or (ii) reduced co-activation of antagonist muscles, and/or (iii) improved co-activation of synergist muscles (synergists are muscles that contribute to a movement). Increased activation of muscles is usually assessed experimentally by the use of EMG, with most training studies showing an increase in overall electrical activity of the trained muscles during maximal contractions. This increase in the quantity of EMG (which, incidentally, may plateau at an earlier stage in the course of a training programme in women than in men) suggests that the number of motor units recruited have increased and/or the motor units are firing at higher rates, or some combination of the two. While these adaptations will increase the maximal contractile force, it is worth noting that a faster rate of force development is an additional neural adaptation which can occur if training involves rapid, maximal effort (so-called 'ballistic') contractions with sub-maximal loads (typically 30–40% RM). This adaptation was referred to earlier (see under 'Force–velocity relationship' and Fig. 6.3) and results from an increased motor-unit firing rate at the onset of movement, perhaps from 60 Hz to 130 Hz (van Outsem et al 1998). As a result of such neural adaptations, peak force is both enhanced and reached more quickly, with obvious implications for power and speed. These changes may become apparent after as little as 2 weeks of resistance training and precede hypertrophic changes in trained muscles (Sale 2003), the latter taking about 16 training sessions to become manifest (equivalent to 4–6 weeks of training in a typical programme). Thus, the athletes who wish to maximize their power:weight ratio might incorporate the following training strategies:

- Resistance training which incorporate a combination of high loads (90–100% 1 RM) with low repetitions (1–3 per set), and lower loads (30–50% 1 RM) with more repetitions (6–10 per set, at very high, 'ballistic' movement velocities), are likely to maximize 'neural' adaptations and minimize hypertrophic adaptations in the trained muscles (Huijing 1992).
- Such resistance training regimes need to be periodized so that breaks of 1–2 weeks are introduced every 4 weeks, to dampen the hypertrophic response.

It should be emphasized that there is only a limited experimental base to support these recommendations, and that such training would be considered as an 'advanced' option, to be undertaken after prolonged (possibly several years) of foundation training.

For athletes in whom maximal strength, irrespective of muscle mass, is the goal, more prolonged 'hypertrophic' resistance training, over several months and characterized by medium to high loads (60–80% 1 RM) and high volumes (typically 4–6 sets of 6–12 repetitions) is required. While the training 'triggers' for increased net protein synthesis in muscle remain largely unknown, the genetic and molecular basis for muscle hypertrophy are being unravelled (in particular the interplay between peptides such as mechano growth factor (MGF) that seems to act as a rapid response mechanism in muscle to promote protein synthesis following training, and myostatin, whose normal function is to limit muscle growth).

Two further scientific observations may be of interest to the power/sprint athlete. (i) A recent study by Bowtell et al (2003) demonstrated that rates of protein synthesis were comparable irrespective of whether subjects lifted weights at 60% or 90% 1 RM. Thus, there may be a lower threshold of resistance beyond which it is unnecessary to go to achieve hypertrophy. (ii) Earlier experiments by Geoffrey and David Goldspink indicated in animal models that prolonged stretch may be a potent anabolic agent for muscle growth, even in the absence of an intact nerve supply. This is particularly true if the muscle stretch is held under tension, as exemplified by resistance training exercises when the limits of the range of motion are approached (for example, the stretching of the pectoralis and triceps muscles as the bar approaches the chest in a bench press exercise). It may be that athletes seeking to maximize muscle mass should emphasize this (stretching) portion of the range through which the muscles must contract. Stretching may, therefore, be about more than simple flexibility for the power athlete (Shrier 2004), although there is some evidence that prolonged stretching can have deleterious acute effects on power output for up to 2 hours post-stretching (Power et al 2004).

## TYPES OF MUSCLE FIBRE

Observe any junior school sports day, and an obvious truth emerges from the running races. In any group of young, untrained children, there is enormous variety in the sprinting speeds of those taking part. What determines this biological variation in speed? It is now accepted that speed of muscle movement is largely determined by the relative proportions of different types of muscle fibre which make up the bulk of the muscle. Muscle fibres differ according to their contractile and metabolic properties and can accordingly be broadly categorized into three types: (i) fast-contracting fibres with a predominantly glycolytic metabolism (commonly known as type IIb fibres); (ii) fast-contracting fibres with a more oxidative metabolism (type IIa fibres), and (iii) slow-contracting, oxidative fibres (type I fibres). A fourth type (type IIc fibres) are thought to be fibres in transition from type II to type I, and are uncommon except in muscle undergoing intensive training, or in young developing muscle.

Most human muscles are made up of the two main types of fibre, I and IIb, depending on the function of the muscle. In a fast-contracting muscle which does not require endurance, such as the blinking muscle of the eye (orbicularis occuli), more than 90% of the fibre population will be type IIb, while at the other extreme, a muscle such as the soleus of the lower leg, which is required primarily to maintain posture over long periods, is composed mainly of slow, type I fibres. The greater fatigue resistance displayed by these slower fibres arises from their oxidative metabolism and greater metabolic efficiency. All muscles however, are composed of a mosaic of fast and slow fibres to deal with the contingencies of everyday existence. A major ambulatory muscle such as the vastus lateralis of the thigh, for example has, in the average individual, approximately equal proportions of type I and II fibres, presumably (in the evolutionary sense) to cope with a range of movement demands from fast, explosive jumping and sprinting, to more prolonged endurance running. However, there is much genetic variation in the make-up of human muscles, and it is clear that an individual at either end of the fibre-type spectrum may possess either 90%+ type I, or 90%+ type II fibres in an important (in the sporting as well as the evolutionary sense) muscle such as the vastus lateralis.

It is possible to biopsy small pieces of human muscle and examine the fibre-type profile. The biopsy procedure is illustrated in Figure 6.5, and micrographs of thin slices of muscle stained to differentiate the two main types of muscle fibre are shown in Figure 6.6. It is abundantly clear that muscle taken from a power lifter (Fig. 6.6A), has a totally different profile (predominantly type IIb) from that of a marathon runner (Fig. 6.6B; predominantly type I). The differences in contractile speed are largely complemented by metabolic structures to support energy production. Fast-contracting, glycolytic fibres are surrounded by few capillaries (normally just one or two), contain relatively few mitochondria (perhaps 2–3% of total cell volume), and have virtually no intracellular myoglobin or fat molecules, while the aerobic type I fibres have more capillaries (up to five or six per fibre) surrounding each fibre, abundant mitochondria (perhaps 4–6% of cell volume), myoglobin and fat molecules to support Krebs cycle and the aerobic supply of ATP. Such differences are illustrated in the electron micrograph of two adjacent muscle fibres of different types (type IIb and type I) in Figure 6.7.

Our observation that performance in power lifting and marathon running is strongly correlated with muscle fibre-type profiles is replicated for other sports along the power–endurance continuum. This is not surprising given that the myosin isoform from fast fibres can split ATP 3–5 times faster than slow fibre myosin, resulting in much faster contraction velocities (a fast fibre is estimated to shorten maximally in about 1/10 seconds, compared with one-third of a second for a slow fibre). Not surprisingly, fast fibres may produce 2.5× more power than slow fibres; thus, a preponderance of fast fibres in ambulatory muscles is a fundamental advantage in speed and power activities. It is therefore of obvious concern to coaches and athletes, as well as scientists, to know whether fibre-type profiles can be altered by training, in particular if slower type I fibres can be transformed into faster type II muscle.

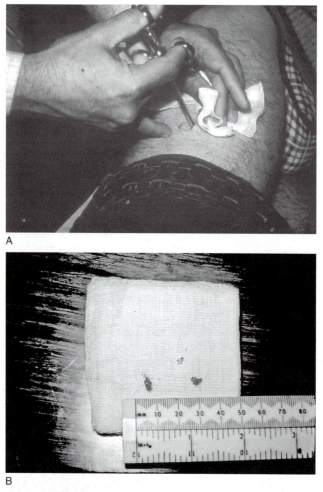

A

B

**Figure 6.5**  Muscle biopsy. A hollow biopsy needle is inserted through an incision in the right thigh under local anaesthetic (A) so that small pieces of muscle from the vastus lateralis can be removed (B) for freezing, transverse sectioning, staining and determination of fibre type proportions.

Unfortunately for sprinters and other power athletes, the available evidence suggests that prolonged training may shift the profile from IIb (fast glycolytic) to IIa (fast oxidative glycolytic) and eventually (given sufficient duration of training) (Izquierdo et al 2002), to type I (slow oxidative), but that conversions in the opposite direction – from slow to fast – are probably not possible (Harris et al 1996, Pette 2001). An exception to the latter assertion was provided by Almeida-Silveira et al (1994) using chronic stretch-shortening cycle exercises in rats to induce a significant increase in type II fibres in the soleus muscle. This training affect has yet to be demonstrated in humans, although interestingly human muscle subjected to prolonged disuse does become faster (Goldspink & Harridge 2003). This latter observation gives a clue to the mechanisms underlying fibre transformations from fast to slower with chronic exercise, irrespective of whether that exercise is associated with strength training, sprinting, or endurance activity. It appears, from the earliest experiments involving the surgical

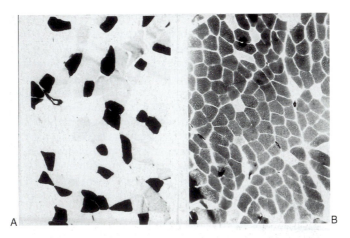

**Figure 6.6**   Muscle fibre type profiles from an elite power-lifter (A) and from an elite marathon runner (B) stained for myosin ATPase (4.2). Approximately 85% of the area of the power-lifter's muscle is composed of fast, type II fibres (here stained lightly), while over 90% of the area of the marathon runner's muscle is composed of slower, oxidative type I fibres (here stained darkly).

cross innervation ('switching') of nerves to fast and slow muscles (and the subsequent transformation of the muscles) that the nerve supply determines the contractile and metabolic properties of the fibres supplied. Further experimentation revealed that the specific quality of the nerve that determined whether its muscle fibres were fast or slow was the total amount of electrical activity delivered to the muscle cells in conjunction with a certain level of mechanical strain (Goldspink & Harridge 2003). Thus the genetic 'switch' to upregulate the production of the slow, type I isoform of myosin

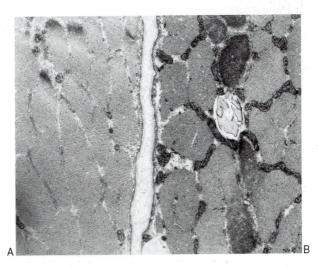

**Figure 6.7**   Electron micrograph of adjacent fast (A) and slow (B) muscle fibres. Note the abundant dark structures (mitochondria) lying between myofibrils, and the pale, fat molecule located in the central portion of the slow fibre. This contrasts with the lack of mitochondria and fat molecules in the faster, glycolytic fibre.

and related proteins seems to be the chronic nerve stimulation experienced by muscles used in posture – or indeed by muscles undergoing heavy training. Similarly, type IIb fibres, which normally receive relatively little nerve stimulation, do not express the slower myosin isoforms unless 'switched on' by increased contractile (and therefore electrical) activity. In this respect genes regulating the expression of fast myosin phenotypes can be seen as 'default' genes in that they are largely expressed in the absence of chronic activity. This is exemplified by the postural soleus muscle, which reverts to expressing fast myosin genes when immobilized in the shortened position or subjected to hypogravity (Goldspink & Harridge 2003).

Interestingly the upregulation of slow myosin in response to increased activity may take longer than other important responses to training in the power athlete, notably the induction of hypertrophy. Thus, short, sharp, intense training sessions may induce muscle hypertrophy (with the attendant advantages for power and speed improvement described previously) without the decided *disadvantage* of increasing the proportion of slower fibres in the muscles. This may be seen as the 'sprinters paradox' – that more (training) may be less (gain).

There is one other advantage in relation to muscle fibre profiles to be gleaned from training in short bursts of intense activity; that of so-called 'selective hypertrophy' of type II fibres. This phenomenon is illustrated in Figure 6.8, illustrating muscle fibres from an international high jumper. In normal untrained muscle, faster type II fibres are marginally larger than their slower type I neighbours. The type II (lighter shaded) fibres in Figure 6.8, however, are up to twice as large as the type I fibres, implying some sort of selective hypertrophy as a result of training. Training for a power event such as the high jump is characterized by a preponderance of explosive, dynamic movements of short duration but maximal intensity. Such activity, according to the 'size principle' of motor unit recruitment (whereby motor units are recruited in an orderly fashion from the smaller, slower motor units to the larger, faster motor units according to the force and velocity requirements of the contraction

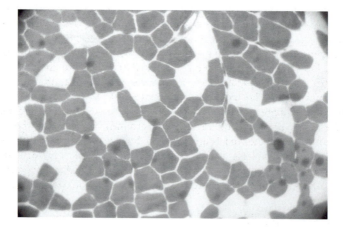

**Figure 6.8** Selective hypertrophy in the muscle of a high jumper. In this section of vastus lateralis from an international high jumper, the selective hypertrophy of the fast, type II fibres (stained lightly here) is apparent. This is probably the result of dynamic, 'ballistic'-type training repeated over a prolonged period. The result is that a greater proportion of the muscle cross-sectional area is composed of type II fibres, creating greater power when these fibres are recruited.

(Moritani 2003)), will recruit all motor units regardless of speed in a well-trained athlete. Fast, type II fibres appear to display greater hypertrophy as a result of regular resistance-type training than type I fibres (Hather et al 1991), possibly due to a selective up-regulation of androgen receptors in the former (Kraemer et al 2003). Thus, intensive, high resistance training of the type performed by high jumpers and other power athletes may lead to selective hypertrophy of type II fibres simply because these fibres are more responsive to such stimuli, when recruited. An alternative explanation is that selective hypertrophy of type II fibres may result from selective recruitment of these faster motor units in dynamic, ballistic-type movements, i.e. a reversal of the 'size principle'. Although there is some evidence that type II motor units may be preferentially recruited in fast concentric (Grimby & Hannertz 1977) and eccentric (Nardone et al 1989) contractions, there is also much evidence to support the inviolability of the 'size principle' (Duchateau & Hainaut 2003).

Whatever the mechanism of selective hypertrophy of type II fibres, the advantage lies in the resultant increased cross-sectional area occupied by these fibres relative to the slower type I fibres. The greater the cross-sectional area occupied by type II fibres the greater the number of fast myosin cross-bridges that can produce force during contraction. Thus, when the type II motor unit pool is recruited to produce explosive, movements, these can be produced with correspondingly greater force, thereby enhancing power output. In the case of our high jumper in Figure 6.8, selective hypertrophy of his fast fibres presumably helped him to achieve competitive success, despite a relatively high proportion (70%) of slower type I fibres.

## MUSCLE ELASTICITY AND THE STRETCH SHORTENING CYCLE (SSC)

The stretch shortening cycle (SSC) was highlighted in the introduction to this chapter, and with good reason. While an enormous amount of research has been carried out in furthering our knowledge about skeletal muscle physiology (mechanisms of contraction, training adaptations, muscle fibre types etc.), only recently has it become clear that muscle contraction per se contributes something less than half of the total work done in many dynamic sporting movements, including sprinting, throwing and jumping; the remainder is derived from the release of elastic energy stored during the SSC. For example, it has been calculated that without the elastic contribution of the SSC to force production, the power produced at the ankle during a one-legged jump would be reduced from about 1700 W to about 750 W (Huijing 1992). Thus, the storage of elastic energy as muscle and tendon are loaded and stretched (as in the sprinters leg striking the ground), followed by the contraction of these structures and the boosting of power by the release of the stored 'energy pool', is of critical importance to sporting performance. It is therefore important to understand both the mechanisms underpinning the SSC and whether training can enhance the catapult effect arising from it for the benefit of performance.

## Mechanisms of the SSC

While a detailed explanation of the SSC has been presented elsewhere, a brief synopsis of this complex phenomenon will be given here (Komi 2003).

The increased production, or 'potentiation', of muscle power by the SSC may be explained by two models, the mechanical and the neurophysiological, both of which are thought to contribute. In the mechanical model, the rapid stretching of muscle and tendon causes elastic energy to be stored in the so-called 'series elastic components'

(SECs) of these tissues. The SECs are thought to reside largely in the tendon (collagen, the main protein of tendon, has a helical or spring-like conformation) but also in the flexible myosin heads of the muscle cross-bridges. When the musculotendinous structures are stretched, as in a rapid eccentric movement, the SECs act as a spring and are lengthened, thereby storing elastic energy. If this lengthening action is rapidly followed by a concentric contraction (i.e. a short 'coupling' time), the elastic energy is fed into and supplements that of the contracting muscle to boost power production. If the coupling time is too long (for example, if there is a pause after bending one's knees prior to a vertical jump), the stored elastic energy will be dissipated and lost as heat. Similarly, if there is no rapid stretching of the structures, subsequent jumping power will not benefit from this source of additional power.

In the neurophysiological model, muscle spindles (proprioceptive organs that are sensitive to rate and magnitude of stretch) are thought to be stimulated by rapid stretch (or even in anticipation of rapid stretch) to both increase the stiffness of muscle during the eccentric phase, and increase the force production of the agonist muscles via the stretch reflex during the concentric phase.

The results of these mechanisms on human power output may be clearly and simply demonstrated in Figure 6.9 (A–C). The first frame depicts the result of a vertical jump to touch a board from a static semi-squatting position, i.e. without a preceding 'countermovement' to stretch the musculotendinous structures. The second frame depicts the athlete preparing to drop down from a low platform prior to his next vertical jump. On landing, the high forces resulting from this drop jump create rapid stretching of the leg muscles and a considerable storage of elastic energy. If the coupling time is short, this elastic energy boosts jumping performance, seen clearly in the final frame (Fig. 6.9C). Before examining the training of the SSC, it is worth emphasizing the complexity of the mechanisms outlined above. For example, work done by Fukunaga et al (2002) have demonstrated that not all stretching of tendon takes place in the eccentric phase of a squat jump. Using real time, ultrasonic imaging, they demonstrated that during the first half of the push-off phase,

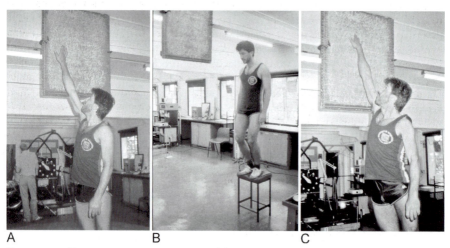

A            B            C

**Figure 6.9** Elastic properties of muscle. In (A) a vertical jump is being performed from a static, semi-squat position. In (B), the athlete performs a drop jump to the semi-squat position, before performing the vertical jump. The resulting improvement in performance (C) is the result of an increase in power arising from the stretch-shortening cycle.

the gastrocnemius muscle shortens by 26%, which in turn causes the stretching (by about 6%) of the Achilles tendon, most of which recoils to boost power at take off. Other recent research from the same group in Tokyo has demonstrated clear differences in the tendon stiffness between men and women, the latter showing a deficit of about one-third. These differences are yet to be satisfactorily explained, although they may clearly have implications for performance.

## TRAINING MUSCLE ELASTICITY: PLYOMETRICS

While the mechanical and neurophysiological mechanisms underlying the SSC may be complex and incompletely understood, the movement pattern which elicits the SSC is relatively straightforward. It consists of three phases. The first of these is the eccentric phase, during which the agonist muscles are loaded, resulting in the storage of elastic energy by the SEC, and the stimulation of the muscle spindles. The second phase is the transition between the eccentric and concentric phases, sometimes called the amortization, or coupling phase; this phase is perhaps the most crucial in facilitating greater power production, particularly, as mentioned previously, the need to minimize delay, or coupling time. The final phase is the concentric phase, during which the energy stored in the SEC is either used to enhance force production or is dissipated as heat. The movement pattern described above forms the basis of a specialized training, plyometrics (from the Greek plio = more, and metric = to measure) which seeks to improve power output arising from the SSC. The majority of plyometric exercises are based on jumping activities and, as such, cater primarily for the lower body, although upper body exercises have been developed also (Potach & Chu 2000). Typical jumping activities would include two-legged and single-leg hopping, jumping over hurdles, bounding activities and drop jumps from various heights. Rapidity of movement needs to be emphasized, with each effort requiring a maximal effort. Experience would indicate that plyometric exercises should not be performed by inexperienced of poorly conditioned athletes, and should not be performed over prolonged periods due to the risk of injury and the rapid onset of fatigue. Due to the high eccentric contration component inherent in plyometrics, delayed onset muscle soreness (DOMS) is invariably experienced, particularly in the early stages of a programme prior to adaptation. Nevertheless, plyometric exercises have become commonplace and invariably form an important element of the power-athlete's training regime. Their efficacy is not only anecdotal but is illustrated by numerous training studies. For example, Toumi et al (2004) reported that, even in well-conditioned handball players, 6 weeks of combined weight and plyometric training increased jumping height (largely as a result of shorter coupling time and increased leg 'stiffness'). Such improvements did not occur in the weight-training-only group. Kyrolainen et al (2004) demonstrated that in untrained subjects, a plyometric programme (2 × weekly for 15 weeks) improved jumping take-off velocity by 8%, with a considerable (24%) improvement in mechanical efficiency of sub-maximal jumping. Other training studies employing plyometrics, have also shown improvements in power performance (Hewett et al 1996, Svantesson et al 1994).

## KEY POINTS AND CONCLUSION

1. Human power production is an important contributor to performance in most sports.
2. Depending on the specific characteristics of the sport, both strength and speed will contribute to human power production.

3. Although intrinsic muscle speed and strength are highly inheritable characteristics, both can be enhanced by training.

4. Skeletal muscles and their tendon structures act together as a unit, such that the stretching of elastic structures in these tissues during limb 'loading' boosts subsequent power production as this energy is released in a catapult-like action as the muscle shortens. This cycle of activity is known as the stretch shortening cycle (SSC).

5. The SSC can be trained to enhance elastic recoil by the use of specific dynamic exercises called plyometrics. These normally involve explosive jumping and bounding activities for the legs, and equivalent actions for the upper body. The main mechanisms of improvement appear to be a shortening of the transition time between stretching and shortening phases, and an enhanced stiffness of musculotendinous structures.

6. Strength training will not only improve maximal voluntary contraction (MVC) force but will also increase the speed of muscle contraction and power output, mainly by shifting the force–velocity curve to the right.

7. Heavy weight-training well tend to shift the slower, 'force' portion of the force–velocity curve, while, lighter, more dynamic weight training will tend to shift the 'velocity' portion of the curve in the same direction. A combination of the two types of strength training will be optimal for most types of sports which require both acceleration and maximal speed enhancement. An increase in maximal strength should precede and form the platform for more dynamic training exercises.

8. Local muscular endurance (repeated, dynamic contractions lasting up to 40–50 seconds) also benefits from enhanced strength.

9. To optimize the power:weight ratio, strength training should incorporate a combination of high loads and low repetitions, with lighter resistances and higher repetitions at very high 'ballistic' velocities. After about 16 strength sessions, a short break of a few weeks may help to minimize hypertrophic adaptations.

10. Muscle speed is largely determined by the proportion of fast-contracting, type II fibres contained in a given muscle. This is largely genetically determined, but there is some evidence that the overall volume of training (irrespective of type) can change fast to slow (type I) fibres. Speed/power athletes should, therefore, concentrate on the quality of training rather than quantity. A further advantage of high intensity training may be the selective hypertrophy of type II fibres, so that they occupy a greater proportion of the overall muscle cross-sectional area. This adaptation should increase power/speed.

11. To conclude, training for power and speed needs firstly to be based around a high level of basic strength and conditioning. Thereafter, training practices need to be characterized by high-quality, dynamic exercises involving both resistance training and plyometrics. Such exercises should not be prolonged in nature, and should always commence in a fully rested state.

## References

Aargaard P, Simonsen EB, Andersen JL et al 2002 Increased rate of force development and neural drive of human skeletal muscle following resistance training. Journal of Applied Physiology 93:1318–1326

Almeida-Silveira MI, Perot C, Pousson F, Goubel F 1994 Effects of stretch-shortening cycle training on mechanical properties and fibre-type transition in the rat soleus muscle. Pflugers Archiv 427:289–294

Blazevitch AJ, Jenkins DG 2002 Effect of movement speed of resistance training exercises on sprint and strength performance in concurrently training elite junior sprinters. Journal of Sports Sciences 20(12):981–990

Bowtell JL, Park DM, Smith et al 2003 Stimulation of human quadriceps protein synthesis after strenuous exercise: no effects of varying intensity between 60 and 90% of one repetition maximum (IRM).

Costill D, Sharp R, Troup J 1980 Muscle strength: contributions to sprint swimming. Swim World 21:29–34

Delecluse C, van Coppenolle H, Willems E et al 1995 Influence of high-resistance and high-velocity training on sprint performance. Medicine and Science in Sports and Exercise 27(8):1203–1209

Duchateau J, Hainaut K 2003 Mechanisms of muscle and motor unit adaptation to explosive power training, ch 16, 2nd edn. In: Komi PV (ed.) Strength and power in sport. Blackwell, Oxford, p 315–330

Fukunaga T, Karvakami Y, Kubo K et al 2002 Muscle and tendon interaction during human movements. Exercise and Sport Science Reviews 30(3):106–110

Goldspink G, Harridge S 2003 Cellular and molecular aspects of adaptation in skeletal muscle, ch 12, 2nd edn. In: Komi PV (ed.) Strength and power in sport. Blackwell, Oxford, p 231–251

Grimby L, Hannertz J 1977 Firing rate and recruitment order of toe extensor motor units in different modes of voluntary contraction. Journal of Physiology 264:865–879

Häkkinen K 2002 Training-specific characteristics of neuromuscular performance, ch 2. In: Kraemer WJ & Häkkinen K (eds) Strength training for sport. Blackwell, Oxford, p 20–37

Harris G, Stone M, O'Bryant H et al 1996 Effects of three weight training programs on measures of athletic performance: maximum strength, power, speed and agility. Journal of Strength and Conditioning Research 10(4):287

Hather BM, Tesch PA, Buchanan P et al 1991 Influence of eccentric actions on skeletal muscle adaptation to resistance. Acta Physiologica Scandinavica 143:177–185

Hewett TE, Stroupe AL, Nance TA et al 1996 Plyometric training in female athletes. American Journal of Sports Medicine 24:765–773

Huijing PA 1992 Elastic potential of muscle, ch 6D. In: Komi P (ed.) Strength and power in sport. Blackwell, Oxford, p 151–168

Izquierdo M, Hakkinen K, Gonzalez-Badillo JJ et al 2002 Effects of long-term training specificity on maximal strength and power of the upper and lower extremities in athletes from different sports. European Journal of Applied Physiology 14:267–273

Komi P 2003 Stretch-shortening cycle, ch 10, 2nd edn. In: Komi PV (ed.) Strength and power in sport. Blackwell, Oxford, p 184–202

Kraemer WJ, Fleck SJ, Evans WJ 2003 Strength and power training: physiological mechanisms of adaptation, ch 12, vol 24. Exercise and sports sciences reviews. Williams & Wilkins, Baltimore, p 363–397

Kyrolainen H, Avela J, McBride JM et al 2004 Effects of power training on mechanical efficiency in jumping. European Journal of Applied Physiology 91(2–3):155–159

Moritani T 2003 Motor unit and motoneurone excitability during explosive movement, ch 3, 2nd edn. In: Komi PV (ed.) Strength and power in sport. Blackwell, Oxford, p 27–49

Nardone A, Romano C, Schieppati M 1989 Selective recruitment of high threshold human motor units during voluntary isotonic lengthening of active muscles. Journal of Physiology 409:451–471

Newton RU, Kraemer WJ, Häkkinen K 1999 Effects of ballistic training on preseason preparation of elite volleyball players. Medicine and Science in Sports and Exercise 31(2):323–330

Pette D 2001 Plasticity in skeletal, cardiac and smooth muscle. Historical perspectives: Plasticity of mammalian skeletal muscle. Journal of Applied Physiology 90:1119–1124

Potach DH, Chu DA 2000 Plyometric training, ch 19, 2nd edn. In: Baechle TR & Earle RW (eds) Essentials of strength training and conditioning. Human Kinetics, Champaign IL, p 427–471

Power K, Behm D, Cahill F et al 2004 An acute bout of static stretching: effects on force and jumping performance. Medicine and Science in Sports and Exercise 36(8):1389–1396

Robinson JM, Perland CM, Stone MH et al 1995 Effects of different weight training exercise rest intervals on strength, power and high intensity endurance. Journal of Strength and Conditioning Research 9(4):216–221

Sale D 2003 Neural adaptation to strength training, ch 15, 2nd edn. In: Komi PV (ed.) Strength and power in sport. Blackwell, Oxford, p 281–314

Shrier I 2004 Does stretching improve performance? A systematic and critical review of the literature. Sports Medicine 14(5):267–273

Svantesson U, Grimby G, Thomée R 1994 Potentiation of concentric plantar flexion torque following eccentric and isometric muscle actions. Acta Physiologica Scandinavica 152:287–293

Tesch PA, Alkner BA 2003 Acute and chronic muscle metabolic adaptations to strength training, ch 14, 2nd edn. In Komi PV (ed.) Strength and power in sport. Blackwell, Oxford, p 265–280

Toumi H, Best TM, Martin A et al 2004 Muscle plasticity after weight and combined (weight & jump) training. Medicine and Science in Sports and Exercise 36(9):1580–1588

van Outsem M, Duchateau J, Hainaut K 1998 Changes in single motor unit behaviour contribute to the increase in contraction speed after dynamic training in humans. Journal of Physiology 513:295–305

Wilson GJ, Newton RU, Murphy AJ et al 1993 The optimal training load for the development of dynamic athletic performance. Medicine and Science in Sports and Exercise 25(11):1279–1286

## Further reading

Baechle TR, Earle RW (eds) 2000 Essentials of strength training and conditioning, 2nd edn. Human Kinetics, Champaign IL

Komi PV (ed.) Strength and power in sport, 2nd edn. Blackwell, Oxford

Kraemer WJ, Häkkinen K (eds) 2002 Strength training for sport. Blackwell, Oxford

Chapter **7**

# The physiology of strength training

Stephen Ingham

## LEARNING OBJECTIVES:

This chapter is intended to ensure that the reader:

1. Appreciates basic philosophy, definitions and quantification of strength performance.
2. Appreciates the role of musculoskeletal properties and neural command to maximum muscular force expression.

3. Comprehends training-induced physiological adaptations to strength training.
4. Recognizes the principles of strength training as categorized by the exercise repetition and exercise set.
5. Appreciates the progression of strength performance through training.

## INTRODUCTION

The development of high muscular forces for the purposes of sporting endeavour has long been a fascination of humankind. However, the development of pertinent strength-training techniques has relied as much upon mythology, hearsay, fads and increasing market pressures as scientific discovery. Nevertheless, the modern strength and conditioning coach has specialist knowledge of how to successfully and systematically blend the many factors associated with strength training, such as type of muscle action, load, number of repetitions and sets, rest periods etc., into a holistic physical training programme eliciting pronounced changes in the neuromusculo-skeletal unit. Resistance training programmes can be specifically tailored to address increases in muscle dimension and/or the upper limit of muscle force generating capability.

## MUSCLE ACTIONS

Muscle actions (as they are not always 'contractions') correspond to the interaction between muscle force development and external resistance. Exertion of force is often associated with the command of body movements, yet muscular actions may take the shape of static or dynamic exercise. Static efforts involve the application of muscle force with no movement or change in the joint angle, i.e. no work is performed, and are termed isometric. Actions that involves movement are broadly termed as concentric, where the muscle shortens, and eccentric, where the muscle lengthens. Conditions of constant muscular force (isotonic) or angular limb velocity (isokinetic) are not involved during sporting activities. Even the control of movements using specialist dynamometry equipment may be at (or as close to as possible) a constant external velocity or force; uniform conditions are unlikely to be achieved within the exercising muscle. Consequently, when referring to dynamic human exercising muscular action, the terms isokinetic and isotonic are not appropriate descriptors. Rather, the human musculoskeletal system operates by way of combining eccentric, concentric and isometric actions of agonist, antagonist and synergist muscle groups during sporting pursuits.

## QUANTIFICATION OF EXERCISE PERFORMANCE

Exercise is defined as any and all activity involving force generation by activated skeletal muscles (Knuttgen & Kraemer 1987). Performance can be assessed in terms of the physical concepts of force, torque, work, power and velocity. Force is that which changes or tends to change the state of rest or motion in matter (SI unit of force: newton (N)). Torque is the effectiveness of a force to produce rotation of an object about an axis and is measured as the product of the force and the perpendicular distance from the line of action of the force to the axis of rotation (SI unit of torque: newton metre (N.m)). Work is the equivalent to a force expressed through a displacement with no limitation on time (SI unit of work: joule (J)). Power is the rate of performing work or the transformation of metabolic potential energy to work and/or heat (SI unit of power: watt (W)). The application of 1 N expressed through

1 m results in 1 J of work. The transformation of 1 J of metabolic energy to work or heat in 1 s results in 1 W of power. Velocity is measured in metres per second.

Therefore, exercise quantification during dynamic exercise situations is possible as the opposition of force, e.g. ergometer, exercise machine, gravitational pull to a free weight; isometric force sustained; power or velocity of progression, e.g. running, swimming etc.

## MEASUREMENT OF LOADING

Strength is defined as the maximal force or torque a muscle or muscle group can generate in a specified movement pattern at a specified velocity (Komi 2002). In the practical sense this very definition pertains to a single maximal lift (one repetition maximum, 1 RM), for example, powerlifting bench press, involving a single repetition of full eccentric and concentric maximal voluntary muscular action, requiring heightened motivational control in order to complete.

In this sense the term 'maximal' truly does mean that no greater effort can be generated. Strength exercise, however, is not confined to single maximal muscular actions. The repetition maximum (RM) is the maximum number of repetitions per set that can be performed at a given resistance with proper exercise form. Strength exercise performance can be measured by a set of repetitions at a given load performed to momentary voluntary muscular fatigue or failure. 1 RM is the highest concentric exercising load. 10 RM is a lighter load that allows performance of 10, but not 11, repetitions. The RM system can be successfully used as a means of quantifying the loading during a bout of strength exercise. The test requires determination of the number of repetitions a person can perform to exhaustion in lifting a certain mass (kg). Characterization of a particular set can be made as a proportion of one's 1 RM for a particular exercise.

**Table 7.1** The approximate relationship between the percentage of 1 RM and the probable maximum number of repetitions

| | Repetition maximum (RM) | | | | | | | | | |
|---|---|---|---|---|---|---|---|---|---|---|
| | 1 | 2 | 3 | 4 | 5 | 6 | 7 | 8 | 9 | 10 |
| Percentage of 1 RM | 100 | 95 | 90 | 85 | 80 | ← | 75 | →← | 70 | → |
| Example load (kg) with 1 RM of 90 kg | 90 | 84 | 82 | 80 | 77 | 75 | 73 | 71 | 68 | 66 |

For example:
Set,    8 repetitions with 75 kg squatting;
        1 RM for squat of 100 kg;
        8 RM = 75% of 1 RM.

Whereas this testing system is useful to provide surface information about an athlete's abilities and permits comparison of like-for-like exercises for the same person, it is one-dimensional and fails to fully define strength output because it discounts the specified or determined velocity of movement and distance. Ideally, when testing muscle function the force and/or torque measurements must be made when the muscle or muscle groups are at a similar length or as the peak force obtained during a dynamic action. Work describes more fully the training volume by encompassing the vertical distance a weight is lifted. For example:

100 kg (or 981 N) lifted vertically 0.8 m during a repetition;
exercise volume = 981 N × 0.8 m = 785 N.m.

If the lift is completed in 0.6 s, the power of the lift equals 785 N.m ÷ 0.6 s = 1308 W. If the lift is near maximal, it may take considerably longer (e.g. 2.5 s, 785 N.m ÷ 2.5 s = 313 W). Thus, 1 RM efforts are unlikely to yield high-power outputs because of the time taken to generate the force required to affect the mass lifted. It is for this reason that near-maximal lifts are considered 'strength oriented' (i.e. high force), whereas during high-velocity efforts movement completion is much shorter, thus becoming 'power orientated'.

The total work or power accomplished can be added for each exercise, body part, exercise session, microcycle, macrocycle and mesocycle etc. to provide a measure of the strength stimulus. A plot of the peak work and peak power attained across time is a useful way of tracking longitudinal periodization of the strength training stimulus.

## HUMAN FORCE EXPRESSION

The expression of muscular force (pulling effect) takes place when the central motor system regulates the contractile operation of the myofilament cross-bridges. The muscle force generated is applied to the attached bone tissue and, if greater than the external resistance, causes a shortening of the contractile tissues and results in a turning effect, or torque, about the joint. Equally, if the external resistance exceeds the muscular force the muscle lengthens and offers a degree of deceleration to the ensuing load (potential).

Maximal muscular tension comes with only the highest motivation and is expensive to the homeostatic milieu and acts as a potent stimulus for reordering motor unit involvement, repair to damage tissues and stimulus for growth.

## HUMAN FORCE EXPRESSION – MUSCLE

Muscle contractile function takes place when availability of calcium ions permit the union of myosin and actin myofilaments by cross-bridge head binding. Hydrolysed ATP provides the energy for the regulation of cross-bridge cycling in order to achieve sarcomere shortening and generation of a tensile force along the myofibril.

The most obvious determining factor of muscle strength is muscle size. As a general principle the cross-sectional area of muscle relates to the force-generating capability because the greater volume of muscle relates to the number of myofibrillar units present. The summation of muscular force, therefore, reflects the manifestation of total sarcomere cross-bridge tension development. However, the tension developed by a motor unit in response to a single action potential operating upon the axon terminal, known as the twitch, can vary distinctly between motor units even belonging to the same muscle. Characterization of motor unit types is based upon their physical properties of contractile speed of shortening, force development, endurance and histochemical profile.

Human muscle exists as a variable continuum of types but can broadly be categorized according to their myosin isoforms that are distinguishable on the basis of the sensitivity of myofibrillar ATPase (the enzyme that catalyses the breakdown of ATP for the liberation of energy for cross-bridge function) to staining, revealing the following types of muscle fibre:

Type I: slow twitch speed (90–140 milliseconds); high aerobic enzyme concentration; high mitochondrial volume; moderate glycogen content: high capillary perfusion; resistant to fatigue; small diameter. Engaged specifically for sustained, low-force activity, e.g. steady cycling.

Type IIa: fast twitch speed (50–100 milliseconds); fatigue resistant; moderate to high glycolytic and oxidative enzyme concentration; moderate to high mitochondrial volume; moderate to high capillary perfusion; moderate to high glycogen content. Engaged during prolonged high-intensity activity, e.g. 400 m track sprint.

Type IIb: fast twitch speed (40–90 milliseconds); fatiguable: high glycolytic enzyme concentration; moderate to high capillary perfusion; moderate to high glycogen content. Engaged during intermittent maximal-force activity, e.g. 1 repetition maximum.

While the types of motor unit differ in their contraction speeds, the force developed during maximum static efforts is more closely related to the cross-sectional area of the contractile tissue and not necessarily the fibre type proportions. Moreover, in elite athlete populations, extreme proportions of muscle fibre types are observed, for example, track sprinters are known to possess about 80% type II motor units and marathon runners 80% of type I motor units of the m. vastus medialis. In the instance of talented sportspersons, the dominance of motor unit type is one of the fundamental discriminating factors, underpinning gross-motor, high-energy sporting events. Motor unit proportions and the total number of fibres are primarily (and literally) born out of ones genetic inheritance.

Muscular force expression, however, is not only determined by the cross-sectional area, type and density of contractile tissue but also by the conductance of muscle by the neurological system. The major factor determining the recruitment pattern of motor units is the amount of force necessary to perform the action. The 'size', principle (Henneman et al 1965) of motor unit recruitment suggests that as the intensity of voluntary contraction increases from near resting, motor unit involvement is hierarchical according to the magnitude of the respective unit, and thus the potential for force generation. That is, the smallest motor units are recruited during low-force muscle action, i.e. slow oxidative, followed by fast oxidative glycolytic (type IIa), then 'low-threshold' fast glycolytic and lastly 'high-threshold' fast-glycolytic (type IIb) as the force of contraction gets closer to the maximal voluntary muscle contraction. In order for type II fibres to be recruited and thus receive a training effect, the exercise must be intense. Also, the recruitment order is specific to the movement executed (Desmedt & Godaux 1977); if the body position is changed, even if the muscle may be acting at the same intensity, the order of recruitment can change. The selection of motor units from the pectoralis major during the flat bench press is different from that chosen for the inclined bench press exercise, for example.

The ensuing force output of a motor unit or muscle can also be modified by the frequency of the nerve impulse transmission to the motor end plate, known as the firing rate. Thus, 'high-threshold' type IIb units are engaged when very high rates of motoneuron impulses are achieved. Indeed, the force-generating capability of a single motor unit can alter tenfold depending upon the excitation of the motoneuron. Therefore, maximum duty of agonist muscle force is determined by the highest possible number of motor units recruited and the highest rate of motoneuron excitation.

For the subconscious co-ordination of body movements and muscular action to approach maximal level there must be a conscious desire to generate maximal force.

Essentially, the neural programme for maximal force production comes from the motor cortex that is stimulated by the higher level brain controller to 'intend to lift'. Thus, maximal strength efforts are ordered with maximum motivation.

The function of the antagonist muscle during the action of an agonist is to provide a supportive environment for the active joints and to prevent damaging consequences of vigorous agonist action. The antagonist acts to stabilize and protect through deceleration of prime mover co-action. The opposing torque expressed by the antagonist typically amounts to about 10% of agonist torque, but in essence acts as an inhibitor by reducing the net torque of the desired movement.

## HUMAN FORCE EXPRESSION – BONE AND CONNECTIVE TISSUE

During movements, the affect of the neural stimulus and the concomitant muscle function only develops into a physical action by transmission of the tensile force to the skeletal system. The force generated by the soft tissues of muscles is harnessed by the collagenous connective tissue sheaths that surrounds and binds the entire muscle (epimysium), groups of muscle fibres (perimysium) and individual muscle fibres (endomysium). The collective and concentrated muscle force is channelled through the strong but pliant extension of the muscle sheaths, the collagenous tendon. The terminal end point of the muscle is the junction with the bone where muscle function turns from potential into a physical action. Bone is a dynamic tissue in its resistance to deformation from compressive, tensile and shear loading. The organic matrix contributes to bone strength and the mineral components give bone its stiffness, both of which adapt to the duty of loading stimuli.

Muscle has the ability to adjust the control of force development in response to the load taken. When the load is high the muscle increases the speed of shortening in order to take time to achieve the necessary force to overcome the load. In turn, if the load is small, the force generated is correspondingly small, but the muscle has the capacity to maintain a relative maximal effort, but decreasing the time taken to accomplish the lift, i.e. increased speed of movement. For example, with maximal motivation and effort, the time taken to perform a 1 RM bench press exercise will be slower than pressing, for a single repetition, half of the 1 RM. The relationship between the velocity of muscle shortening and the maximal possible force demonstrates a hyperbolic shape. The maximum velocity attainable can occur with maximum effort against zero loading. The maximum concentric load is produced when muscle shortening velocity is zero, e.g. while the muscle is stationary and exercising isometrically. If the load exceeds the applied force of a maximal muscular effort the muscle must lengthen, as indicated by a negative velocity. Under eccentric conditions greater forces are possible at increasing velocities, which is thought to be due to the elastic properties of the muscle tissue. The resilience of muscle and thus sarcomere action is demonstrated by the transition from near-maximal concentric contractions to isometric actions through to sub-maximal eccentric actions, in response to incremental loading. The muscle is capable of withstanding up to 40% increases in loading and only yield about 2% of maximum velocity. This flat portion to the force–velocity relation provides a broad ranging ability to comfortably withstand loads in excess of the maximum concentric/isometric force, e.g. walking down stairs, landing from a jump.

The force–velocity relationship is increasingly recognized as a diagnostic tool for both the assessment of functional performance and the periodization of strength-oriented training.

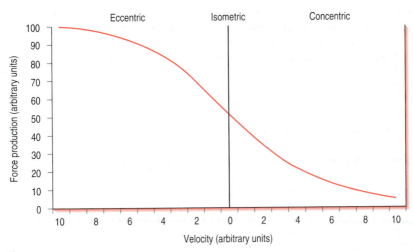

**Figure 7.1**  Theoretical force–velocity curve for eccentric, isometric and concentric muscle actions.

## TRAINING AND ADAPTATION

Resistance exercise dedicated to the advancement of maximal force expression acts as a physical stimulus for the musculoskeletal system to respond by reordering the control and architecture of active tissues. The term adaptation (accommodation is a more passive term also sometimes used) describes the reaction to the strength training stimulus, such that if the same resistance training regime were performed again within a reasonable amount of time that the impact of the stimulus upon the integrity of the cellular milieu would be smaller. An increased potential for even greater functional ability would exist.

There are several mechanisms of how strength can increase. These will be generally discussed in the following sections, with reference to the targeting of specific adaptative responses in later sections.

### Hypertrophy

A muscle undergoes enlargement in response to a chronic strength training stimulus. The degree of training induced growth can be assessed simply by means of girth measurements or more accurately by analysing the cross-sectional area as quantified by direct muscle biopsy, ultrasound, computed tomography imaging (CT) or magnetic resonance imaging (MRI).

The growth in muscle is thought to be due primarily to an increase in the size of muscle fibres, known as hypertrophy. Numerous studies have demonstrated the extent to which muscle fibres increase in response to a programme of resistance training. MacDougall et al (1979) followed unconditioned young men who trained their triceps brachii for 6 months. Fibre areas increased by 33% for type II units and 27% for type I units. In older men a 3-month biceps brachii training programme increased type II units by 30% and type I units by 14% (Brown et al 1988). In a cross-sectional study, MacDougall et al (1984) noted the muscle fibres of bodybuilders to be 58% (type II) and 39% (type I) larger than untrained. Komi et al (1982) demonstrated a change in fibre area diameter of type I and type II units following 16 weeks of either heavy resistance or power-oriented training. Both types I and II units increased fibre diameter in response to heavy resistance training, but only type II units underwent hypertrophy following power training.

The stimulus for muscle growth appears to originate from a loss of sarcomere integrity. A minor level of strain to individual filaments leads to the addition of actin and myosin filaments to the periphery of the myofibril. In this process, a larger myofibril is formed because packing density and cross-bridge spacing is left unchanged. More wholesale changes to myofibrillar architecture occur when the Z line end plates of the sarcomere experience displacement, also known as streaming. The mechanical stresses generated during high force activity create an oblique pull, causing the Z line lattice of actin filaments to tear at the centre, resulting in longitudinal myofibril splitting (not to be confused with muscle fibre splitting) into two or more daughter myofibrils. As the myofibrillar mass increases in volume, the sarcoplasmic reticulum, T-tubule system and associated sarcoplasm are generated in and around the myofilaments, indeed adding to muscle mass. Thus, muscle mass size increases due to an increase in myofibril area and number with no change in myofibril packing density.

## Muscle growth

The ultrastructural damage experienced following high tensile loading of the muscle tissue acts as the stimulus for active repair and subsequent adaptive growth. Muscle satellite cells are said to regulate the regeneration of injured tissue by undergoing mitotic proliferation and migrating to the site of repair. The satellite cells then form a multinucleated myotube from which the transcriptions of new proteins serve to construct myofilaments.

The induction of messenger RNA (mRNA) species and subsequent nature of gene expression acts in accordance with the type of mechanical signal developed. For example, persistent mechanical stimuli are known to encourage the expression of slow adult genes and repression of fat genes, whereas myosin heavy chain and other fast contractile protein isoform gene expression is more completely achieved when active tension development is high. The switching of muscle genes may be related to changes in metabolites and/or calcium levels, for which the nature of physical activity is a major stimulus.

The composite stimulus of metabolic and mechanical loads that a muscle experiences is thus the primary modulator of muscle fibre adaptation and phenotype expression. Because muscle fibres do not exist as distinct types, but are positioned on a sliding continuum of fast to slow twitch properties, and that motor units are made up of mixed muscle fibre types, phenotypical expression of the fibre twitch property is adaptable.

Hence the maximal force-generating capability of a muscle fibre is, in turn, dependent upon pre-existing contractile protein isoforms and the extent to which genes progress toward expression of fast genes and regression of slow genes.

Several studies have demonstrated fibre sub-type conversions following resistance training. Staron et al (1994) recruited male and female subjects to performed 2 days of resistance training, of 6–8 RM or 10–12 RM, for 8 weeks. Maximal strength levels increased without changes in muscle fibre size or fat free mass. Type IIb fibres, however, were decreased from 21% to approximately 7%. Similar studies of longer duration (32 weeks, Staron et al 1991; 19 weeks, Dudley et al 1991) have observed that conversions from type IIb can be almost complete (16–1%, Staron et al 1991), but that the transformation is completely to type IIa fibres. It would appear that as soon as a type IIb unit is activated, it begins a conversion to type IIa properties.

The full extent of motor unit translation, particularly in response to a full career of physical training is relatively unknown. It would appear, however, that the rate of motor unit conversions, in response to a particular type of training, would not nearly fully explain the divergence observed between elite, sub-elite and enthusiast strength athlete that may indeed train to equivalent volumes.

## Hyperplasia

The question of whether muscle fibres are able to increase in number is one that has been keenly debated in the literature in the late 20th Century. It has been generally accepted that fibre number remains constant and that changes in muscle sizes occur from the adaptation of existing fibres. Satellite cell proliferation and the ensuing presence of developing myotubes in humans has been used as evidence that new fibre formation (hyperplasia) is possible, in response to intense exercise training. The satellite cell proliferation, however, may simply be acting upon necrotic fibres, following damaging, perhaps eccentric, exercise. Several studies have indicated that muscle growth following training in chicken, cat and rat was accounted for by hypertrophy and hyperplasia. Numerous observers point to limitations in the methodology underpinning the treatment of muscle sections and counting procedures, as a way of overestimating total fibre number. As several studies have reasoned that, because elite strength athletes possess no more muscle fibres than untrained or part-trained counterparts, fibre number must be constant, eliminating hyperplasia as an adaptive mechanism. Moreover, an association between pre-existing muscle size and muscle fibre number is evidence that, although muscle size is predetermined by the size of muscle fibres, it is also influenced by the genetically established fibre number (MacDougall et al 1984).

## Neurological changes

Subjects that are not familiar with strength training are initially unlikely to be able to fully engage the highest threshold motor units, for maximal efforts. As a consequence the potential for agonist muscle force generation is not achieved. During the early phases of resistance exercise training the reordering of neural control begins to allow the recruitment of high-threshold motor units, conferring greater force development by reordering and adding to the number and functional force-generating capabilities of the motor unit pool. Increased activation of muscle may also come from a greater rate of neural firing of an individual unit with training, providing higher force from the same recruited fibre pool.

Electromyography (EMG) is a method of recording the magnitude of electrical conductance of a muscle. Although, the actual form of neural adaptation is difficult to fully elucidate from EMG data, the integrated (IEMG) signal recorded from an agonist muscle increases following strength training can provide information relating to whether more motor units are being recruited and/or that motor units are being innervated at a higher rate. The EMG activity-to-muscular force ratio can provide information relating to the recruitment order utilized during an action. Moritani & DeVries (1980) noted, following 8 weeks of resistance training, a reduction in EMG activity for a greater force production. Therefore, the reduced EMG:force ratio led authors to believe that more selective and effective recruitment order contributes to increased force production with training. Several studies have also shown that a total increase in neural drive is associated with increased strength levels. Häkkinen & Komi (1983) reported an immediate and pronounced increase of 14–35% in IEMG in the first few weeks of training of the quadriceps muscles. It appears that increased efferent drive, increased motoneuron excitability and a down-regulation of inhibitory pathways contribute to the excitation of the agonistic muscle.

Training of an agonist is also shown to reduce the EMG activity of the antagonist muscle. Häkkinen et al (1998) demonstrated that, while leg extensors increased strength by 20–30% following 6 months of strength training, a concomitant 5–10% reduction of bicep femoris EMG activity was observed during leg maximal extension exercise in older people. The authors reasoned that deactivation of the antagonistic muscle following agonist training decreases the opposing pulling force of antagonist coactivation. Absolute coactivation of the antagonist during agonist muscle contraction is not completely removed with training as it is necessary to assist stability of the joint and acts as a protective mechanism. Antagonist deactivation, however, enables the tension of the agonist to take a greater net effect. In addition, Lee et al (1999) demonstrated that greater activation of synergistic muscles of the arm enabled improved wrist stability and exercise performance. Together, greater force production capability of the agonist, coupled with less inhibition from the antagonist acting around a more stable platform established from the greater coactivation of synergistic muscle action, allowed expression of greater strength capability.

## TIME COURSE OF MUSCLE AND NEURAL ADAPTATION

Maximal force expression is a product of neural conductance and recruitment of muscle and of the mass of muscle and their twitch properties. With training, however, the contribution of neural and hypertrophic changes to the increase in maximal force production do not occur in tandem. Häkkinen et al (1981) demonstrated that the increased force production in the first 8 weeks of concentric and eccentric training was paralleled closely with an increase in IEMG. Further, when non-strength-trained athletes begin resistance training, the relationship between the increases in strength and increases in muscle fibre cross-sectional area (Ploutz et al 1994) or muscle girth (Moritani & DeVries 1979), is poor. It is suggested that an enhancement of the neural firing rate and engagement of high threshold units make the greatest contribution to increased force production, above that of muscle hypertrophy (Sale 1992). It is proposed that during the early stages of strength training (2–8 weeks) the neuromusculoskeletal system 'learns' how to exert force. Changes in protein quality, as shown by alterations in the type of myosin heavy chains and type of myosin ATPase enzymes, are observed from the beginning of resistance training programmes. It is suggested that 16 workouts are required before significant improvements in muscle fibre hypertrophy is experienced (Staron et al 1994).

## IMPROVEMENTS IN STRENGTH

The literature reflects a wide variety of responses to resistance programmes, mostly depending upon the age of the group, pre-training status and potential for improvement. The average improvement in strength for sedentary young and middle-aged participants for up to 6 months of training is 25–30%. Fleck & Kraemer (1997) reviewed 20 training studies that examined the effect of dynamic constant external resistance training and testing of 1 or multiple ($\leq 10$) RM performance with the equipment on which they trained. The 20 studies that were reviewed for bench press performance (for a mean of $12 \pm 4$ weeks, $3.3 \pm 1$ days per week) demonstrated a mean increase of $19.8 \pm 13.5\%$ increase in strength. The 10 studies involving leg press exercise (for a mean of 14.5 ± 5.8 weeks, 2.8 ± 0.4 days per week) showed improvements in strength of 30.9 ± 17.5%.

Improvements in isometric strength as a result of isometric training have also been reviewed (Fleck & Kraemer 1993). The 10 studies included assessments of elbow flexors, quadriceps, triceps surae and triceps brachii muscles exercised for 19.1 ± 14.7 contractions per day each of 5.1 ± 2.7 s duration (totalling 73.6 ± 43.7 s isometric contraction time per day) for a period of 41 ± 22 days resulted in an increase of maximum voluntary isometric action of 31.3 ± 24.4%.

## ENDOCRINE RESPONSES TO STRENGTH TRAINING

The endocrine system is key to many aspects of training-induced increases in strength. In general, early improvements in strength are dominated by neuromuscular changes. The stimulus provided by strength training induces hormonal secretion from the initiation of training and many of these are responsible for protein synthesis leading to muscle hypertrophy. In evolutionary terms, however, muscle is costly, requiring a good supply of energy and if food is short muscle is one of the first tissues to be reduced in size. Accordingly, there is a certain resistance to greatly increase muscle-derived protein synthesis until constant demand (i.e. a regular stimulus) dictates that it is required. For this reason, early increases in strength are dominated by neuromuscular adaptation (which does not require increased protein synthesis), while later increases in strength are related to muscle hypertrophy.

There are a number of hormones associated with increased muscle protein synthesis whose secretion is stimulated by resistance exercise. These include testosterone (the primary male sex hormone), growth hormone (hGH) and insulin-like growth factor-1 (IGF-1).

With respect to growth at puberty, testosterone and hGH play a key role. In terms of muscle hypertrophy, testosterone acts as a classic steroid hormone. Being lipid-based, testosterone is easily diffused through the lipid-bilayer membrane of the cell and is also therefore able to diffuse through the membrane of the cell's nucleus. Steroid hormones interact with receptors in the nucleus and encourage the formation of a copy or transcript of the appropriate section of DNA. This transcript is made of RNA and can be transferred from the nucleus to the cytoplasm of the cell (known as sarcoplasm in the muscle cell). In the sarcoplasm the RNA transcript is used by organelles known as ribosomes that construct the appropriate proteins from amino acids, hence, more muscle is constructed.

hGH is a peptide hormone whose secretion is also stimulated by resistance exercise. It has a more minor direct effect on muscle cell protein synthesis. Peptide hormones act by interacting with receptors on cell membranes. When the hormone and receptor bind it causes a 'second messenger' to be released inside the cell. This second messenger initiates a cascade of reactions involving transcription factors which interact with receptors in the cytoplasm and nucleus. Until recently, however, hGH was recognized as having only an indirect role in muscle hypertrophy. hGH interacts with liver membrane receptors to stimulate the release of IGF-1 from liver and it is this IGF-1 of hepatic origin that was deemed to be the most important initiator of muscle hypertrophy. This central role for IGF-1 is encapsulated in the somatomedin hypothesis (Daughaday 2000). Recently, IGF-1 has been shown to have a number of splice variants and IGF-1 is produced in liver and locally in muscle. Currently, it is suggested that muscle derived IGF-1 will be renamed 'mechano growth factor' (MGF) in recognition of the fact that its major stimulus is muscle contraction per se.

With respect to GH, a more direct effect on muscle hypertophy has been recently demonstrated. GH appears to directly inhibit the muscle protein somatostatin. Somatostatin normally acts to inhibit muscle growth and so ensure that muscle development does not exceed what is functionally required. By inhibiting somatostatin GH directly facilitates muscle hypertrophy.

In summary, it is obvious from a considerable volume of research literature that there are a number of routes by which endocrine function directly, indirectly, in isolation and by interaction, can affect muscle hypertrophy and ultimately, therefore, strength.

## STRENGTH TRAINING PRINCIPLES

### Overload

When a muscle is required to respond to a load to which it is not accustomed in normal daily activity, the muscle is 'overloaded'. The overloading event acts as a discrete stimulus for the biological mechanisms of adaptation (see Ch. 1).

A stimulus for muscle strength development can take many forms. Simplistically, the muscle increases in strength to time under tension. To this extent, various combinations of exercise mode, type, and intensity of muscle actions are effective at developing maximal force production capability. Current understanding is a long way from being able to categorically prescribe accurate loading for the multitude of requirements for everyday functionality to sporting endeavour; maximum to minimum strength adaptation; for untrained or trained; young or old; male or female. Further, pre-training status determines the extent to which athletes are able to make proportional improvements. Well trained athletes will be closer to their genetic ceiling of strength development potential than untrained subjects. Studies that have examined the responses of untrained young, middle-aged (Pollock et al 1989) and elderly (Fiatarone et al 1994) participants using lumbar extension strengthening exercises have observed greater than 100% increases in strength in just 8–12 weeks. Likewise, Häkkinen et al (1981) observed improvements in back squat, following 24 weeks of strength training of about 100% for non-athletes, compared with about 50% in athlete populations. It appears also that untrained participants require much lighter loading in order to experience hypertrophy and strength gains.

At one end of the loading spectrum, high-volume, low-tension exercises such as those undertaken during endurance training will induce hypertrophy of type I units. Equally, multiple isometric actions will result in moderate hypertrophy and gains in strength but not of the same magnitude as dynamic strength exercise. It has been suggested that the threshold training stimulus for strength adaptation should not be less than one-third of the maximal strength. As adaptation occurs and strength increases, however, the proportional intensity at which resistance exercise is levelled in order to constitute a stimulus must increase. Strong evidence from the literature, coaching, and athlete experience show that light loading regimes are far less effective in developing strength than programmes that involve maximum athlete exertion.

### Full range of movement

No study has adequately examined whether exercises are best performed through the full range of movement or partial range to optimize strength gains. A number of studies have considered the strength adaptations to maximal isometric exercise training, however, and concluded that whereas hypertrophic gains are moderate, the improvements in strength are specific to a limited joint angle and not throughout the full range of motion. Resistance training movements are typically performed through the full possible range of motion allowed by the body positioning and joints involved, with the greatest consideration to safety of the athlete. Positioning the muscle so that it acts through a large range of movement requires the muscle to experience tensile loading along a greater length of its entirety leading to uniformity of loading stimuli and requiring greater forces at the start (long) position. It may be argued that a greater range of motion is possible for a host of exercises when using dumbbells versus barbells (e.g. dumbbell bench press versus barbell bench press), therefore applying the tensile force through a greater range. Indeed, studies have demonstrated that muscle actions involving greater range of movement (e.g. seated incline dumbbell bicep curl versus preacher dumbbell bicep curl) result in greater muscle damage and thus a more potent strength stimulus. In contrast, greater loads (and thus tensile forces) can be lifted for an equivalent number of repetitions when using barbells over dumbbells, therefore creating a greater level of work and thus enhancing the overall stimulus. Movements involving partial range of motion can be useful for rehabilitation or sports-specific training.

## Good form

Exercise form refers to the practice of implementing recommended movement patterns, maintenance of postural control, use of full range of motion and regulation of breathing. For example, swaying of the torso or excessive movement of the elbow during barbell bicep curls would be considered a lack of good form. Therefore, good form allows a muscle or muscle group to be isolated well and to minimize potential injury. Good form tends to be easier to maintain if the contraction and lengthening phases of an exercise are performed at a slow velocity because momentum developed by fast moving body parts is minimized.

## Stability and kinaesthetic control

Even the most basic exercise, whether involving the control of free weight, body resistance or machine system, requires a high level of co-ordination and control. The level of proprioceptive control afforded for a given exercise depends greatly upon the experience of the type of movement performed and the refinement of the hierarchical control of fine and gross motor unit pattern recruitment. The novice practitioner may struggle, for example, to hold the hips in line with the torso and legs during a press up; or to control the descent of a weight during the eccentric phase of a triceps extension with a resistance that required only moderate effort during the concentric phase. A further example, commonly observed, is the lack of movement control exhibited by experienced weight training athletes when asked to perform dumbbell bench press, when all previous experience has been of barbell bench press. Furthermore, there is a heavy dependence of exercises that involve actions exclusively through the sagittal and frontal planes, but few that are either in the transverse plane or that combine one or more planes of movement.

Whereas the preponderance for traditional, big, compound exercises such as the power clean, barbell bench press and back squat is warranted as extremely productive movements for strength development – as they allow for the greatest force production, muscle mass involvement, hormonal release etc. (see later section on exercise choice) – they are often chosen for these very reasons over more functional, kinaesthetic, multi-directional oriented movements that may have greater cross-transfer to sports-specific movement techniques. Strength and conditioning coaches should give serious programme space to exercises that provide greater kinaesthetic and therefore, globally valid exercise movements that can be creatively constructed rather than simple, one-dimensional replication of the customary exercises.

## Velocity of action

Training at a low action velocity for strength movements appears to greatly enhance strength at low action velocities but has a minimal effect upon high-velocity strength. While high velocity entrainment greatly improves high-velocity strength, in contrast it has a greater transfer to low-velocity strength than does low-velocity training on high-velocity strength. Because high-velocity training does not allow enough time for the development of high forces, however, full development of muscular hypertrophy through application of high volumes of tensile loading will only be possible with low-velocity training. Likewise, low-velocity training may fail to stimulate neural activation sufficiently, owing to the reduced velocity of contractile excitation. Therefore, one would consider low-velocity training is more oriented to hypertrophy and high-velocity training to neural strength adaptation.

It is thus clear that resistance training produces the greatest strength gains at the velocity at which training is performed. More importantly, numerous studies have shown that the effect of fast isokinetic training upon power-based tests of performance such as jump and sprint ability is much greater than slow isokinetic training. It has been recommended, however, that medium velocity strength training has the greatest effect of any one particular velocity of training upon a rightward shift of the force velocity curve and thus optimal but generic strength performance.

## The set

A series of repetitions is termed the set. As the set progresses the neuromuscular system will fatigue, resulting in an increasing perceptual effort required to perform an exercise at a given resistance.

## The repetition

The basic unit of resistance training is the repetition, defined as the performance of a complete cycle from start position, through the end of the movement and back to the start. For isometric training, the repetition refers to a muscle action or effort at a specified joint angle. For dynamic constant external resistance exercise, one single number or range of repetitions does not present the optimal stimulus for maximal strength adaptation. The number of repetitions that is intended for a given exercise set should depend upon the desired physiological adaptive response. Numerous studies have examined the effect of varying repetition number upon the strength gains of novice strength athletes. Many studies that have attempted to standardize the total work performed have concluded that improvements in strength adaptation is independent of repetition number (typically between 2 and 12 RM).

## VOLUNTARY MAXIMAL MUSCULAR FORCE PRODUCTION

Several studies have shown that a crucial aspect of the impact of multiple repetitions at a given exercise load is the degree of maximal effort involved. Maximum effort strength exercise (a voluntary maximal muscular action) is the most effective means of developing maximal force generating ability (Fleck & Schutt 1985). Perhaps the most obvious means of maximal exercise is the performance of a 1 RM effort. However, strength-training programmes, even for competitive lifters, do not commonly involve 1 RM efforts in isolation. A set of multiple continuous repetitions require near maximal muscular actions. Multiple repetitions are performed with a moderately heavy resistance in which the acting muscle experiences progressive fatigue until momentary concentric failure (which needs to be overseen or 'spotted' in order to assist the completion of the final repetition or remove the resistance from the fatigued athlete) or just before momentary concentric failure. Thus the final repetition of a multiple repetition exercise set is performed as a voluntary maximal muscular action. Compared with a single maximal action, the performance of multiple repetitions presents a greater volume of high tension dynamic actions, which in turn act as a stimulus for adaptation.

## RESISTANCE

The most important factor for strength training is the amount of resistance used. It is the major stimulus for strength adaptation and, assuming maximal voluntary muscular failure, will decide the number of repetitions possible. Thus, $n$RM or %RM is the simplest method of assessing load. Research supports varying training effects derived from exercise on a continuum of RM. The use of percentage RM for power exercises such as power clean, clean and jerk and snatch may not be appropriate because the emphasis for performance of these exercises is velocity of movement and technique rather than maximal muscular fatigue and thus slowing of movement velocity.

## EXERCISING AT PROPORTIONS OF 1 RM

The fatigue rate associated with exercises performed at heavy loads means that as the weight increases the number of repetitions decreases. Consequently, a number of investigators have developed equations or charts to facilitate the prediction of maximal or sub-maximal performance. For many, these charts are integral to the development of training plans and progression; however, there are a number of limitations to these extrapolations that the strength training athlete and coach should be aware of. Firstly, many predictions assume a linear relationship between repetition number and load, whereas this has been shown not to be the case. Secondly, for exercises involving a large muscle mass (e.g. leg press), the strength athlete will be able to perform a higher number of repetitions for a given percentage of 1 RM than possible with a small muscle mass (e.g. bicep curl). Therefore, the strength athlete should seek to maintain a repetition number in a strength zone, for large muscle mass exercises, by increasing intensity to a higher percentage of 1 RM (Kraemer & Häkkinen 2002).

Strength appears to increase in the early stages of training consistently regardless of the nature of the loading. Equivalent rates of improvement are observed when loads of 20, 40, 60 and 80% of 1 RM are used for participants with no background in resistance work. Thus, intricate prescription based upon loading, velocity of movement and rest interval is only warranted for athletes with several months of resistance training experience.

Studies have demonstrated that RM resistances of 6 or less result in the greatest increases in strength measures and maximal power outputs. Resistances of 20 RM or above are shown to improve muscular endurance to the greatest degree, but strength gains experienced from such high number repetitions are minimal. Table 7.2 outlines

Table 7.2   Differentiation in 'neural' and 'hypertrophic' stimuli with training repetition ranges

|  | Adaptation | Neural system stimulation | Hypertrophy stimulation |
|---|---|---|---|
| 1–3 RM | Strength/power | High | Moderate |
| 3–6 RM | Strength/power | High | Moderate–high |
| 6–12 RM | Moderate- to high-intensity strength | Moderate | High |
| 12+ RM | High-intensity endurance | Low | Moderate |

the programme goals that are classically attached to the most popular configurations of exercise repetitions (Häkkinen, 2002).

A 'neural' oriented heavy resistance session involves efforts at 80–90–100% of 1 RM, for less than six repetitions per set. During such high loading the neuromuscular system undergoes acute fatigue, as measured by reduced maximal voluntary neural activation (~20%, for 20 × 1 RM lifts), a reduction in maximal force generating ability (~25%, for multiple 20 × 1 RM lifts) and a reduction in the force–time curve characteristics of force application (~one-third, for 20 × 1 RM lifts). Performance of a few maximal repetitions requires the generation of maximal muscular forces, and thus maximum motivation. Maximal force performance takes a greater amount of time to develop than lighter power oriented movements (> 600 milliseconds to reach maximum force). The power development during 1–6 RM efforts is unlikely to be maximal owing to the longer time taken to develop maximal force. Indeed, maximal force development during 100% 1 RM efforts may not reach absolute maximal force generating abilities because acceleration is compromised by the high resistance (mass) used. In this way, absolute external mass loading is at its highest during 'neural' sessions which should be considered as the primary stimuli for strength adaptation.

The 'hypertrophic' model involves medium to high loads, such as 60–80% of 1 RM, for multiple sequential repetitions until maximal voluntary concentric failure. The classic hypertrophy workout involving sets of 10 RM is the bedrock of bodybuilding and recreational athlete programmes. Features of such loading lead to severe acute fatigue of the neuromuscular unit (~30%, for 10 × 10 RM lifts), reduction in maximal force generating ability (~50%, for 10 × 10 RM lifts), pronounced accumulation of blood lactate and considerable acute hormonal responses. The common emphasis for this type of training is to maximize the stimulus to the muscle by balancing the period of time that the muscle is exposed while ensuring that the load creates sufficiently high tensile stresses to cause ensuing concentric failure, for example within 10 repetitions. Therefore, the combination of moderate-to-high tensile stresses applied over a significant time period creates the stimulus of tension induced myofibrillar streaming and high volumes of anaerobic energy release from the prolonged nature of high-intensity efforts.

A traditional, hypertrophy oriented technique for repetition performance involves the active deliberation of concentric and eccentric phases during dynamic constant external resistance exercise. The, 'up-for-two, down-for-three' method of repetition control, accentuates the 'time-under-tension' principle, in order to ensure a quality tensile and metabolic stimulus. For example, for a barbell bent-over row movement, the bar is pulled up from the start position to the abdomen for a count of two, and then returns from the finish to the start position for a count of three.

The emphasis placed upon the eccentric component of this training method reinforces the uniquely important role that eccentric muscle lengthening has on strength development. During eccentric actions the IEMG per unit of force is lower than during concentric actions, meaning that motor unit recruitment per unit of force is lower and that the tension placed upon each motor unit is greater for eccentric versus concentric actions. Eccentrically biased activities (such as downhill running) are often discussed in relation to delayed onset of muscular soreness (DOMS), associated Z-line disruption, inflammation, creatine kinase enzyme release, reduced range of motion and loss of muscle force during the period of days of recovery.

Observers and practitioners alike often place too much emphasis upon the seemingly deleterious damage response that results from eccentric activity, citing soreness, injury and loss (albeit transient) of strength as reasons to avoid this type of training. This view overlooks the most rudimentary mechanistic understanding of the importance of inducing micro-morphological damage, as the very essence of the neural and myofibrillar adaptive stimuli development. The greater tensile stresses that motor units undergo during eccentric actions are often magnified beyond the simple premise that when a sarcomere is loaded excessively its component structure becomes compromised and thus repairs to a more robust setting.

Studies have demonstrated that the degree of strength development that occurs in response to concentric training alone is inferior to concentric plus eccentric cyclic training. Because eccentric actions are integrally involved in many sporting activities, dynamic constant external resistance exercise involving eccentric actions are fundamentally important to functional strength development.

Therefore, eccentric work would appear to be a potent stressor of the tensile properties of muscle tissue and thus should be used as an effective training stimuli when incorporated into dynamic overloading. An obvious weakness of attempts to create a muscle loading stimulus without undue strains to the skeletal system, such as isokinetic or isometric training, is a neglect of eccentric modality that frequently results in less functional kinematic capability, for predominantly land based sports.

Overall, the strength training response is very specific to the type, mode and loading combinations applied to the neuromuscular system. In this way, adaptation is precise. However, due attention should be given to the requirement for variety and holistic transfer of training effects to the sporting movement. For example, a particular exercise, such as bench press, may be considered a bedrock exercise for many sports' resistance training programmes and continual use will lead to improved performance but may not facilitate greater force production in a host of movement patterns, in proportion to the amount of time spent exercising with it.

## MANIPULATION OF FORCE DEVELOPMENT CHARACTERISTICS

The criteria for maximal muscular force production need not only involve the performance of exercises to failure or maximal loading. Newton's Second Law of Motion states that 'The change of motion is proportional to the motive force impressed; and is made in the direction of the straight line in which that force is impressed', such that the rate of change of velocity is proportional to the resultant force acting on the body and is in the same direction as the force or:

force = mass × acceleration (F = m.a)

Therefore, if the goal of strength training is to utilize the generation of the level of force during a repetition/set, then the magnitude of force (F) can be manipulated in several ways:

(i) $F = M.a$    where mass M is large and the acceleration is small;
(ii) $F = m.A$    where the mass is small and the acceleration A is large;
(iii) $F = m.a$    where mass and acceleration are moderate.

Thus, in theory, training can be manipulated using a variety of loading and velocity combinations to achieve 'force training'. However, when an athlete trains with high resistance (i.e. high mass), as does a powerlifter, or trains with high acceleration and small mass, as does a track sprinter or arguably an Olympic lifter, or trains with moderate mass and acceleration, as does a bodybuilder, very different physical and importantly performance responses are experienced. This is because the loading and accelerative components of high force generation act as highly specific stimuli for neural, muscular and metabolic adaptations (Siff 2003).

The force–velocity characteristics of muscle performance dictate that the maximal force development potential is determined by the velocity of the movement. During high-velocity movements there is little time for the development of force, e.g. during the rapid foot contact during a long jump take off. In contrast, during low-velocity movements, such as a rugby scrum, there is much more time for the attainment of greater force levels. Likewise, during strength exercises the maximum movement velocity possible will depend largely on the magnitude of the load used. Whereas, a 1 RM bench press performance may require maximal effort and is indeed categorized as maximum strength, the load is so high that it can only be completed slowly. Likewise, multiple repetition sets may also be voluntarily performed at slow speeds for a particular training adaptation. If the athlete chooses to perform all movements slowly either due to maximal loading or repetition deliberation; however, improvements in maximal force (high force end of the force–velocity curve) production will occur but little improvements in the velocity of movement (velocity end of force–velocity curve) will take place. In resistance training, it is common for athletes who are interested in power training to choose lighter resistances, typically 30–60% of 1 RM, for which the load will not feel 'heavy' per se, but the athlete will be able to turn his/her attentions to performing the movement at maximum possible velocity. Furthermore, ballistic movements will make only small improvements in maximal force ability yet will greatly enhance rapid development of lower forces (see Ch. 6). Therefore, the characteristics of force generation adaptation are specific to the rate of force development training undertaken.

As a general principle, training at a specific velocity will carry over adaptation to force production ability for velocities ± 20–30% either side of that trained. To this extent, training between 30 and 60% of 1 RM has been shown to facilitate improvements to all portions of the force–velocity curve. However, continually training at a fixed intensity and velocity of movement will result in limited improvements in high force or high velocity generating ability.

## PROGRESSIVE OVERLOAD

At the start of a training programme a person will be able to complete a certain number of repetitions with a given load or be able to lift a certain load for a single repetition, i.e. an athlete's strength is definable. If that person undertakes just one training session (the configuration of which would typically involve multiple repetitions and sets, of a variety of given exercises specific to the intended muscle groups, at a given exercise intensity), the subsequent compensation and adaptation means that the muscle then becomes capable of producing greater force. Therefore, if the same training session were repeated exactly, the overall impact of the training stimulus and subsequent provocation of adaptation would be reduced. Subsequently, if the same training session continues to be repeated, with time, strength gains would inexorably approach a plateau. If it is the goal of exciting the appropriate systems into continuous adaptation, the stimulus, i.e. the configuration of loading, must increase.

For example, an athlete at the start of the training programme may be able to bench press 40 kg for 10 repetitions and press 53 kg for a 1 RM. The 10 RM load represents a proportional load of 75% of 1 RM. Using the average responses observed by Fleck & Kraemer (1997), if the athlete trained for 12 weeks, three times per week and experienced a 20% increase in strength performance, the athlete would then be able to perform 10 repetitions with 48 kg and be able to press 64 kg for a 1 RM effort. Following training, the original 10 RM loading of 40 kg would then represent a proportional load of 63% of 1 RM.

- Pre-training bench press performance:
  10 RM = 40 kg
  1 RM = 53 kg
- Following 12 weeks of 3 training sessions per week:
  10 RM = 48 kg (40 × 1.2 (+ 20% improvement))
  1 RM = 64 kg (53 × 1.2 (+ 20% improvement))
  Previous 10 RM of 40 kg = 63% (40/64 × 100) of training enhanced 1 RM

Overload can be progressed in all manner of ways, but perhaps the most obvious means is to increase the resistance (amount of weight) used for a given number of repetitions. One of the first steps in the adaptation process is likely to be that the athlete is able to perform more repetitions with a particular weight. In this circumstance, for overload to be progressive an athlete may decide to alter subsequent training sessions by:

- increasing the weight used;
- attempting to perform further repetitions with the same weight;
- reducing the rest interval between sets;
- increasing the number of sets performed.

In most circumstances the resistance chosen must be predetermined before a set of repetitions begins. Given that individual progression, over time, is highly variable, a fixed increment in resistance for each subsequent training session is likely to produce unpredictable performances. Assuming that an athlete intends to perform the set of exercises to voluntary maximal muscular failure, the athlete should select a weight that will induce fatigue within the prescribed repetition range. In the example outlined below, the athlete overloads the elbow flexor muscles by exercising at 70% of 1 RM, resulting in 8–10 repetitions per set. Overload progresses by an increase in the resistance only when an increase in repetition number is observed. Thus, the athlete aims to increase resistance while maintaining intensity. This stepwise method of progression is a logical way of advancing the resistance appropriately and in accordance with the ability of the active muscle group unit. Detailed record taking of training performance greatly facilitates step-wise progression, as the athlete is able to refer back to previous efforts and present reasonable but challenging feats for current or future workouts.

## Example of training progression

Week 1 able to perform barbell curls for 8 repetitions with 30 kg;
Week 2 able to perform barbell curls for 10 repetitions with 30 kg;
Week 3 able to perform barbell curls for 11 repetitions with 30 kg;
Week 4 able to perform barbell curls for 9 repetitions with 32.5 kg.

## NUMBER OF SETS

Increases in maximal strength have been reported in response to a single set of an exercise per training session (American College of Sports Medicine 1998). Strength gains are not different between programmes that use 1, 2 or 3 sets of 10–12 RM during the first few weeks of resistance training. Single-set systems are also useful for the maintenance of strength during heavy competitive schedules. It is well understood, however, that multiple (3–6 per body part) sets produce significantly superior results over longer term programmes. In more highly trained athletes strength gains are very small with low volume, single-set training regimes. It is recommended, therefore, that the use of one or two sets of an exercise are useful for novice athletes, for circuit training or for maintenance phases (Fleck & Kraemer 1997).

## REST PERIODS

Recently it has been shown that the period of rest provided between sets greatly influences the nature of the workout stress. Following the performance of an exercise set, a reduction in neuromuscular excitation ability, an increase in local metabolic acidosis and the replenishment of ATP and PC energy sources, occurs. Longer rest period protocols (3–5 minutes) are more appropriate for 'neural' or strength/power orientated sessions in order to facilitate more complete recovery of neural performance. Progressive fatigue across sets, resulting from inadequate rest, will lead to either a reduction in the velocity of the speed of movement for a fixed load or a reduction in the load in order to maintain movement velocity. Studies demonstrate that when comparing responses to a strength/neural protocol (5 RM, 3 minutes rest) versus a hypertrophy protocol (10 RM, 1 minute rest), blood lactate concentration was 50–100% greater and growth hormone response 30–90% greater, for the latter regime. Thus, metabolic responses are not related to the magnitude of the resistance used but to the amount of work and the duration of muscle loading. In simple terms, the intensity, as indicated by the severity of effort or psychological anxiety expressed rather than an index of load, can be dramatically increased with the reduction of rest between sets. Such high-volume–low-rest regimes should be phased gradually into a novice strength programme in order for the acid–base balance to progress. One of the common themes that emerges from the literature is that the degree of lactic acid accumulation in the muscle and blood may be related to the growth hormone response observed during strength workouts and so may indeed be an underpinning pre-cursor for muscle growth.

Rest periods of less than 60 seconds are not considered optimal for maximal strength adaptation and are more indicative of 'circuit' training. Where numerous resistance exercises, often including actions of varying body parts are performed in rotation or in repetitions, with minimal rest between sets, the loading resistance tends to be lower than conventional strength loads in order to accomplish many 'stations' and 'circuits', There is also a marked cardiovascular effort due to the relatively short period of rest between sets. Circuit training tends to be used by athletes whose primary source of energy is from the glycolytic/lactate pathway; for added variety to resistance training; or when a gym is not freely available and only body-weight resistance exercises can be performed.

Table 7.3    The effect of differing rest periods upon loading and programme goals during resistance training

| Rest period | Comments | Loading | Programme goals |
| --- | --- | --- | --- |
| 0–30 s | Very, very short rest | Light resistance: 15–25 RM | Fatigue resistance, muscular endurance |
| 31–60 s | Very short rest | Light resistance: 10–20 RM | High glycolytic stress, anaerobic endurance, hypertrophy |
| 61–120 s | Short–moderate rest | Moderate resistance: 8–12 RM | Muscular strength, hypertrophy |
| 120–180 s | Moderate–long rest | Moderate–heavy: 6–10 RM | Muscular strength, hypertrophy, moderate velocity of movement |
| 180–300 s | Long rest | Heavy | Absolute strength, power, high velocity of movement |
| 300–420 s | Very long rest | Very heavy–maximal resistance | Maximal RM and power |

The novice strength athlete can take many approaches to controlling the rest periods between sets, depending upon the desired goal. It is not recommended that the novice use rest periods of more than 3 minutes in duration in order to develop fundamental anaerobic biochemical, ultrastructural and morphological adaptations. In the early stages of training, even moderate to long rest periods may not prevent a naïve muscle from fatiguing across multiple sets. In this instance, the regime should control rest periods to 60–120 seconds, and let the adaptive response be the achievement of consistent performance across multiple sets. Alternatively, the novice may begin resistance training with very short rest periods and light loading, experiencing adaptations in muscular endurance before, progressing to heavier loads and increasing the rest between sets.

## TRAINING FREQUENCY

The frequency of strength-training stimulus will depend upon the intensity of the muscle stimuli, number of muscle groups worked, and recovery potential. Research shows that muscles should be trained at least 1 day per week in order to initiate strength gains and to maintain strength adaptations. A number of medium-term longitudinal studies show that two or three training sessions per muscle group elicit near-optimal improvements in strength. However, professional strength/hypertrophy oriented athletes, such as bodybuilders, rugby players, weightlifters are likely to conduct 4–6 strength workouts per week, with some conducting two training sessions per day. The configuration of these weekly workout regimes are developed in order to 'split' bodyparts, and accrue rest between workouts in order to increase training volume.

## WORKOUT COMPOSITION

Once the resistance, velocity of movement, number of repetitions, number of sets and amount of rest between sets have been decided, there are still a multitude of choices to be made relating to the exercising movements to be performed. Yet commonly, despite having thousands of resistance movements to choose from, workout composition is frighteningly familiar for all, given the equally infinite individual factors such as gender, age, body dimension, functional ability and sport. It is

**Table 7.4** Classification of exercise according to number of joints involved and complexity of movement[a]

| Categories | Classification – Joint number – Complexity of movement | |
| | Example movements (joints involved) | Weight/force |
| --- | --- | --- |
| Single joint (also referred to as isolation) | Calf raise (ankle) Knee raise (hip) Tricep extension (elbow) Pec flye (shoulder) | Low–moderate |
| Multi-joint (also referred to as compound combination) | Bench press (shoulder, elbow) Chin-up/Lat pull down (elbow, shoulder) Lunge (ankle, knee, hip, back) | Moderate–high |
| Complex multi-joint (also referred to as power lift, compound lift) | Snatch (ankle, knee, hip, back, shoulder, elbow, wrist) Power clean (ankle, knee, hip, back, shoulder, elbow, wrist) | High–maximal possible weight |

[a]*Comments.* Exercises are categorized according to whether a single joint or multiple joints are involved, and whether the action requires a high level of complexity to perform. This categorization is used to facilitate decisions about the magnitude of physical loading, i.e. heavier absolute loads are possible with multi-joint exercises, whereas greater emphasis is possible for a selected muscle with isolation exercises. Olympic and power lifting athletes tend to perform a large majority of resistance training with complex multi-joint movements, with a moderate amount of multi-joint actions, with little or no use of single joint movements. Body building athletes, on the other hand, will use multi-joint and single-joint exercises almost exclusively with very little use of complex multi-joint exercises. Strength training for athletic sports tends to involve a combination of all three categories of training, in order to address power (complex multi-joint), functional strength (multi-joint) and specialized muscle development (single joint) components of an activity. Complex multi-joint and multi-joint exercises are best performed at the beginning of the workout, i.e. before isolation, because isolation work may pre-fatigue a particular body part.

**Table 7.5**    Classification of exercise according to the priority or specificity of the exercise movement[a]

| Classification – Priority | |
| --- | --- |
| Categories | Example for sprinter |
| Primary (also referred to as specifics) | Power clean |
| | Snatch |
| | Front squat |
| | Hamstring curls |
| | Calf raise |
| | Push press |
| | Bent over row |
| Supplementary (also referred to as cross training) | Bench press |
| | Front dumbbell raise |
| | Reverse dumbbell raise |
| | Dumbbell bicep curl |
| | Tricep kickbacks |
| | Outer range leg extension |

[a]*Comments.* The priority system places emphasis upon the selected exercises based upon one or more of the following:

- Muscle groups heavily involved in sporting action
- Actions requiring maximum motivation, effort and/or velocity of movement
- Weak muscle groups

The priority system is widely used by athletes participating in a variety of sports primarily as a means of attaching a hierarchy of importance to what amounts to auxiliary training to event-specific preparation. Bodybuilders and weightlifters will also use this system to prioritize certain movments. Sports persons typically use the priority system as it categorizes resistance training. This system can be applied to a prioritization of neuromuscular patterning, for exercise movements that may be used to prevent injury or recover from injury, or to present a new movement pattern. Primary exercises are typically performed at the start of a workout, while the athlete is fresh and free from fatigue, enabling the performance of high-quality technical and maximum effort movements.

beyond the scope of this text to explore all the possible movements that may be useful for strength training. It is perhaps more pertinent to present the various classifications of exercises because decisions of workout composition are primarily informed by the discrimination of movements based upon its merits for a particular situation.

The categories shown in Tables 7.4 and 7.5 are among the most commonly used in Western contemporary strength training.

## TRAINING ORGANIZATION

Constant monitoring and adjustment of the imposed load in relation to current abilities is an essential component of training programme effectiveness. However, if an athlete maintains the same routine with only manipulations in weight used, a plateau in training adaptation will occur. The simple stress/training–adaptation response dictates that the human body will respond by altering its function according to the nature of the stress imposed. The adaptive response is both dynamic and specific.

The adaptive response is an expensive process, in terms of energy and resources, one which the human system performs only under coercion. Therefore, it is not surprising that the body will, with time, be able to minimize adaptation by maintaining the current homeostatic cellular milieu by attempting to accommodate a persistent stressor. In this respect, all the fundamental constituents of the training stimulus must continuously evolve in order to create an incentive for physiological change. All too frequently a programme is set in stone during the early stages of a strength-training programme implementation (often based upon the practices of others) and may deviate only slightly over a long period of time.

In reality, the human system must be exposed to variety in training in order to 'shock' the body into change. Variety can only be achieved with constant renovation of the content, style and nature of the training programme. Perhaps the most established form of organized variation is what has become known as periodization, termed to reflect the periodical adjustment of programme variables (see Ch. 1). Periodization is largely based upon the Eastern European observations that increasing training volume in the early and middle phases of a training season followed by a decreased training volume, while increasing intensity, in later phases of training resulted in the greatest adaptive response. Prior to peaking intensity reaches a peak, while volume reaches its lowest level. Enhancement of the recovery processes and consequent supercompensation is enhanced by a reduction in intensity just prior to peaking. The classic periodization programme underpins the development of power for sporting performance. In this context, the training season can be broken into five mesocycles:

- hypertrophy – high volume, moderate resistance, little rest between sets, increase in muscle mass;
- strength – high volume, high resistance, build upon muscle mass gained, develop neural component;
- power – moderate volume, high levels of rest, high velocity of movement, peak neural activation and development;
- peaking – reduced volume, increased intensity, maximum rest = enhanced performance;
- rest – low volume, low intensity, minimize deconditioning.

The typical periodization method utilizes a linear approach, where each subsequent microcycle builds upon the progressive intensity of the predecessor. Typically, the greater volume of repetitions in the first microcycle is progressed to fewer repetitions at a higher load in the following microcycles, depending upon the objectives of the training phase. For example (4-week microcycle):

- Week 1–4:        3–4 sets of 12–15 reps
- Week 5–8:        3–5 sets of 8–12 reps
- Week 9–12:       3–4 sets of 4–8 reps
- Week 13–16:      3–5 sets of 1–4 reps

The linear model fits well for sports that have a competitive schedule containing few, selected competitions, typically with one or two major competitions per year, for example, athletics, rowing, cycling.

A more recent strength training model has been formalized in which the athlete trains all of the different training components (repetition ranges) within a microcycle of 1–2 weeks, known as undulating periodization. The undulating strength programme accounts for sports with more frequent and perhaps unpredictable competition patterns, such as football, hockey and netball. An example of an undulating programme (7–10 day microcycle):

- Monday:       3–4 sets of 12–15 reps
- Wednesday:    3–5 sets of 8–12 reps
- Friday:       3–4 sets of 4–8 reps
- Monday:       3–5 sets of 1–5 reps

Whereas research into the effects of periodization versus non-varied programmes is relatively limited it would appear that periodized programmes (both linear and undulating) yield greater results in strength performance. Linear and undulating models of periodization do not show a clear benefit above each other. The practitioner should apply or adapt the periodized model that best suits the training and competitive needs of the athlete or team.

## KEY POINTS AND OVERVIEW

When the musculoskeletal system is presented with high-level loading it responds dynamically by adapting the command, architecture, morphology and biochemistry of its tissues in order to be better equipped to withstand and generate high level forces. Appropriate mechanical overload is achieved with a maximal or near-maximal resistance that can only performed for few repetitions, with full volitional effort.

1. Muscular hypertrophy seems best achieved by performing multiple sets of 8–12 repetitions with a moderate to high resistance, with 1–3 minutes of recovery between sets.
2. Enhanced neural command is best stimulated by the use of multiple sets of 1–6 repetitions with a very high resistance, with 3–6 minutes of recovery between sets.
3. For continuous strength development strength workouts should be performed two or three times per week. For maximum, long-term strength development, resistance training should be performed 3–6 times per week in a progressive periodized plan.
4. Sports that have infrequent competitions may best utilize a linear periodized programme, whereas unpredictable and/or frequent competition sports would be advised to use an undulating periodization plan for maximum strength training gains.

## References

American College of Sports Medicine Position Stand 1998 The recommended quantity and quality of exercise for developing and maintaining cardiorespiratory and muscular fitness in healthy adults. Medicine and Science in Sports and Exercise 30:975–991

Brown AB, McCartney N, Moroz D et al 1988 Strength training effects in aging. Medicine and Science in Sports and Exercise 20:S80

Daughaday WH 2000 Growth hormone axis overview – somatomedin hypothesis. Pediatric Nephrology 14(7):537–540

Desmedt JE, Godaux E 1977 Ballistic contractions in man: characteristic recruitment pattern of single motor units of the tibialis muscle. Journal of Physiology 264:673–694

Dudley GA, Tesch PA, Miller BJ, Buchannan P 1991 Importance of eccentric actions in performance adaptations to resistance training. Aviation, Space and Environmental Medicine 62:543–550

Fiatarone MA, O'Neill EF, Ryan ND et al 1994 Exercise training and nutritional supplementation for physical frailty in very elderly people. New England Journal of Medicine 330:1819–1820

Fleck SJ, Kraemer WJ 1997 Designing resistance training programs, 2nd edn. Human Kinetics, Leeds, p 21–24

Fleck SJ, Schutt RC 1985 Types of strength training. Clinics in Sports Medicine 4:150–169

Häkkinen K 2002 Training specific characteristics of neuromuscular performance. In: Kraemer WJ & Häkkinen K (eds) Strength training for sport. Blackwell Scientific, Oxford

Häkkinen K, Komi PV 1983 Electromyographic changes during strength training and detraining. Medicine and Science in Sports and Exercise 15:455–460

Häkkinen K, Komi PV, Tesch P 1981 Effect of combined concentric and eccentric strength training on force-time, muscle fiber and metabolic characteristics of leg extensor muscles. Scandanavian Journal of Sports Sciences 3:50–58

Häkkinen K, Kallinen M, Izquierdo M et al 1998 Changes in agonist-antagonist EMG, muscle CSA, and force during strength training in middle-aged and older people. Journal of Applied Physiology 84:1341–1349

Henneman E, Somjen G, Carpenter DO 1965 Functional significance of cell size in spinal motoneurones. Journal of Neurophysiology 28:560–580

Knuttgen HG, Kraemer WJ 1987 Terminology and measurement in exercise performance. Journal of Applied Sports Science Research 1:1–10

Komi PV, Souminen H, Heikkinen E et al 1982 Effects of heavy resistance and explosive-type strength training methods on mechanical, functional and metabolic aspects of performance. In: Komi PV et al (eds) Exercise and sport biology. Human Kinetics, Leeds, p 90–102

Kraemer WJ, Häkkinen K 2002 Strength training for sport. Blackwell Scientific, Oxford

Lee JB, Matsumoto T, Othman T et al 1999 Coactivation of the flexor muscles as a synergist with the extensors during ballistic finger extension movement in trained kendo and karate athletes. International Journal of Sport Medicine 20:7–11

MacDougall JD, Sale DG, Moroz JR et al 1979 Mitochondrial volume density in human skeletal muscle following heavy resistance training. Medicine and Science in Sports 11:164–166

MacDougall JD, Sale DG, Elder GCB et al 1984 Muscle fiber number in biceps brachii in bodybuilders and control subjects. Journal of Applied Physiology 57:1399–1403

Moritani T, DeVries HA 1980 Neural factors versus hypertrophy in the time course of muscle strength gains. American Journal of Physical Medicine 82:521–524

Moritani T, deVries HA 1979 Neural factors versus hypertrophy in the time course of muscle strength gain. American Journal of Physical Medicine 58(3):115–130

Ploutz LL, Tesch PA, Biro RL, Dudley GA 1994 Effect of resistance training on muscle use during exercise. Journal of Applied Physiology 76:1675–1681

Pollock ML, Leggett SH, Graves JE et al 1989 Effect of resistance training on lumbar extension strength. American Journal of Sports Medicine 17:624–629

Sale DG 1992 Neural adaptation to strength training. In: Komi PV (ed.) Strength and power in sport. Blackwell Scientific, Oxford, p 249–265

Staron RS, Leonardi MJ, Karapondo DL et al 1991 Strength and skeletal muscle adaptation in heavy resistance-trained women after detraining and retraining. Journal of Applied Physiology 70:631–640

Staron RS, Karapondo DL, Kraemer WJ et al 1994 Skeletal muscle adaptations during the early phase of heavy resistance training in men and women. Journal of Applied Physiology 76:1247–1255

## Further reading

Dudley GA, Fleck SJ 1987 Strength and endurance training: Are they mutually exclusive? Sports Medicine 4:79–85

Fleck SJ, Kraemer WJ 1997 Designing resistance training programs, 2nd edn. Human Kinetics, Leeds, p 21–24

Komi PV 2002 Strength and power in sport, 2nd edn. Blackwell Scientific, Oxford

Siff MC 2003 Supertraining, 6th edn. Supertraining Institute, Denver

# Chapter 8

# The physiology of training and the environment

Gregory Whyte

## CHAPTER CONTENTS

## LEARNING OBJECTIVES:

This chapter is intended to ensure that the reader:

1. Comprehends the heat balance equation.
2. Appreciates the physiological responses to exercise in the cold.

3. Appreciates the impact of exercise in the cold on health.
4. Recognizes the signs of cold injury.
5. Recognizes the impact of exercise in the cold on performance.
6. Appreciates the impact of exercise in the cold on special populations.
7. Appreciates the physiological responses to exercise in the heat.
8. Appreciates the impact of exercise in the heat on health.
9. Recognizes the signs of heat illness.
10. Recognizes the impact of exercise in the heat on performance.
11. Comprehends ways in which heat stress can be minimized.
12. Understands the physiological responses to acute hypoxia.
13. Understands the physiological adaptations to chronic hypoxia.
14. Appreciates the different methods of altitude training.
15. Understands the role of hypoxic training in training.
16. Recognizes the adverse effects of hypoxia on performance and health.

## INTRODUCTION

While the limit of human performance remains the subject of much conjecture and debate, what is irrefutable is the impact of the environment upon athletic performance. Environmental conditions not only have a profound effect on performance but can also be potentially detrimental to health. Despite the known effects of environmental extremes on performance, sporting events are often programmed in some of the planet's most inhospitable venues, at the most inappropriate time. An historical review of the Olympic marathon suggested that not only have times been affected by environmental factors, but also that drop-out rates and health have been the product of environmental extremes. Early Olympic marathons saw a drop-out rate of up to 56%; however, despite advancing knowledge regarding the environment and performance, the drop out rate remains at about 20%. These data suggest that, despite advances in coaching and sports science, we remain at the mercy of the environment (Pfeisser & Reilly 2004).

This chapter examines the main environmental conditions experienced during training and competition: heat, cold and altitude. Each section discusses the physiological and performance impact of each environment and reviews the strategies employed to reduce their impact.

## TRAINING AND THE COLD

### INTRODUCTION

Athletes competing in the traditional winter sports, including the skiing sports (alpine, cross-country, biathlon, jumping), ice sports (figure and speed skating, curling) and sliding sports (bobsleigh, luge, skeleton), regularly train in cold environments for prolonged periods of time. In addition, most non-winter sport athletes spend a great deal of time throughout the year training in cold conditions that often approach those experienced by winter sport athletes. As previously mentioned, environmental conditions can have a profound effect on performance. It appears, however, that the optimum temperature for endurance performance is between 10 and 15°C. As temperatures decline below this point performance and health are affected negatively.

## TRAINING IN THE COLD AND HEALTH

Cold environmental conditions impose a significant challenge in the maintenance of core temperature. If core temperature falls significantly enough to affect physiological function, 'hypothermia' (defined as a 20°C fall in core temperature) may result, leading to a variety of complications (see Summary box 8.1). In addition, skin temperature may be reduced dramatically, and if this is not carefully monitored cold injury, including frostbite, can occur.

---

**Summary box 8.1**

Risk factors and treatment of hypothermia. Reproduced with permission from Tipton M (2005) Environmental factors. In: Whyte G et al (eds) *ABC of Sports Medicine*, BMJ Books, London.

**Hypothermia**
Hypothermia exists when deep body temperature falls below 35°C. Risk factors for hypothermia include:
- Cold air/water temperature
- Air/water movement: faster moving fluids increase convective heat loss
- Age: children cool faster than adults due to their lower levels of subcutaneous fat and higher surface area to mass ratio
- Body stature: tall thin individuals cool faster than short fat people
- Body morphology: body fat and unperfused muscle are good insulators
- Gender: females tend to have more subcutaneous fat than men
- Fitness: high fitness enables higher heat production
- Fatigue: exhaustion results in decreased heat production
- Nutritional state: hypoglycaemia attenuates shivering and accentuates cooling
- Intoxication: drug or alcohol depressant effects on metabolism
- Lack of appropriate clothing

**Out of hospital treatment of hypothermia**
- Lay casualty flat, give essential first aid, enquire about coexisting illness.
- Prevent further heat loss (blankets/sleeping bag) – cover head, leave airway clear.
- Insulate from the ground.
- If possible provide shelter from the wind and rain.
- Allow slow spontaneous re-warming to occur; re-warming too quickly can result in re-warming collapse.
- Maintain close observation of pulse and respiration.
- Obtain help as soon as possible and transport the casualty to hospital.
- If breathing is absent, becomes obstructed or stops, standard expired air ventilation should be instituted.
- Chest compression should be started only if:
  - There is not carotid pulse detectable after palpating for at least 1 minute (the pulse is slow and weak in hypothermia), AND
  - Cardiac arrest is observed, or there is a reasonable possibility that a cardiac arrest occurred within the previous 2 hours, AND
  - There is a reasonable expectation that effective CPR can be provided continuously until the casualty reaches more advanced life support. This is likely to mean being within 2 hours of a suitable hospital.
- The rates of expired air ventilation and chest compression should be the same as for normothermic casualties. Hypothermia may cause stiffness of the chest wall.

The impact of cold on an exercising individual is dependent upon whether the exercise is undertaken in air or water. Water is 25 times more conductive than air, leading to a 3–5 times faster heat loss compared with air at the same temperature (Nimmo 2004). The body will also cool quicker when air or water is moved across the skin due to increased convection. Therefore, if the water/air is moving over the skin, or the body is moving through water/air, the rate of heat loss will be greater. Obviously, the temperature has a marked effect on the rate of heat loss; however, in air, wind speed, body composition and body size play a significant role in the rate of heat loss. In air, an increasing wind speed will increase the rate of heat loss, resulting in wind chill (see Fig. 8.1). Rapid skin cooling on immersion in cold water evokes a set of cardiorespiratory responses that include uncontrollable hyperventilation, hypertension and increased cardiac workload, which can be precursors to cardiovascular accidents and drowning (Tipton 2005).

Individuals with a high body surface area to body mass ratio will lose heat at a faster rate. In other words, tall individuals with low body weight will lose heat faster

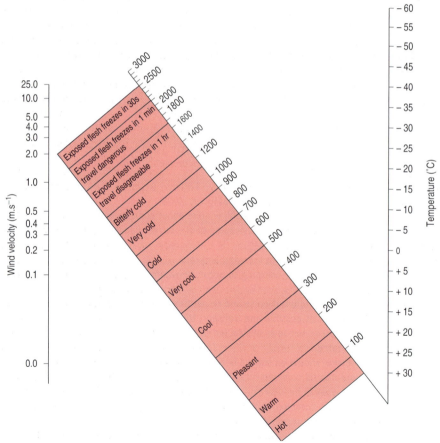

**Figure 8.1** Relationship between ambient temperature and wind speed, and perception of cold and risk of cold injury. Reproduced from Siple P & Pasel C (1945) Measurement of dry atmospheric cooling in subfreezing temperatures. *Proceedings of the American Philosophical Society* 89:177–199.

than short, heavy individuals. Body fat is the key insulator, and those individuals with high body fat will lose heat at a slower rate than thin individuals. It is important to note that in air a wet individual will lose heat at a greater rate than if they were dry. Therefore, care should be taken in cold weather if it is snowing/raining, or the individual is sweating excessively due to inappropriate clothing.

## PERFORMANCE IN THE COLD

The skin is the first tissue to cool on exposure to low environmental temperatures. The next tissues to cool are the superficial nerves and muscles. As a result the conduction of action potentials is slowed (15 m.s$^{-1}$ per 10°C fall in local temperature) and their amplitude reduced. Below a muscle temperature of 27°C the contractile force and rate of force application is reduced and fatigue occurs earlier – maximum power output falls by 3% per °C fall in muscle temperature (Reilly & Waterhouse 2004). As a consequence, speed of movement, dexterity, strength and mechanical efficiency are all reduced with cooling, potentially leading to incapacitation.

During low-intensity exercise in air, including walking, there is a danger that heat production will not be sufficient to counteract heat loss. However, if precautions are taken to combat the cold low-intensity exercise can be safely undertaken. Appropriate clothing is of key importance. Finding a balance, however, may be a difficult task. A balance must be sought between maintaining core/skin temperature and excessive insulation leading to a rise in core temperature and resultant sweat production. This sweat production can lead to wet clothing that may effect heat balance, particularly if exercise intensity falls, or the individual rests. Of greater concern is the potential for cold injury to the extremities (i.e. hands, face and feet). In air or water, the first tissue to be affected on exposure to cold is the skin. Skin cooling is accentuated by the peripheral vasoconstriction initiated by the body in order to reduce heat loss. It is the extremities that are most likely to be affected due to their high surface area to mass ratio, and the fact that their major source of heat, blood flow, has been restricted by vasoconstriction. This, in part, explains why it is the extremities that normally receive cold injuries (Tipton 2005).

During moderate and high-intensity exercise in air i.e. running or cycling, while performance may be reduced at temperatures below 10°C there is little concern for core temperature irrespective of clothing. Obviously care must be taken to avoid cold injury of the extremities. Similar findings have been observed for maximal and supra-maximal exercise in the cold (Nimmo 2004). When training in the cold, however, care is warranted during recovery between reps and sets and immediately following the session. During these periods of light exercise rapid cooling of the periphery and core may occur as a result of sweat accumulation and limited clothing. If training in cold water cooling will be exacerbated. Training prescription should account for low environmental temperatures. A thorough warm-up performed indoors where possible immediately prior to training, limiting the period of inactivity prior to starting the session. Care should be taken in the choice of clothing for training sessions, with the aim to balance heat production with heat loss. Reducing recovery periods and tailoring warm-down for indoor/sheltered spaces helps to avoid cooling during and post-training.

In cold water, a fall in deep body temperature intensifies shivering, which raises oxygen consumption during sub-maximal exercise (9% in water at 25°C; 25.3% in water at 18°C) (Tipton 2005). Thus, the energy cost of sub-maximal exercise is increased in water cooler than 26°C; this can result in a more rapid depletion of carbohydrate and lipid energy sources and earlier onset of fatigue. $\dot{V}O_2$max, during ergometry or swimming, and maximum performance are reduced during cold water immersion. This reduction occurs in water temperature as high as 25°C and is approximately linearly related to deep body temperature, with a 10–30% reduction observed following a 0.5–2°C fall in deep body temperature. Associated with this reduction in $\dot{V}O_2$max, lactate appears in the blood at lower workloads and accumulates at a more rapid rate suggesting a decreased oxygen supply to the muscle and greater reliance on anaerobic metabolism. A decrease in deep body temperature of 0.5–1.5°C results in a reduction of 10–40% in the capacity to supply oxygen to meet the increased requirements of activity. With more profound cooling, anaerobic metabolism is also reduced due to muscle cooling and direct impairment of the processes responsible for the anaerobic production of energy.

## POST-EXERCISE

Irrespective of exercise intensity care must be taken following exercise due to the potential for rapid post-exercise cooling. Exercise-induced heat production is reduced post-exercise and heat is lost to the environment. In response to this negative thermal balance the body responds in two ways. First, vasoconstriction of the peripheral vasculature occurs, reducing blood flow to the skin and increasing central blood volume and central venous pressure. The reduction in blood flow is variable across different body parts, leaving some areas of skin more susceptible to cold injury. In response to this increased venous pressure, mean blood pressure increases and, despite a cold-induced reduction in heart rate, cardiac output rises. Second, involuntary metabolic heat production occurs leading initially to an increased skeletal muscle tone (pre-shivering) and eventually shivering (muscular thermogenesis). The degree of shivering is related to the individual's aerobic capacity ($\dot{V}O_2$max). At maximum shivering, resting metabolic rate is increased fourfold and equates to approximately 40% of $\dot{V}O_2$max. The response to cold exposure is individual specific and, therefore, some individuals will be affected to a much greater extent than others. It is important to reduce heat loss following exercise in cold environments to avoid possible cold injury. Get out of the cold environment as quickly as possible, remove wet clothing and replace with dry clothing adding extra layers taking care to cover high-risk areas, i.e. hands, feet and head.

It is worthy of note that when exercising in the cold energy consumption increases, primarily in the form of carbohydrates. Therefore, higher quantities of carbohydrate ingestion are recommended when exercising in the cold. Further, the rate of dehydration in the cold can be the same or greater than that experienced in warm conditions. The reasons underpinning this fluid loss are threefold. First, inappropriate clothing can lead to an excessive rise in core temperature leading to high sweat rates (a problem not only for hydration status, but also rapid post-exercise cooling rates). Second, an increased blood pressure associated with peripheral vasoconstriction can lead to an increased diuresis (urine excretion). Third, because cold air tends to be dry (low relative humidity) large volumes of fluid are lost through respiration (Nimmo 2004). These three factors combined result in significant dehydration during prolonged exercise in the cold. It is, therefore, important to increase fluid and carbohydrate intake in the cold, similar to or greater than warm conditions (Reilly & Waterhouse 2004).

Acclimatization to the cold is limited in comparison to that of heat with limited physiological adaptations. Within 5–6 hours of acute cold exposure thyroxine, adrenaline and adrenocorticoid output is elevated, resulting in an increased metabolic rate. The observed perturbations of peripheral vasoconstriction and vasodilation are altered in cold habituated individuals leading to a reduction in the initial vasoconstrictor response and longer, more frequent episodes of vasodilation. The 'cold shock' response to cold water emersion is reduced in habituated individuals. The adaptations are small in magnitude and are unlikely to occur following transient exposure to the cold. It is, therefore, imperative that behavioural adjustments are made to avoid the deleterious effects of the cold when training.

## COLD INJURY

Due to the pronounced peripheral vasoconstriction during cold exposure, the temperature of the skin and extremities may fall rapidly to temperatures that may lead to cold injuries. Early warning signs of cold injury include tingling, numbness and/or a burning sensation in the extremities (fingers, toes, ears and nose). If action is not taken at this point tissue damage resulting in cold injuries may occur. Cold injuries can be of the 'freezing' (frostbite; FCI) or non-freezing variety (non-freezing cold injury, NFCI).

Human tissue freezes at about $-0.55°C$. Rapid cooling leading to the formation of intracellular crystals results in direct mechanical disruption of the tissues. In contrast, slow cooling and freezing results in extracellular water crystallization that increases plasma and interstitial fluid osmotic pressure. The resulting osmotic outflow of intracellular fluid raises intracellular osmotic pressure and can cause damage to capillary walls. This, along with the local reduction in plasma volume, causes ooedema, reduced local blood flow and encourages capillary sludging. These changes can produce thrombosis and a gangrenous extremity. The risk of frostbite is low above air temperatures of $-7°C$, irrespective of wind speed, and becomes pronounced when ambient temperature is below $-25°C$, even at low wind speeds (Tipton 2005).

Non-freezing cold injury (NFCI) describes a condition that results from protracted exposure to low ambient thermal conditions, in the absence of freezing. Immobility, posture, dehydration, low fitness, inadequate nutrition, constricting footwear, fatigue, stress or anxiety, concurrent illness or injury can all increase the likelihood of NFCI. The precise pathophysiology of NFCI is poorly understood but appears to be related to the neuro-endothelio-muscular components of the walls of local blood vessels. Debate continues as to whether the primary damage is vascular or neural in origin; or, whether the aetiology is primarily thermal, ischaemic, post-ischaemic reperfusion, or hypoxic in origin (Tipton 2005).

Treatment depends on whether the dominant injury is FCI or NFCI. All cases of FCI should be thoroughly re-warmed by immersion of all the chilled part in stirred water at $38–42°C$. A topical antibacterial should also be diluted into the water bath. Re-warming should be delayed if there is a chance that re-freezing may occur. Thawing an FCI can be intensely painful and conventional narcotic analgesics should be provided as necessary. Continuing treatment for FCI is a twice daily, 30-minute immersion of the affected part in a $38–42°C$ whirlpool bath containing an appropriate antibacterial. In contrast to those with FCI, patients with NFCI should have their affected extremities re-warmed slowly, by exposure to warm air alone, and must not be immersed in warm water. The early period after re-warming can be very painful in NFCI, even in those without any obvious tissue damage. With either form of injury, once re-warmed, the affected extremities should be treated by exposure to air and early mobilization (Tipton 2005).

It is unusual for the respiratory tract and lungs to be in danger of damage when training in the cold. The air is warmed and moistened rapidly during inspiration to avoid potential damage. This moistening/humidification of the inspired air can result in airway drying; however, that may lead to respiratory complaints, including dryness of the mouth, a burning sensation in the throat, and general irritation of the respiratory tract. Cold air inhalation may worsen asthma symptoms in those that suffer from the disease, and may even lead to the development of exercise-induced asthma in an otherwise normal individual. In order to reduce these symptoms, the wearing of a scarf or face mask will improve humidification of the inspired air and reduce water loss.

## SPECIAL POPULATIONS

Elderly individuals are less able to maintain core temperature, and as such are at higher risk of hypothermia and cold injury. Children are also less able to maintain core temperature due to a higher body surface area to body mass ratio. Children counteract this in part by increasing peripheral vasoconstriction; however, this results in an increased potential for cold injury. Additional precautions for the young and elderly should be taken when training in cold environments.

## CONCLUSIONS

In general, cold presents less of an immediate threat to the exercising individual than hot/humid conditions. Rarely is it too cold to train if the correct precautions are taken to avoid hypothermia and cold injury. In general, however, when the temperature falls to below −20°C (−5°F) extreme caution should be taken, and exercise avoided (Fig. 8.2). The most significant problems associated with training in the cold are cold injury and hypothermia. Take careful note of environmental conditions, including wind chill, and take steps to avoid excessive heat loss before, during and after exercise, and protect the extremities from cold injury.

## KEY POINTS

1. Cold environments have a limited impact on performance when the correct precautions are taken to avoid hypothermia and cold injury.
2. Water is 25 times more conductive than air leading to a 3–5 times faster heat loss compared with air at the same temperature.

| Wind speed (mph) | Thermometer reading (°F) | | | | | | | | | | |
|---|---|---|---|---|---|---|---|---|---|---|---|
| | 50 | 40 | 30 | 20 | 10 | 0 | −10 | −20 | −30 | −40 | −50 |
| | Equivalent temperature (°F) | | | | | | | | | | |
| 5 | 48 | 37 | 27 | 16 | 6 | −5 | −15 | −26 | −36 | −47 | −57 |
| 10 | 40 | 28 | 16 | 4 | −9 | −24 | −33 | −46 | −58 | −70 | −83 |
| 15 | 36 | 22 | 9 | −5 | −18 | −32 | −45 | −58 | −72 | −85 | −99 |
| 20 | 32 | 18 | 4 | −10 | −25 | −39 | −53 | −67 | −82 | −96 | −110 |
| 25 | 30 | 16 | 0 | −15 | −29 | −44 | −59 | −74 | −88 | −104 | −118 |
| 30 | 28 | 13 | −2 | −18 | −33 | −48 | −63 | −79 | −94 | −109 | −125 |
| 35 | 27 | 11 | −4 | −20 | −35 | −51 | −67 | −82 | −98 | −113 | −129 |
| 40 | 26 | 10 | −6 | −21 | −37 | −53 | −69 | −85 | −100 | −115 | −132 |
| | Minimal risk | | | | Increasing risk | | | Great risk | | | |

Figure 8.2  Wind chill index.

3. Individuals with a high body surface area to body mass ratio will lose heat at a faster rate.
4. A balance must be sought between maintaining core/skin temperature and excessive insulation leading to a rise in core temperature and resultant sweat production.
5. Care should be taken after exercise to avoid hypothermia and cold injury.
6. There are limited physiological adaptations to the cold.
7. Of greatest concern in cold environments is the potential for cold injury to the extremities (i.e. hands, face and feet), including non-freezing and freezing cold injury.

## TRAINING AND THE HEAT

### INTRODUCTION

Core temperature is tightly controlled within about 1°C of 37°C and skin temperatures of about 33°C. Humans can survive a fall in core temperature of about 10°C and an increase of about 6°C (Tipton 2005). The balance between heat gained and heat lost is tightly regulated to maintain thermal homeostasis. During exercise the two most potent stimuli challenging thermal homeostasis are metabolic heat production (M), directly associated with measurable external work (W), and environmental conditions. The exchange of heat between the body and the environment is achieved through convection (C), conduction (K), radiation (R) and evaporation (E) and the relationship between heat gain and heat loss is represented by the heat balance equation: $M - W = R \pm C \pm K - E$.

The most potent stimulus to variations in metabolic heat production (M) is muscle activity including exercise or shivering. The human is only 25% efficient with 75% of the chemical energy produced during muscular contraction being lost as heat. During sustained vigorous exercise heat production can reach in excess of 20 kJ. If the body were prevented from losing any of the heat it produced a fatal level of heat storage would be reached in about 4 hours at rest, and after just 25 minutes with moderate exercise (Tipton 2005).

The primary aim of the thermoregulatory system is to maintain body temperature within safe limits. This is achieved by a complex combination of cold and warm receptors, afferent and efferent pathways, central nervous system integrating and controlling centres, and effectors. In air at 25–28°C, or water at 35°C, a naked, resting individual can maintain body temperature by varying the amount of heat delivered to the skin via the circulation, in this situation cutaneous blood flow averages 250 mL.min$^{-1}$. As air/water temperature falls, or increases, the physiological responses of shivering or sweating are initiated in an attempt to defend body temperature. These autonomic responses have only a limited capability to defend body temperature and are costly in terms of substrate and fluid.

Training in cold and hot environments can have a profound effect on performance and health. Recognition of the physiological mechanisms associated with exercise in the cold and heat are crucial to avoid the deleterious effects of these environments. Identification and implementation of strategies to ameliorate their impact will enhance training performance and reduce the risk of injury.

Training in high ambient temperatures can have a profound effect on performance and health. The impact of heat on training performance is highly dependent on the ambient temperature, humidity and radiant heat, combined with the intensity, duration and mode of exercise and whether the event takes place outdoors or indoors.

During exercise metabolic heat production may increase 25-fold compared with resting conditions. Core temperature rises in association with the balance of heat production and dissipation and the metabolic heat produced during exercise, together with heat gained by convection, conduction and radiation, must be matched by the heat loss to maintain homeostasis. The primary mechanism for heat dissipation is through evaporative sweat loss. In order to facilitate evaporative sweat loss during exercise the cardiovascular system responds by re-directing blood flow (cardiac output) from the splanchnic and renal beds to the skin. The sweat glands are activated within seconds of commencing exercise and reach maximum output after 30 minutes. The rate of evaporative sweat loss depends on skin surface area that is wet, the difference between the water vapour pressure at the skin surface and that in the air, and air movement around the body (Tipton 2005). It is sweat evaporation that is fundamental to the dissipation of heat, not sweat production. In humid conditions the increase in water vapour pressure in the air reduces the potential for evaporative sweat loss and therefore impedes heat dissipation. When relative humidity is 100% no sweat will evaporate. The use of wet bulb globe temperature (WBGT) is more effective in determining heat stress as it takes into account humidity and radiant heat (Summary box 8.2):

$$WBGT = 0.1\, T_{db} + 0.7\, T_{wb} + 0.2\, T_g$$

in which $T_{db}$ = dry bulb temperature, $T_{wb}$ = wet bulb temperature, and $T_g$ = globe temperature.

The associated body fluid loss during training in the heat due to increased sweating can lead to hypohydration if fluid loss outweighs fluid intake and absorption. Daily water turnover for sedentary individuals living in a temperate environment is typically about 2–3 L.day$^{-1}$. In contrast, athletes training intensively in the heat can lose up to 10–15 L of fluid per day, with most of the increase coming from sweat losses (Maughan & Shirreffs 2004). Hypohydration can lead to a lowered plasma volume resulting in a reduced venous return. In response to a reduced venous return, heart rate will rise to maintain cardiac output in the face of the reduced stroke volume. This progressive rise in heart rate, independent of exercise intensity is termed 'cardiovascular drift'. It is important to account for heat-related rises in heart rate during training to maintain the appropriate training workloads.

In addition to performance, exercise in the heat can lead to a spectrum of health issues termed 'heat illness'. The risk of heat illness is increased if exercise is undertaken in the heat in a dehydrated condition.

## TRAINING PERFORMANCE AND THE HEAT

It is well recognized that outdoor endurance events and team sports are negatively affected by the heat. The observed decrement in performance becomes progressively

---

**Summary box 8.2**

The American College of Sports Medicine (ACSM) WBGT recommendations for continuous activities such as running and cycling.

| | |
|---|---|
| < 18°C | Low risk |
| 18–23°C | Moderate risk |
| 23–28°C | High risk. Those with predisposing factors for heat illness should not compete |
| > 28°C | Very high risk. Postpone competition |

greater as heat rises (Galloway & Maughan 1997). In outdoor, short-duration, high-intensity events, i.e. sprinting, there may be no loss of functional capacity when individuals are acutely exposed to a hot environment. Indeed, performance may be improved. While short-duration and indoor events may be unaffected by environmental heat stress in the short term there is a real risk that a chronic fluid deficit associated with prolonged periods of time spent exercising at low intensities during training or at rest in the heat will result from a failure to increase fluid intake sufficiently to match fluid losses (Shirreffs & Maughan 1998). The effect of hypohydration on training performance will depend on the degree of hypohydration and the nature of the activity. During endurance activity hypohydration causes an increased reliance on muscle glycogen as fuel for exercise as evidenced by elevated blood lactate values for the same absolute workload and a reduced anaerobic threshold (Reilly & Waterhouse 2005). A pre-exercise fluid deficit of as little as 1.5–2% of body mass is likely to reduce performance and has been shown to cause substantial loss of performance in running events lasting from 4 to 30 minutes (Shirreffs & Maughan 1998). In high-intensity short-duration activity the distance travelled in each effort is reduced in the heat. Thus, sprint and team game training is likely to be affected in the heat.

The reduction in performance in the heat is in part due to the progressive dehydration that results from sweat losses, with negative consequences for cardiovascular capacity and thermoregulatory function (Gonzalez-Alonso et al 1999a). Recent evidence suggests that the central nervous system (CNS) may play a key role in the fatigue process in the heat, and that the fundamental limitation to performance in the heat may be localized to the CNS rather than the muscles evidenced by a critical brain temperature in addition to core body temperature (Nielsen et al 2001, Nielsen & Nybo 2003).

## ACCLIMATION, ACCLIMATIZATION AND HEAT EXPERIENCE

Repeated exposure to the heat produces increases in core and skin temperature and profuse sweating resulting in physiological (and behavioural) adaptations that reduce the impact of heat on exercise performance. The magnitude of the adaptation to heat that occurs is closely related to the degree of heat strain to which the individual is exposed. Exercise during heat exposure is important in optimizing the adaptations as resting in heat only provides partial acclimatization. The adaptations observed following chronic training in the heat include the following:

- increased plasma volume;
- less cardiovascular strain;
- more effective distribution of cardiac output;
- improved cutaneous blood flow;
- earlier onset and increased rate of sweating;
- lowered salt content in sweat;
- more effective distribution of sweat over the skin surface;
- lower skin and deep body temperatures for same absolute intensity;
- improved physical work capacity;
- increased comfort;
- decreased reliance on carbohydrate metabolism;
- decreased pre-exercise core temperature.

Adaptation to heat can be achieved in two ways: (i) train and live in a hot climate (acclimatization), and (ii) train in an artificial climate (acclimation). Often athletes travel to hot environments for 'warm weather training camps' during the winter months. The reduction in exercise capacity following acute exposure to the heat often means that training intensity and volumes are reduced for at least the first few days of the training camp while acclimatization occurs. In order to avoid this loss in training volume and reduce the impact of other environmental stressors, including jet lag and travel fatigue associated with travel to the camp, acclimation to the heat prior to departure may be advantageous.

Acclimatization/acclimation is best achieved by performing moderate intensity exercise for 60–100 minutes per day in conditions similar to those expected during training. There appears to be no advantage in spending longer periods of exposure to the heat (Lind & Bass 1963). Indeed, recent evidence suggests that shorter duration exercise (30 minutes) at higher intensities (75% $\dot{V}O_2$max) may be as effective (Houmard et al 1990). Intermittent exercise may also be an effective alternative to continuous exercise for team game and sprint-based athletes. The total exposure time, including short breaks, should again be 100 minutes for the optimal adaptation.

Within the first few days of training in the heat some adaptations are observed and adaptation is complete for most individuals within 7–14 days. It is not necessary to train every day in the heat, but no more than 2–3 days should elapse between exposures. Adaptations to heat persist for some time following exposure. In athletes who are fully acclimatized the major benefits are maintained for up to 7 days and some of the improved responses are still present after as long as 21 days in a cool climate (Pichan et al 1985).

It is important to note that every athlete responds differently to the heat, and the extent and duration of adaptation required will vary between individuals. There appears to be no way to predict the response of individual athletes (Montain et al 1996). Care is warranted in the use of heat acclimation/acclimatization if acute heat injury is to be avoided (Sutton 1990). The fatalities that have occurred in recent years in pre-season training in American football serve as a reminder of the possible consequences of trying to adapt too quickly.

## Heat experience

Repeated exposure to the heat during training allows athletes to develop a variety of strategies that can significantly enhance performance. The use of training sessions to help the coach and athlete identify, adapt and implement these strategies is an important role of heat exposure. Strategies developed to reduce the deleterious effects of heat on performance include the identification of optimal volume, composition and timing of fluid ingestion; clothing; and pacing strategies. In team games, identifying strategies specific to individual player responses and capabilities in the heat is an important part of heat experience.

## HEAT ILLNESS

Hyperthermia (overheating) and hypohydration (loss of body water) lead to a spectrum of conditions termed heat illness. The conditions range from simple heat cramps to heat stroke and death (Summary box 8.3).

The problems caused by training in the heat result from a decreased circulating blood volume and consequent alterations in regional blood flow, an increased blood viscosity, and a direct effect of temperature on the respiratory centres and proteins. High ambient temperatures are not always necessary to cause heat illness. Cool or

## Summary box 8.3

Heat illness. Adapted from Tipton M (2005) Environmental factors. In: Whyte G et al (eds) *ABC of Sports Medicine*, BMJ Books, London.

### Heat illness

**Heat cramps:** usually occur in the specific muscles exercised due to an imbalance in the body's fluid volume and electrolyte concentration, and low energy stores. Core temperature remains in normal range. Aetiology unknown. Can be prevented by an appropriate rehydration strategy and treated by stretching and massage.

**Heat exhaustion:** the most common form of heat illness, defined as the inability to continue exercise in the heat. Usually seen in unacclimatized individuals. Caused by ineffective circulatory adjustments and reduced blood volume. Characterized by breathlessness, hyperventilation, weak and rapid pulse, low blood pressure, dizziness, headache, flushed skin, nausea, paradoxical chills, irritability, lethargy and general weakness. Deep body temperature is raised, but not excessively, sweating persists and there is no organ damage. Heat exhausted individuals should stop exercising, lie down, control breathing if hyperventilating and rehydrate; failure to do so can result in progression to severe heat illness. Heat exhaustion is a predominant problem when body water loss exceeds 7% of body mass.

**Heat stroke:** medical emergency resulting from failure of the thermoregulatory system as a result of a high deep body temperature ($>40.5°C$). Characterized by confusion, absence of sweating, hot and dry skin, circulatory instability. If not treated by immediate cooling, results in death from circulatory collapse and multi-organ damage. Aggressive steps should be taken to cool the casualty as mortality is related to the degree and duration of hyperthermia. Consider using 'artificial sweat' (spraying with tepid water/alcohol) and fanning; fluid replacement (do not over-infuse/overload; can result in pulmonary oedema). Consider colder water immersion/ice packs for those without a peripheral circulation.

Heat stroke should be the working diagnosis in anyone who has an altered mental state. Deep body temperature should be monitored every 5 minutes; deep (15 cm) rectal temperature is preferable to mouth or ear canal as these may be influenced by hyperventilation and/or the active cooling strategy employed. Heat exhausted individuals should improve rapidly with appropriate immediate care. Any individuals who do not improve quickly should be evacuated to the next level of medical care. Recovery from exertional heat stroke is idiosyncratic and in severe cases may take up to a year.

**Exertional rhabdomyolysis:** is caused by muscle damage resulting in the release of cellular contents (e.g. myoglobin, potassium, phosphate, creatine kinase and uric acid) into the circulation. More likely if dehydrated or taking non-steroidal anti-inflammatory drugs. Overt signs include muscle pain, tenderness and weakness, very dark urine. Treat by giving fluids, evacuate to intensive medical care, kidney function should be assessed.

temperate conditions can lead to heat illness if humidity is high, or individuals are unable to dissipate the heat produced from high work rates due to clothing. There are a large number of factors that influence an athlete's ability to thermoregulate and alter their susceptibility to heat illness (Summary box 8.4). Because some of these factors can operate acutely (e.g. infection), an individual may suffer heat illness in circumstances in which they were previously unaffected (Tipton 2005).

### Summary box 8.4

Factors influencing thermoregulation and an individual's susceptibility to heat illness. Adapted from Tipton M (2005) Environmental factors. In: Whyte G et al (eds) *ABC of Sports Medicine*, BMJ Books, London.

- Air temperature, humidity, movement, radiant heat load
- Body size (mass, skinfold thickness) – heat stroke occurs 3.5 times more frequently in excessively overweight young adults than in individuals of average body mass.
- State of training/sudden increase in training (military recruits with low aerobic fitness (>12 mins for 1.5 mile run) and a high body mass index (>26 kg.m$^{-2}$) have a ninefold greater risk of heat illness).
- Degree of acclimatization
- Hydration status
- Heat production (exercise intensity/duration)
- Clothing worn (vapour permeability, fit, colour)
- State of health (e.g. fever – viral illness, cold, flu; diabetes mellitus, cardiovascular disease, gastroenteritis/diarrhoea)
- Genetic disorders (e.g. mutations for cystic fibrosis, malignant hyperthermia)
- Skin disorders, including sunburn over 5% of body surface area
- Use of medication (e.g. diuretics; antihistamines; ergogenic stimulants)
- Sweat gland dysfunction (e.g. prickly heat)
- Salt depletion
- Age
- Sleep deprivation
- Glycogen or glucose depletion
- Acute/chronic alcohol/drug abuse

## MAINTAINING PERFORMANCE AND AVOIDING HEAT ILLNESS

### Rehydration

Replacing sweat losses during and between training sessions is crucial if performance is to be maintained. Sweat is a hypotonic saline solution (0.3–0.6% NaCl) and as a result there may also be associated salt losses when sweat rates are high (Maughan et al 2004). This has implications for the composition of fluids to be consumed as well as the amount of fluid that is necessary. Because of the increased sweat rate observed in acclimatized athletes the need for fluid replacement is greater (Sawka & Pandolf 1990).

When encouraging an increased fluid intake, palatability (taste) is a key factor (Passe 2001). Care must be taken to avoid excessive fluid consumption as there is a danger of developing dilutional hyponatraemia resulting in collapse and even death if electrolyte-containing foods or drinks are not consumed (Hew et al 2003, Smith 2002). This problem seems to affect only slower runners during prolonged exercise (>4–6 hours). Athletes should be aware of this and of the need to ensure an adequate salt intake (Bergeron 1996). Fluids consumed during training can usefully contain some carbohydrate and electrolytes, especially sodium (Murray & Stofan 2001) and a properly formulated sports drink containing 2–8% carbohydrate and up to 50 mmol.L$^{-1}$ of sodium is likely to be the best option in most situations (Maughan 2001). The volume and composition of human sweat varies widely between individuals, and the need for fluid and electrolyte replacement therefore varies accordingly.

Where rapid replacement of fluid losses is a priority after training or competition, athletes should aim to drink sufficient fluid to replace about 1.5 times the amount of sweat lost: if this fluid contains no electrolytes, foods containing salt should be consumed at this time (Shirreffs et al 1996). This recommendation may be especially important when multiple training sessions are undertaken in a single day.

Monitoring of body mass changes before and after training can give some indication as to the extent of sweat loss in training. Further, monitoring of urine parameters, including volume, colour, conductivity, specific gravity or osmolality may help to identify individuals suffering from dehydration (Shirreffs & Maughan 1998) and can provide feedback that athletes find helpful in establishing their fluid requirements.

## Selection of clothing

During training the type and amount of clothing worn can have a major effect on thermal balance. There are a number of key considerations in the selection of clothing for training in the heat. The key factor is to avoid developing a local micro-climate that is restrictive to evaporative sweat loss (Gonzalez 1988). Clothing should be light coloured to reflect more radiant heat and lightweight to minimize insulation and increase exchange of air between the microclimate (beneath the clothing) and environment with body movement ('bellows effect'). To assist the 'bellows effect' the clothing should be loose fitting. Vapour-permeable material that readily absorbs water will enhance the evaporative heat loss. Protection of the head and neck may be especially important when prolonged exposures to direct sunlight are unavoidable. When training in direct sunlight for prolonged periods care should also be taken to avoid sunburn. While some degree of tanning of the skin can be beneficial in reducing the risk of sunburn, even mild sunburn sufficient to cause redness of the skin can impair thermoregulatory capacity and exercise performance for up to 21 days (Pandolf et al 1980). A high factor sunscreen should be used during training.

For some sports, for example fencing and equestrian, wearing protective clothing can exacerbate the thermal load on the athlete, resulting in significantly higher skin and deep body temperatures. The combination of insulating clothing and high levels of metabolic heat production has resulted in cases of fatal heat stroke – the most publicized of which are among American Football players during pre-season training (Tipton 2005).

## Warm-up and pre-cooling

The role of warm-up in temperate climates is to elevate body temperature and increase blood flow to the muscles and associated soft tissues. In hot climates, however, dramatic increases in core temperature should be avoided to reduce the negative impact of hyperthermia on performance. Indeed, there is evidence to suggest that pre-cooling the body may enhance performance in the heat, with time to exhaustion being inversely related to initial body temperature (Gonzalez-Alonso et al 1999b). While whole-body pre-cooling may not be a practical solution during training, improved performance has been reported following skin cooling in the absence of changes in core temperature. Returning body temperature to normal levels between repeated bouts of exercise during training in the heat helps to maintain performance and decreases physiological strain. A quick and simple way of achieving this is by hand immersion in cold water (10°C). The large surface area and high cutaneous blood flow of the hands make them ideal for heat exchange. The rates of heat exchange achieved by this method are similar to those achieved by the use of ice vests or forced convective cooling.

The mechanisms responsible for improved performance following pre-cooling appear to be associated with an increased time to critical temperature during exercise and an enhanced thermal comfort. This is consistent with recent evidence that high core and brain temperatures are a major factor in the aetiology of fatigue during prolonged exercise in the heat (Nybo et al 2002).

Modifications to the warm-up in the heat are required to optimize training. This must be well practised in training, however, to avoid any undue psychological impact of altering warm-up rituals on competition performance. Simple modifications include warming up in the shade and reducing the duration and intensity of exercise.

## KEY POINTS

1. During exercise metabolic heat production may increase 25-fold compared with resting conditions.
2. Evaporative sweat loss is the most effective mechanism in core temperature regulation in the heat.
3. Training in high ambient temperatures can have a profound effect on performance and health dependent on ambient temperature, humidity, radiant heat, and the intensity, duration and mode of exercise.
4. There are a number of physiological adaptations to hot environments termed 'acclimatization' that result in improved performance in the heat.
5. Experience of hot environments can enhance performance.
6. In addition to performance, exercise in the heat can lead to a spectrum of health issues termed 'heat illness'.

## ALTITUDE AND TRAINING

### INTRODUCTION

The recent sporting success of high land natives has resulted in an increased interest in the role of living and training at altitude on performance. The primary aim of altitude training for endurance athletes is to increase the red cell mass (RCM) and haemoglobin mass (Hb) resulting in an increased arterial blood $O_2$-carrying capacity, and $\dot{V}O_2$max, with the aim of improving performance at both sea level and altitude. For sprint/power-based athletes, recent studies have reported performance gains following an altitude sojourn probably associated with alterations in acid–base balance.

Rapid ascent to moderate (<3000 m) and high (>3000 m) altitude causes a cascade of physiological responses triggered by hypobaric hypoxia associated with a reduction in barometric pressure (reducing in a curvilinear relationship with increasing altitude) leading to a reduced partial pressure of oxygen. This cascade of physiological responses to hypoxia acts to increase oxygen supply to body tissues with the greatest effect observed in those body systems directly associated with oxygen delivery, i.e. the cardiorespiratory system. Following a period of time these physiological responses lead to adaptation and consequent acclimatization. The time course and success of acclimatization is a function of the interaction between the physiological characteristics of the individual and the magnitude of the hypoxic stress (elevation and speed of ascent). The time course of the physiological responses and adaptations to hypoxia are listed in Figure 8.1 on page 166.

Altitude training currently takes a number of forms including: living high, training high (HiHi); living high, training low (HiLo); living low, training high (LoHi). The development of 'hypoxic hotels', 'altitude tents', and special breathing apparatus have allowed the generation of a hypoxic stimulus at sea level (normobaric) by altering the fraction of inspired oxygen ($FiO_2$).

The benefits of living and training at altitude for an improved altitude performance are clear. Research examining the efficacy of living and training at altitude on low land natives is equivocal, however, with most controlled studies failing to observe a positive effect of hypoxic training on sea-level performance (Rusko et al 2004). The reason for the lack of clarity surrounding the role of altitude training on sea level performance is associated with the equivocal research findings associated with: (i) the use of insufficient altitude (<2000 m) or inadequate period of time at altitude (<3 weeks) to elicit an adaptive response; (ii) de-training at altitude as a result of reduced training volume; (iii) immunosuppression leading to illness and under performance (Rusko et al 2004).

## THE PHYSIOLOGICAL EFFECT OF HYPOXIA

The reduced pressure of inspired oxygen ($P_iO_2$), observed following a reduction in barometric pressure (hypobaric hypoxia) or reduced $FiO_2$ (normobaric hypoxia) results in a decreased $O_2$ partial pressure in arterial blood ($P_aO_2$) and arterial oxygen saturation ($S_aO_2\%$). The observed reduction in $S_aO_2\%$ results in a cascade of acute physiological responses that affect all phases of the oxygen delivery from lung to muscle. The reduced $S_aO_2\%$ stimulates the peripheral and central chemoreceptors causing an immediate increase in ventilation, termed the hypoxic ventilatory response (HVR). This hyperventilation causes a respiratory alkalosis that limits the increase in ventilation during the early stages of altitude exposure. Within several days an increased bicarbonate secretion is observed that compensates for the respiratory alkalosis allowing resting ventilation to increase reaching a maximum in 7–10 days. This increased ventilation is the principal mechanism responsible for improving oxygen availability at the cellular level during acclimatization. Concomitant to an increased ventilation, a decreased plasma volume of 10–20% is observed within hours of altitude exposure. This decrease in plasma volume is related to a shift of fluid from intravascular to interstitial and intracellular compartments. This fluid shift results in an increased urine output (diuresis). The decreased plasma volume leads to an increased haemoglobin concentration and resultant oxygen-carrying capacity in the absence of an absolute increase in red cell mass (RCM). The acute decrease in plasma volume leads to a concomitant decrease in stroke volume (SV). To combat this decrease in SV, resting and sub-maximal exercise heart rate is increased associated with an increased sympathetic activity.

The decreased $S_aO_2\%$ induces an increase in the renal release of erythropoietin (EPO) within a few hours. An altitude of >2100 m is required to induce EPO release (Ri-Li et al 2001) above which the increase in EPO-concentration in blood is negatively associated with changes in $S_aO_2\%$ (Piehl-Aulin et al 1998). Despite the immediate increase in the secretion of erythropoietin (EPO) observed during hypoxic exposure, increases in RCM are not observed for several weeks.

Following prolonged hypoxic exposure an increase in plasma volume and RCM result in an increased oxygen-carrying capacity. Tissue oxygen delivery is further

Table 8.1  Physiological advantages and disadvantages of hypobaric hypoxic (natural altitude) exposure and response times adapted from Bailey & Davies (1997)

| Physiological advantages | Response time | Physiological disadvantages | Response time |
|---|---|---|---|
| Increased free fatty acid mobilization | Weeks Days/months | Increased ventilation | Immediate |
| | | Decreased Q | Days |
| Increased Hb | Months/years | Decreased blood flow | Days |
| Increased capillarity density | Weeks | Increased oxidative stress and damage | Immediate |
| Increased oxidative enzyme activity | Weeks | Increased dehydration | Immediate |
| | | Decreased training intensity | Immediate |
| Increased mito-chondrial density | | Jet lag | Immediate |
| | | AMS/HAPE/HACE | Immediate |
| | | Sunburn | Immediate |
| | | Catecholamine-induced glycogen depletion | Immediate |
| | | Increased haemolysis | Immediate |

enhanced by an increase in red blood cell 2,3-diphosphoglycerate (2,3-DPG) that shifts the $O_2$-dissociation curve to the right. An increased SV and decrease in sympathetic activity result in a reduction in resting and sub-maximal exercise heart rate towards sea-level values. As the tissue level increases in capillary density, mitochondrial size and density and changes in enzymatic pathways are all adaptations to chronic hypoxia that result in an improved oxygen consumption (see Table 8.1).

## ALTITUDE ACCLIMATIZATION AND ENDURANCE PERFORMANCE

It is well accepted that living high and training high (HiHi) improves performance at moderate altitude (>1500 m). In contrast, the role of HiHi for improved sea level performance is equivocal.

Because of the potential detrimental effects of residing at altitude for prolonged periods of time (see later), however, scientists have investigated the role of combining periods of hypoxic exposure with normoxic training; living high–training low (HiLo). The development of HiLo allows the maintenance of the normoxic training stimulus combined with the benefits altitude acclimatization. Only a limited number of training venues exist where HiLo training regimes can be employed using natural altitude (hypobaric hypoxia). A number of techniques have been developed to overcome this problem, including (i) using an increased oxygen concentration of inspired air during training at natural altitude, and (ii) reducing the $FiO_2$ (normobaric hypoxic) by way of nitrogen dilution often employed in altitude houses/hotels or tents (Wilber 2001). Despite the equivocal evidence supporting the efficacy of HiLo training, athletic populations are increasingly using nocturnal hypoxia in an attempt to gain some physiological benefit. The principle method used by athletes to achieve a HiLo training regime is to live and train at sea level and sleep in a normobaric hypoxic environment artificially simulating an altitude of ~2500 m for periods of 12–20 hours.

The primary goal of hypoxic exposure is to increase RCM and/or haemoglobin mass (HbM) through an increased EPO secretion. During HiLo training, morning EPO concentration appears to be at a higher level after 2–5 days compared with HiHi. During the day, however, EPO concentration decreases significantly from the morning values due to short half-time of EPO elimination following HiLo exposure.

A number of studies have reported an increased sea level $\dot{V}O_2$max and improved sea level endurance performance following HiLo (Rusko et al 2004). Levine & Stray-Gundersen (1997) demonstrated an improved $\dot{V}O_2$max, ventilatory threshold and 5000 m track running performance at sea following HiLo that was not observed following HiHi or LoLo. The authors postulated that the maintenance of a high training velocity, cardiac output and oxygen flush primarily during interval training was the key factor underpinning the observed performance gains following HiLo. Similarly, Rusko et al (1999) showed a significant increase (~5%) in maximal treadmill performance after 25 days of HiLo, and Piehl-Aulin (1999) reported a significant increase (~3%) in treadmill performance following 21–28 days of HiLo. Not all studies have demonstrated an improved sea level performance following HiLo (Hahn et al 2001). However, the low total duration of exposure to hypoxia and lack of RCM/HbM increase in these studies may be responsible for the absence of change observed. In those studies reporting an improved sea level performance a minimum of 3 weeks HiLo exposure was employed, suggesting that a threshold duration may exist below which no improvement is observed. Thus, HiHi and HiLo may induce an acclimatization effect and increase RCM/HbM. Importantly, however, the minimum dose to attain acclimatization effect appears to be > 12 hours.day$^{-1}$ at an altitude > 2000 m for at least 3 weeks.

Irrespective of outcome, all studies reported considerable individual variation in response to altitude training. In those studies that reported an improved performance following HiLo the responders, defined as a greater than mean improvement in sea level running performance, had greater EPO response at altitude than non-responders, and responders also showed significant increase in RCM and $\dot{V}O_2$max that was not observed in non-responders. In addition, the responders were better able to maintain normal training velocities and oxygen flux than the non-responders.

## ALTITUDE ACCLIMATIZATION AND ANAEROBIC PERFORMANCE

The decreased air resistance at altitude results in increased maximal sprinting speeds. Thus, the detrimental effect of reduced training intensities observed for endurance exercise in hypoxia leading to a reduced neuromuscular training load and resultant de-training may not effect sprint/power-based sports.

Anaerobic endurance may be affected during hypoxic exposure, probably associated with a loss of bicarbonate and a plasma volume decrease (Hahn & Gore 2001). In contrast, however, acute hypoxia does not impair a single short-term (<1 minute) maximal performance despite a reduced $\dot{V}O_2$max during performance, and an increased muscle lactate and glycogen decrease following performance.

A number of studies have failed to demonstrate an improved supramaximal anaerobic performance at sea level following HiHi for 3–4 weeks (Bailey et al 1998, Levine Stray-Gundersen 1997). In contrast, studies have reported increases in running time to exhaustion (range 240–380 seconds) during sea level $\dot{V}O_2$max measurement without an increase in $\dot{V}O_2$max, and an increased maximal accumulated oxygen deficit (MAOD) and muscle buffer capacity after return to sea level following HiHi training above 2000 m for 2 weeks.

Nummela & Rusko (2000) demonstrated an improved sea level 400-m race time in elite sprint-runners as well as a decreased blood lactate concentration during submaximal sprinting on a treadmill following 2 weeks with 14–18 hours daily exposure to normobaric hypoxia ($FiO_2$ 15.8%). The limited available evidence suggests that HiHi and HiLo with sprint-type training may improve subsequent anaerobic performance at sea-level.

## SLEEPING IN NORMOBARIC HYPOXIA

Recently, concern has been raised regarding the impact of hypoxia on sleep quality. The key area of concern is the impact of disturbed sleep, often observed at altitude, on recovery and performance.

In a recent study Kinsman et al (2002) attempted to quantify the effect of normobaric hypoxia (2650 m) upon markers of sleep quality. This study investigated respiratory events in cyclists participating in a HiLo programme using a nitrogen-enriched facility. Results suggested a substantial increase in respiratory events during sleep, present in nearly 25% of the athletes studied. In a similar study, Pedlar et al (2005) examined the impact of sleeping in a normobaric hypoxic tent (2500 m) in eight recreational athletes. Results demonstrated that normobaric hypoxia resulted in significant sleep disturbance. The observed sleep disturbance manifested as an increased respiratory disturbance was associated with an increased prevalence of apnoeas (a cessation of airflow for longer than 10 seconds) and hypopnoeas (a 50% reduction in airflow for longer than 10 seconds with a 3% reduction in $SpO_2$). As a result, the subjective analysis of sleep quality, based upon assessment of the ease of 'getting to sleep' (GTS), 'behaviour following waking' (BFW) and 'quality of sleep' (QS), measured using the Leeds sleep evaluation questionnaire (LSEQ), was significantly reduced. The practical implications of these findings may be that early morning performance may be impaired by sleep in normobaric hypoxia, and an overall reduction in the quality of rest experienced during sleep. It is widely believed that the quality of rest and recovery of the athlete between training bouts is an essential part of the adaptation process (the restorative hypothesis of sleep; Shapiro 1981). Therefore, inadequate recovery may lead to symptoms of overtraining and ultimately underperformance. It must be noted, however, that the impact of normobaric hypoxia on sleep was highly heterogeneous with some athletes responding very poorly while others remained unaffected. These findings suggest that significant implications exist for individuals wishing to commence a HiLo training programme using nocturnal normobaric hypoxia, in order to avoid the detrimental effects of poor sleep upon training and recovery. The analysis of sleep variables in normobaric hypoxia may assist in the early identification of poorly responding individuals to altitude environments prior to ascent. Further study is required to fully elucidate the efficacy of normobaric hypoxic environments on sleep in trained athletes. It would appear, however, that establishing individual sleep responses to hypoxia is required to limit the impact of hypoxia on sleep and resultant recovery and performance.

The potential detrimental effects associated with sleeping in hypoxia has led to an increased interest in the use of hypoxia for training while living at sea level. The following section examines the effect of living low and training high (LoHi).

## EFFECTS OF LoHi TRAINING

The aim of LoHi training is to induce muscle-specific adaptations to hypoxic exposure while avoiding the detrimental effects of prolonged altitude sojourns or sleep disturbance associated with nocturnal normobaric hypoxic exposure (Pedlar et al 2005). Further, recent work has examined the role of LoHi training to accelerate altitude acclimatization (Whyte et al 2002), and in injury rehabilitation.

The majority of studies examining the use of LoHi have failed to demonstrate a positive performance effect, despite observing increases in EPO. In contrast, however, LoHi training has been shown to increase the work capacity of athletes in hypoxia. Recent studies have reported an accelerated acclimatization to altitude (hypobaric hypoxia) in elite biathletes (Whyte et al 2002). Therefore, while LoHi training appears to have a limited effect on sea level performance it may be valuable in the pre-acclimation of athletes prior to altitude ascent.

Interest in the role of LoHi training for injury rehabilitation is based on studies that have demonstrated improved sea level performance and increased myoglobin and oxidative capacity when absolute training intensities in hypoxia is equal to that in normoxia. Therefore, when an athlete is injured and there is a concomitant reduction in training intensity, LoHi offers an additional physiological stimulus to the maintenance/improvement of aerobic capacity.

## SHORT–TERM INTERMITTENT HYPOXIC TRAINING AT REST (IHT)

Short-term IHT, originally developed in the former Soviet Union, consists of breathing hypoxic air (9–11%) through a mask or mouthpiece for repeated periods of 5–7 minutes, interrupted by equal periods of recovery in normoxia totalling 1–3 hours for one or two sessions a day (Serebrovskaya 2002).

A number of studies have demonstrated a variety of benefits of short-term IHT (3–5 hours daily for 2–4 weeks) including improved altitude acclimatization, and increase performance, Hb-concentration, haematocrit and reticulocytes. Care is warranted in interpreting these results, however, as they failed to employ a control group. Further, a number of studies have failed to demonstrate positive effects of IHT. The effect of IHT on subsequent performance remains unclear; however, it may improve adaptation to subsequent exposure and training at altitude (Rusko et al 2004).

## DETRIMENTAL EFFECTS OF HYPOXIA ON EXERCISE

Training at natural altitude (hypobaric hypoxia) may induce some negative effects on performance that may mask and prevent the use of benefits obtained from an increased oxygen carrying capacity (see Table 8.1). Exercise performance and $\dot{V}O_2max$ as well as training response at sea level and at altitude may not only be dependent on the $O_2$ delivery and utilization, but also on other factors linked to the ability of the central nervous system to recruit muscle. According to the suggested central governor hypothesis, the CNS regulates muscle recruitment and force production. Potentially, both feedback (e.g. chemo- and baroreceptors, proprioceptors) and feed forward mechanisms could affect the function of the CNS. With optimal training, the continued increased recruitment of the muscles results in a new higher-level $\dot{Q}max$, $\dot{V}O_2max$, and exercise performance (Rusko 2003). Therefore, one possible reason for the absence of a positive altitude training effect following an altitude sojourn is that even moderate hypoxia during exercise may substantially compromise training pace and decrease mechanical and neuromuscular stimuli, leading to gradual weakening of some specific determinants of performance.

Concomitant to the observed decrease in $S_aO_2\%$ is a reduction in $\dot{V}O_2max$ that is directly associated with the degree of hypoxic stimulus. For every 1% decrease in $S_aO_2\%$ below the 95% level a 1–2% decrement in $\dot{V}O_2max$ is observed (Dempsey & Wagner 1999). As a result, athletes are obliged to train at lower $\dot{V}O_2max$ values and at lower maximal, sub-maximal and interval training velocities in hypoxia than in normoxia (Hahn et al 2001). The reduced training velocities in hypoxia may decrease the physical and neural stimuli to muscles compared to training in normoxia resulting in a possible de-training effect (Peltonen et al 1997).

During exercise hypoxia a leftward shift in the ventilation (VE), heart rate (HR) and blood lactate (bLA) versus velocity curves is observed. Further, the bLA versus HR curve is shifted leftwards especially at high HR and, consequently, training HR may be decreased during training in hypoxia (Levine & Stray-Gundersen 1997). The paradox in lactate production at altitude, however, dictates a lower maximum bLA ($bLA_{max}$), probably associated with a reduced maximum exercise capacity. Concomitant to the reduced $bLA_{max}$, maximum heart rate ($HR_{max}$) is reduced at altitudes above 3100 m (Hahn & Gore 2001). The decrease in $HR_{max}$ is linearly related to the decrease in $S_aO_2\%$ and as a result the greater decrease in $S_aO_2\%$ often observed in highly trained athletes at altitude may result in a decreased $HR_{max}$ occurring at altitudes <3100 m.

In addition to the deleterious effects of hypoxia on performance a number of clinical conditions termed 'altitude illness syndromes' exist that range in severity from mildly debilitating to death. The following section examines the syndromes in more detail.

## CLINICAL ISSUES ASSOCIATED WITH HYPOXIA

Rapid accent to moderate altitude (c. 2500 m) and high-altitude environments causes a spectrum of physiological responses in unacclimatized athletes. This spectrum is associated with hypobaric hypoxia and often develops into pathological conditions requiring medical intervention. These conditions include; acute mountain sickness syndrome (AMS), high-altitude pulmonary oedema (HAPE) and high-altitude cerebral oedema (HACE) (Summary box 8.5). The impact of these altitude illness syndromes is heterogeneous, ranging from mild self-limiting discomfort to death. While the majority of studies examining the incidence of these pathological conditions have focused on hypobaric hypoxia (HiHi) it is possible to induce these conditions in normobaric hypoxia (HiLo). The frequency and severity of these problems depend on altitude, rate of ascent and degree of individual susceptibility.

Acute mountain sickness (AMS) is a benign, self-limited system complex. The cause of AMS was thought to be associated with hypoxia-induced subclinical cerebral oedema. Recent evidence, however, suggests that oxidative stress may play a key role in the aetiology of AMS (Bärtsch et al 2004). Symptoms of AMS include headaches, anorexia, nausea, vomiting, weakness, malaise, decreased co-ordination and dizziness. Sleep disturbance associated with an increased incidence of apnoeas and periodic breathing is common following acute exposure to hypoxia (Pedlar et al 2005). While symptoms appear to intensify at altitudes above 2500 m, AMS may be experienced at lower altitudes, and may occur during HiLo periods in normobaric hypoxia. Allowing sufficient time for acclimatization by using graded ascent and staging are the most effective methods for preventing AMS. Further, pre-acclimation may diminish AMS symptoms (Bärtsch & Roach 2001) with previous studies demonstrating the

## Summary box 8.5

Summary of key points for AMS, HAPE and HACE.

### Acute mountain sickness (AMS)
- All athletes are suseptible
- Directly related to rate and magnitude of ascent
- Headache is the most common symptom
- Acclimatization using graded ascent, staging and pre-acclimation reduces AMS
- Can evolve to HAPE and HACE

### High-altitude pulmonary oedema (HAPE)
- Non-cardiogenic pulmonary oedema
- Most common cause of death among the altitude illness syndromes
- Risk factors include moderate to severe exertion, cold exposure, anxiety, young age, male gender and obesity
- High rate of recurrence in individuals who have had a prior episode of HAPE
- Best treatment is immediate descent

### High altitude cerebral oedema (HACE)
- Rarely occurs below altitudes < 3600 m
- Less common that AMS and HAPE
- Often a complication of AMS and HAPE
- Distinguished by disturbances in consciousness that may progress to coma, confusion and ataxia of gate.
- Immediate descent is required for treatment

use of HiLo as a successful pre-acclimatization measure (Pedlar et al 2005). AMS can be treated with pharmacological prophylaxis using acetazolamide (a carbonic anhydrase inhibitor). At present, however, acetazolamide is currently on the WADA banned drug list and care should be taken when using pharmacological agents in the treatment of AMS.

High-altitude pulmonary oedema (HAPE) is a non-cardiogenic pulmonary oedema caused by a combination of hypoxia induced pulmonary hypertension and an increased permeability of the pulmonary capillary endothelium. If left untreated, HAPE can be rapidly fatal. Symptoms and signs of HAPE are associated with a progressive pulmonary oedema resulting in a worsening hypoxaemia. Early signs are often difficult to distinguish from a normal acute response to hypoxia. As pulmonary oedema progresses, however, a productive cough of frothy, pink/blood streaked sputum is common with wheezing and audible gurgling (especially when supine). Treatment should be initiated immediately as a delay in treating progressive pulmonary oedema at altitude usually results in death. Drug therapy has been used successfully in preventing and treating HAPE, in particular nifedipine, however the best treatment for HAPE is immediate descent.

High-altitude cerebral oedema (HACE) is caused by a hypoxic induced increase in permeability of the blood–brain barrier (vasogenic oedema) and/or a hypoxic induced alteration in cellular fluid regulation with an intracellular fluid shift (cytotoxic oedema).While HACE has been reported at altitudes as low as 2500 m the vast majority of cases occur above 3600 m, well above those altitudes normally experienced by athletes on training camp or during competition.

Another key problem associated with training at altitude is an increased hypoxic stress leading to possible overtraining symptoms associated with an increased sympathetic activation, oxidative damage mediated by free radicals and glycolytic metabolism (Gore et al 1998). A significant increase in resting serum cortisol and decrease in serum testosterone has been observed following altitude training in elite endurance athletes. Further, hypoxia decreases immunoreactivity, specifically by suppressing T-cell mediated immunity. A 50–100% increase in the frequency of upper respiratory tract and gastrointestinal tract infections during or immediately after altitude sojourns has been reported (Bailey et al 1998).

Air temperature falls by about 1°C with every 150 m of ascent. Therefore, low air temperatures experienced at altitude increase the likelihood of cold-related injuries (see Training and the cold). The reduction in humidity together with the increased ventilation rates (HVR) observed at altitude predisposes to dehydration, as a large volume of body water can be lost through the respiratory tract as dry cold air is warmed and humidified during breathing. An additional problem associated with altitude is the increased solar radiation leading to sunburn. Care should be taken by athletes training at altitude to increase fluid intake and wear sunscreen to avoid excessive dehydration and sunburn. Clothing choices at altitude are also of key importance in avoiding cold injury while minimizing the potential for dehydration (see Training and the cold).

## CONCLUSIONS

The benefits of living and training at altitude (HiHi) for an improved altitude performance of athletes are clear but controlled studies for an improved sea level performance are less clear. Current evidence suggests that to obtain a positive acclimatization effect a hypoxic exposure above 2000 m for a minimum of 12 hours per day for at least 3 weeks is required. Athlete response to hypoxia, however, is heterogenic, with some individuals failing to respond, 'non-responders'. Adopting an individualized approach to the use of hypoxia will optimize acclimatization and avoid unnecessary performance decrements.

A decrement in performance may be observed following a period of exposure to hypoxia associated with a decreased mechanical, neuromuscular and cardiovascular stimuli associated with a reduction in training velocities. Further, a rapid accent to altitude in unacclimatized individuals may result in altitude illness syndromes, including AMS, HAPE and HACE. These syndromes are all specific to altitude environments and are related to sustained hypoxia. Immediate medical care should be sought for these syndromes to avoid possible fatalities. Raising the oxygen levels to the body tissues is the primary treatment and can be achieved by using supplemental oxygen. The preferred treatment, however, is to move the athlete to a lower altitude as rapidly as possible.

## KEY POINTS

1. Altitude causes a cascade of physiological responses triggered by hypobaric hypoxia resulting in a reduced arterial oxygen saturation ($S_aO_2$%).
2. For every 1% decrease in $S_aO_2$% below the 95% level a 1–2% decrement in $\dot{V}O_2$max is observed.
3. Acclimatization results in adaptations leading to an improved oxygen delivery and consumption.

4. The benefits of hypoxic living and training for improved altitude performance are clear; however, evidence for an improved sea level performance are less clear.
5. Full acclimatization requires hypoxic exposure for a minimum of 12 hours.day$^{-1}$ for at least 3 weeks.
6. Altitude training takes a number of forms, including living high, training high (HiHi); living high, training low (HiLo); living low, training high (LoHi).
7. Rapid accent to altitude can result in medical conditions requiring medical intervention, including AMS, HAPE and HACE.
8. Considerable individual variation occurs in response to altitude training.

# References

## Training and the cold

Francis TJR, Oakley EHN 1996 Cold injury, ch 23. In: Tooke JE & Lowe GDO (eds) A textbook of vascular medicine. Arnold, London, p 353–370
Golden FStC, Tipton MJ 2002 Essentials of sea survival. Human Kinetics, Champaign IL
Nimmo M 2004 Exercise in the cold. Journal of Sports Sciences 22:898–916
Pfeiser B, Reilly T 2004 Environmental factors in the summer Olympics in historical perspective. Journal of Sports Sciences 22:981–1002
Reilly T, Waterhouse J 2004 Exercise in the cold. In: Sport, exercise and environmental physiology. Elsevier, London, p 33–49
Tipton M 2005 Environmental factors. In: Whyte G et al (eds) ABC of sports and exercise medicine. BMJ Books, London

## Training and the heat

Bergeron MF 1996 Heat cramps during tennis. International Journal of Sports Nutrition 6:62–68
Galloway SDR, Maughan RJ 1997 Effects of ambient temperature on the capacity to perform prolonged cycle exercise in man. Medicine and Science in Sports and Exercise 29:1240–1249
Gonzalez RR 1988 Biophysics of heat transfer and clothing considerations. In: Pandolf KB (eds) Human performance physiology and environmental medicine at terrestrial extremes. Cooper, Carmel, p 45–95
Gonzalez-Alonso J, Calbet JA, Nielsen B 1999a Metabolic and thermodynamic responses to dehydration-induced reductions in muscle blood flow in exercising humans. Journal of Physiology 520:577–589
Gonzalez-Alonso J, Teller C, Andersen SL et al 1999b Influence of body temperature on the development of fatigue during prolonged exercise in the heat. Journal of Applied Physiology 86:1032–1039
Hew TD, Chorley JN, Cianca JC, Divine JG 2003 The incidence, risk factors and clinical manifestations of hyponatremia in marathon runners. Clinical Journal of Sports Medicine 13:41–47
Houmard JA, Costill DL, Davis JA et al 1990 The influence of exercise intensity on heat acclimation in trained subjects. Medicine and Science in Sports and Exercise 22:615–620
Lind AR, Bass DE 1963 Optimal exposure time for development of heat acclimation. Federation Proceedings 22:704–708

Maughan RJ 2001 Physiological responses to fluid intake during exercise. In: Maughan RJ & Murray R (eds) Sports drinks. CRC Press, Boca Raton, p 129–152

Maughan RJ, Shirreffs S 2004 Exercise in the heat: challenges and opportunities. Journal of Sports Sciences 22:917–927

Maughan RJ, Merson SJ, Broad NP, Shirreffs SM 2004 Fluid and electrolyte intake and loss in elite soccer players during training. International Journal of Sports Nutrition and Exercise Metabolism (in press)

Montain SJ, Maughan RJ, Sawka MN 1996 Heat acclimatization strategies for the 1996 Summer Olympics. Athletic Therapy Today 1:42–46

Murray R, Stofan J 2001 Formulating carbohydrate-electrolyte drinks for optimal efficacy. In: Maughan RJ & Murray R (eds) Sports drinks. CRC Press, Boca Raton, p 197–224

Nielsen B, Hyldig T, Bidstrup F et al 2001 Brain activity and fatigue during prolonged exercise in the heat. Pflugers Archiv 442:41–48

Nielsen B, Nybo L 2003 Cerebral changes during exercise in the heat. Sports Medicine 33:1–11

Noakes TD 2003 Overconsumption of fluids by athletes. British Medical Journal 237:113–114

Nybo L, Secher N, Neilson B 2002 Inadequate heat loss from the human brain during prolonged exercise with hyperthermia. Journal of Physiology 545:697–704

Pandolf KB, Griffin TB, Munro EH, Goldman RF 1980 Persistence of impaired heat tolerance from artificially induced miliaria rubra. American Journal of Physiology 239:R226–R232

Passe DH 2001 Physiological and psychological determinants of fluid intake. In: Maughan RJ & Murray R (eds) Sports drinks. CRC Press, Boca Raton, p 45–88

Pichan G, Sridharan K, Swamy VY et al 1985 Physiological acclimatization to heat after a spell of cold conditioning in tropical subjects. Aviations, Space and Environmental Medicine 56:436–440

Reilly T, Waterhouse J 2005 Exercise in the heat. In: Reilly T & Waterhouse J (eds) Exercise and environmental physiology. Elsevier, London, p 13–31

Sawka MN, Pandolf KB 1990 Effects of body water loss on physiological function and exercise performance. In: Gisolfi CV & Lamb DR (eds) Perspectives in exercise science and sports medicine, vol 3. Benchmark Press, Indianapolis, p 1–38

Shirreffs SM, Maughan RJ 1998 Urine osmolality and conductivity as markers of hydration status. Medicine and Science in Sports and Exercise 30:1598–1602

Shirreffs SM, Taylor AJ, Leiper JB, Maughan RJ 1996 Post-exercise rehydration in man: effects of volume consumed and sodium content of ingested fluids. Medicine and Science in Sports and Exercise 28:1260–1271

Smith S 2002 Marathon runner's death linked to excessive fluid intake. New York Times. August 13.

Sutton JR 1990 Clinical implications of fluid imbalance. In: Gisolfi CV & Lamb DR (eds) Perspectives in exercise science and sports medicine, vol 3. Fluid homeostasis during exercise. Benchmark Press, Indianapolis, p 425–448

Tipton M 2005 Environmental factors. In: Whyte G et al (eds) ABC of sports medicine. BMJ Books, London

## Altitude and training

Bailey DM, Davies B 1997 Physiological implications of altitude training for endurance performance at sea level: a review. British Journal of Sports Medicine 31:183–190

Bailey DM, Davies B, Romer L et al 1998 Implications of moderate altitude training for sea-level endurance in elite distance runners. European Journal of Applied Physiology 78:360–368

Bärtsch P, Roach R 2001 Acute mountain sickness and high-altitude cerebral oedema. In: Hornbein TF & Schoene RB (eds) High altitude. An exploration of human adaptation. Marcel Dekker Inc, New York, p 731–776

Bärtsch P, Bailey D, Berger M et al 2004 Acute mountain sickness: controversies and advances. High Altitude Medicine and Biology 5:110–124

Dempsey JA, Wagner PD 1999 Exercise-induced arterial hypoxemia. Journal of Applied Physiology 87:1997–2006

Gore C, Craig N, Hahn A et al 1998 Altitude training at 2690 m does not increase total haemoglobin mass or sea level $VO_2$max in world champion track cyclists. Journal of Science and Medicine in Sport 1:156–170.

Hahn AG, Gore CJ 2001 The effect of altitude on cycling performance: a challenge to traditional concepts. Sports Medicine 31:533–557

Hahn AG, Gore CJ, Martin DT et al 2001 An evaluation of the concept of living at moderate altitude and training at sea level. Comparative Biochemistry and Physiology. Part A 128:777–789

Kinsman TA, Hahn AG, Gore CJ et al 2002 Respiratory events and periodic breathing in cyclists sleeping at 2650 m simulated altitude. Journal of Applied Physiology 92:2114–2118

Levine BD, Stray-Gundersen J 1997 Living high-training low: effect of moderate-altitude acclimatization with low altitude training on performance. Journal of Applied Physiology 83:102–112

Nummela AT, Rusko H 2000 Acclimatization to altitude and normoxic training improve 400-m running performance at sea level. Journal of Sports Sciences 18:411–419

Pedlar C, Whyte G, Emegbo S et al 2005 Acute sleep responses in a normobaric hypoxic tent. Medicine and Science in Sports and Exercise 37(6):1075–1079

Peltonen J, Rusko H, Rantamäki J et al 1997 Effects of oxygen fraction in inspired air on force production and electromyogram activity during ergometer rowing. European Journal of Applied Physiology 76:495–503

Piehl-Aulin K 1999 Normobaric hypoxia – physical performance. Journal of Sports Sciences 12:478–479.

Piehl-Aulin K, Svedenhag J, Wide L et al 1998 Short-term intermittent normobaric hypoxia-hematological, physiological and mental effects. Scandinavian Journal of Medicine and Science in Sports 8:132–137

Ri-Li, G, Witkowski S, Zhang Y et al 2001 Determinants of erythropoietin release in response to short-term hypobaric hypoxia. Journal of Applied Physiology 92:2361–2367

Rusko H, Tikkanen H, Peltonen J 2004 Altitude training and performance. Journal of Sports Sciences 22:928–944

Rusko H 2003 Handbook of sports medicine and science: cross country skiing. Blackwell Science, Oxford

Rusko H, Tikkanen H, Paavolainen L et al 1999 Effect of living in hypoxia and training in normoxia on sea level $VO_2$max and red cell mass. Medicine and Science in Sports and Exercise 31:S86

Rusko H, Tikkanen H, Peltonen J 2004 Altitude training and performance. Journal of Sports Sciences 22:928–944

Serebrovskaya TV 2002 Intermittent hypoxia research in the former Soviet Union and the Commonwealth of Independent States: History and review of the concept and selected applications. High Altitude Medicine & Biology 3:205–221

Shapiro C 1981 Sleep and the athlete. British Journal of Sports Medicine 15:51–55

Whyte G, Lane A, Pedlar C, Godfrey R 2002 The physiological and psychological impact of intermittent hypoxic training (IHT) in the preparation of the GB biathlon team for the 2002 Olympic Games. High Altitude Medicine and Biology 3(4):457

Wilber RL 2001 Current trends in altitude training. Sports Medicine 31:249–265

## Further reading

Armstrong L (ed.) 1999 Performing in extreme environments. Human Kinetics, Champaign IL

Pandolf KB et al (eds) 1988 Human performance physiology and environmental medicine at terrestrial extremes. Cooper, Carmel

Reilly T & Waterhouse J (eds) 2004 Sport, exercise and environmental physiology. Elsevier Ltd, London

Ward M et al (eds) 2000 High altitude medicine and physiology. Hodder Arnold, London

Whyte G et al (eds) 2005 ABC of sports and exercise medicine. BMJ Books, London

# Chapter 9

# Medical conditions and training

**Roslyn J. Carbon** (Reproductive health in exercising women)
**Gregory Whyte** (The athlete's heart)
**Richard Budgett** (The unexplained underperformance
syndrome (UUPS))
**Alison K. McConnell** (Asthma and exercise-induced asthma)

## CHAPTER CONTENTS

## INTRODUCTION

Optimal performance is not only associated with optimizing the training stimulus, it is also associated with the ability to maintain optimal health throughout training and competition while placing significant physiological demands on the body (Fig. 9.1).

It is beyond the scope of this text to examine, in detail, the health-related factors related to performance. The reader is directed to a number of key texts offering comprehensive coverage of sports medicine, including *The ABC of Sports Medicine* (edited by Whyte G, Harries M & Williams C), BMJ Books, London (2005).

This chapter examines four key areas that can have profound effects on the health and performance of an athlete: (i) reproductive health and the female athlete, (ii) the athlete's heart, (iii) asthma and exercise-induced asthma, and (iv) unexplained underperformance.

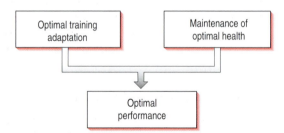

**Figure 9.1**    The balance between optimizing the training stimulus and maintaining optimal health in the attainment of performance.

## REPRODUCTIVE HEALTH IN EXERCISING WOMEN

### LEARNING OBJECTIVES:

This section is intended to ensure that the reader:

1. Understands that exercise has many positive health benefits for women.
2. Recognizes that some women may require management of menstrual symptoms in order to train and compete successfully.
3. Has an understanding of the endocrine changes that occur with exercise and the effect these can have on reproductive function.
4. Acknowledges that athletes may have other significant medical conditions which present as menstrual disturbance and require formal medical diagnosis.

5. Understands the mechanisms behind menstrual disruption in exercising women and the secondary health consequences.
6. Appreciates the rationale behind the management of amenorrhoea in athletes.

## INTRODUCTION

For most girls and women regular physical exercise has a positive impact on general and reproductive health. Regular training improves psychological wellbeing, limits obesity, improves muscle strength and bone density, and is associated with improved cardiovascular health and lipid profiles.

Physical exercise stimulates the endocrine system. However, in general, the effect of regular training is to moderate hormonal flux such that the menstrual cycle tends to be less problematic in active women. In particular, premenstrual symptoms can be ameliorated by regular aerobic training. Some active sports women, however, continue to be troubled by dysmenorrhoea (painful periods) and menorrhagia (heavy bleeding) that may interfere with training and competition. Management of these problems includes modification of training patterns where possible but, as this is often not practical, medication may be necessary. Simple analgesia (paracetamol) may suffice for pain, although mefenamic acid is often more potent and also controls menstrual flow. These medications and other non-steroidal pain relief such as ibuprofen are available 'over the counter' and should be instituted immediately symptoms occur. More significant menorrhagia and pain requires medical consultation to exclude significant pathology. Medication must always be checked against current doping guidelines to avoid use of banned drugs.

For some women use of the combined oral contraceptive (OCP) may be indicated to control menstrual symptoms, with possible manipulation of the cycle around competition. There is very little evidence that this may have any negative effect on performance and many elite performers have competed at their best when taking the OCP.

## EXERCISE–RELATED MENSTRUAL IRREGULARITY

Some highly trained athletes experience disturbance of the menstrual cycle such that menses become irregular or may cease altogether (amenorrhoea). This 'exercise-related amenorrhoea' is the result of a centrally mediated neuro-endocrine adaptation whereby hypothalamic control of the pituitary–ovarian hormone axis is disrupted.

The menstrual cycle is initiated from the hypothalamus at the base of the brain with pulsatile release of the gonadotrophin releasing hormone (GnRH) resulting in the release of follicle-stimulating hormone (FSH) and luteinizing hormone (LH) from the anterior pituitary, which in turn control the function of the ovary and secretion of oestrogen and progesterone. Intricate feedback loops control a finely balanced hormonal interplay which ultimately results in regular ovulation from the ovary and subsequent menstrual flow from the uterus.

The system may be disrupted when stresses alter the central control mechanism in the hypothalamus – so-called hypothalamic hypogonadism. Subsequent diminution of gonadotrophin secretion leads to ovarian shutdown with low-level oestrogen secretion. These changes are essentially an adaptive process rather than an organic disease process and are reversible should the factors responsible for the onset of menstrual disruption be addressed.

A similar situation also occurs in highly trained endurance male athletes where lower testosterone levels have been measured. Menstrual disruption of women, however, appears to be more common and may have more significant sequelae for reproductive and musculoskeletal health.

Hypothalamic disturbance of the menstrual cycle may take the form of delayed onset of menarche (primary amenorrhoea). Athletic girls often start menstruation later than their peers but this may reflect self selection in that late developers often excel in sport. Should menses not have commenced by the age of 16 the girl should be referred for medical evaluation as this may also indicate significant organic pathology, including chromosomal or endocrine defects.

Hypothalamic amenorrhoea may take various forms, depending on the severity of the suppression of the reproductive axis. Some girls may have an unusually short cycle (polymenorrhoea) which is related to an inadequate luteal (post-ovulation) phase of the cycle. In contrast, anovulation may result in cycles longer than the normal 28–35 days (oligomenorrhoea). Amenorrhoea is generally defined as no menses for 6 months, although the International Olympic Committee has recently defined it as no more than one mense per year.

Menstrual disruption occurs in about 5% of the general population but may be much more common in some athletic groups. It is rare in team sports such as netball, hockey and football but common in gymnasts, distance runners and ballet dancers. An interesting example is rowing where the heavy-weight crews typically have normal cycles but the light-weight crews have a high incidence of amenorrhoea.

Athletic girls may also experience menarche but not establish a normal, regular cycle for some years. Most amenorrhoeic athletes are younger, may never have established a regular cycle and are unlikely to have been pregnant. It appears that once hormonal patterning is established it is less likely to be disrupted in the future.

Most sports require a low body fat to optimize performance. Some sports have weight categories and others, such as gymnastics and ballet, encourage a thin appearance for aesthetic reasons. Women, however, naturally carry about twice the body fat of men because the physiology of ovarian hormones favours fat deposition: Higher levels of testosterone in men favour an increased lean mass of muscle and bone. Consequently many female athletes constantly strive to maintain a low body fat while at the same time needing to ensure adequate nutrition for their sport and health.

It is becoming increasingly evident that exercise-related amenorrhoea is due to a chronic negative energy balance whereby athletes do not consume enough energy for the needs of their sport (Zanker & Swaine 1998). Many of these girls have high-volume aerobic training programmes and stressful competition schedules. While they may be able to maintain their training level at a relatively stable body mass, often at a very low level of body fat, they do so as a result of a complex neuroendocrine adaptation which includes hypothalamic amenorrhoea (Kaiserauer et al 1989).

Research indicates that these girls have serum markers of energy deprivation, including altered thyroid function (low T3 levels), low insulin-like growth factor (IGF1) and high IGF-binding protein (IGF-BP) levels and low leptin levels (Kaufman et al 2002, Loucks et al 1992, Musey et al 1993). IGF1 is the peripheral metabolite of growth hormone and is necessary for normal growth and development and maintenance of lean body mass in adulthood. Leptin is produced by adipocytes and is an indicator of fat stores. These athletes also have high levels of cortisol (hypercortisolaemia), indicating chronic stress. High levels of cortisol are associated with low bone mass and poor tissue repair in patients with adrenal hyperplasia (Cushing's disease).

It must be remembered that amenorrhoea is a symptom and not a diagnosis and an athlete with menstrual disturbance requires a medical assessment to determine the cause. Amenorrhoea may herald significant diseases, including malignancy and endocrine disorders, which may require urgent intervention. Similarly, a diagnosis of pregnancy must always be entertained and tested early. True ovarian failure (premature menopause) may also occur in women under thirty.

There are two other causes of amenorrhoea that are important differential diagnoses to the athlete: polycystic ovarian disease and eating disorders.

## POLYCYSTIC OVARIAN DISEASE (PCOD)

Polycystic ovarian disease is characterized by infertility, hirsutism, obesity and amenorrhoea or oligomenorrhoea. On investigation many patients will have enlarged cystic ovaries. The pathogenesis of the PCOD is also related to inappropriate signals (feedback mechanisms) to the hypothalamus and pituitary. In this case it is the release of elevated androgens from the adrenal gland at puberty in an obese girl that lead to increased peripheral aromatization to oestrogen from adipocytes. Feedback loops to the pituitary result in increased LH and decreased FSH levels. This leads to anovulation in the presence of oestrogen that can cause irregular and severe bleeding. Eventually as the hormonal imbalance deteriorates amenorrhoea ensues.

This condition is very variable and the classic finding of obesity may not be evident in an athletic girl. It may present in a somewhat endomorphic athlete in a power sport. Alternatively, PCOD may persist in athletic girls in whom the initial pubescent obesity has resolved, and indeed elements of PCOD and athletic amenorrhoea may co-exist in the same individual. Careful medical evaluation and hormonal profiling is necessary to diagnose and manage these girls.

## EATING DISORDERS AND SPORT

Anorexia nervosa and bulimia are severe psychological disturbances that often require long-term psychiatric care and, especially in the case of anorexia, carry significant morbidity and mortality. Anorexia is characterized by fasting (<1200 calories.day$^{-1}$), weight loss, and amenorrhoea, while bulimia involves food binges and purging, often with fairly normal body weight. Patients with eating disorders have an extreme disturbance of their own body image and/or perception of self-worth that is akin to a psychosis. In western adolescent populations the prevalence of eating disorders is increasing, with a sex ratio approaching 9:1 toward girls.

There is unlikely to be a greater incidence of true eating disorders in athletes compared with the general population (Bale et al 1996), but the stresses of sporting success (coupled with ignorance of the importance of good nutrition in sport) may lead a susceptible individual to develop the condition. Furthermore, some true anorectics may exercise as part of their obsession with thinness. Eating disorder is not compatible with sporting excellence; these girls may attain competitive standard for a brief time only for their health and performance to subsequently deteriorate.

Professionals involved in sport, as well as coaches and managers, need to be alert to signs of eating disorder such as gross weight loss or food avoidance. Nutritional advice should be given to athletes without undue pressure for unrealistic and unnecessary weight control. Body fat should be seen as just one variable of health and training assessment rather than a 'performance target' in itself. As in any form of medical examination, sensitivity and confidentiality must be exercised when measuring body weight and fat. Should there be a suspicion of a true eating disorder in an athlete this must be addressed quickly and management sought from a specialist (psychiatrist) in the field.

# SECONDARY EFFECTS OF HYPOTHALAMIC DYSFUNCTION IN ATHLETES

While absence of menses to a competitive athlete may seem a benign event, there are significant ramifications for the short- and long-term health of the athlete. These include changes in fertility, altered bone metabolism and an increased risk of injury.

## FERTILITY

Obviously, if an athlete is anovulatory due to hypothalamic dysfunction she will be infertile. Most women in heavy training, however, are not seeking pregnancy, and reproductive function will almost always resume with improved nutrition, higher body weight, and lower training load. In a very small minority, especially those with prolonged amenorrhoea since adolescence, infertility remains a problem and requires specialist fertility treatment to induce ovulation. It is important for athletes, their coaches and family to understand that reproductive patterning is most likely to occur in the teenage years. When amenorrhoea persists untreated into the twenties it becomes increasingly difficult to reverse the adaptations.

Athletes should also be warned that ovulatory function can sometimes return without warning and there are several reports of high-level athletes being several months pregnant before they realized their condition. Hence, despite amenorrhoea, contraception should be used if an athlete is sexually active.

## BONE MINERAL DENSITY

Athletes with altered menstrual function have been shown, on average, to have lower bone mineral density than their eumenorrhoic counterparts. This is particularly so for those parts of the skeleton with normally high bone turnover such as the spine. Weight-bearing physical activity is, however, a potent stimulator of bone deposition and hence athletes generally have higher bone density than the general population. There is a site-specific effect of exercise on those parts of the skeleton regularly exercised, so that the long bones of the lower limb may have normal bone density even in long-term amenorrhoeic runners. Interestingly, amenorrhoeic rowers have been shown to have normal spinal bone density commensurate with the strength of their trunk muscles in response to the repetitive rowing action (Wolman et al 1990).

Measured bone mineral content in the skeleton is the combination of bone formation by active osteoblasts, minus the effect of bone loss from osteoclastic activity.

Research on the pathogenesis of low bone mineral content in athletes is limited but it appears that, unlike the high turnover bone loss that results from oestrogen deficiency in post-menopausal women, hypothalamic amenorrhoea is associated with low bone formation (Stacey et al 1998).

Amenorrhoeic athletes should not be labelled as having 'osteoporosis' in terms of the condition of elderly women in whom minimal trauma is likely to cause acute fractures of the spine, wrist, and neck of the femur. Such fractures do not occur in young athletes. It is likely that bone quality, or collagen matrix, is superior in young athletes. Unlike postmenopausal women, young women have the capacity to increase bone mass once amenorrhoea is reversed (Drinkwater et al 1996). There appears to be a 'window of opportunity', however, during late adolescence when bone mass accretion is greatest, and it is likely that optimal bone mass may never be achieved after prolonged amenorrhoea.

True osteoporosis is quantitatively defined as a bone mineral density more than two standard deviations below the age-matched normal values. Athletes very rarely record these levels and it is more accurate and relevant to term their bone mass as 'osteopenia' that is defined as 1–2 standard deviations below normal. Similarly, it is not appropriate to define the decreased bone mass of young women as 'bone loss' unless sequential measurements indicate a true decrease over time.

Of significance to long-term management is the probability that women who continue to exercise are more likely to maintain bone mass into old age beyond the menopause.

## INCIDENCE OF INJURY

Of more immediate relevance to the athlete than infertility and lower bone mass measurements is the observation that amenorrhoeic athletes have a greater injury incidence than those with a normal menstrual cycle. Interpretation of injury statistics is difficult because there are often confounding factors that cannot be controlled such as training load and poor training techniques. However, several reports indicate that total trauma incidence, including acute as well as chronic overuse injuries, is greater in amenorrhoeics (Lloyd et al 1986).

Stress fractures have been shown to be more common in amenorrhoeics and this is evident even in prospective studies that control for the amount of training undertaken (Bennell et al 1995, Carbon et al 1990). Clinically, it is common for amenorrhoeic athletes to have multiple fractures that are slow to heal. However, these fractures often occur in weightbearing bones which have been shown to have normal bone density. It is likely that these women have limited bone repair in the presence of low bone turnover.

## MANAGEMENT OF EXERCISE-RELATED AMENORRHOEA

If a clear diagnosis of exercise-related amenorrhoea has been made, and other conditions excluded, the athlete should be counselled on the adaptive processes associated with chronic energy drain. Athletes and coaches must be made aware that such endocrine changes are an indication that the current training/nutrition/stress paradigm is counterproductive and must be reversed. Certainly, the benefits of improved health and strength on physical performance should be emphasized.

Menstrual disturbance must not be allowed to persist in an athlete for more than 6 months without remedy because of the known health consequences for the athlete. It has been suggested that a minimum of four menses per year is required to confer adequate bone health.

Young athletes in particular should not be allowed to continue training with ongoing oligo-amenorrhoea, especially if normal menses have never been established, as it becomes increasingly difficult to reverse the problem as it is prolonged. Long-term amenorrhoeics rarely remain healthy or injury-free long enough to enjoy success from their hard training. Certainly, there can be little to be gained by being a junior champion whose career does not survive into senior ranks because of injury and illness.

Formal nutritional advice may be required to ensure adequate energy consumption to balance energy output. Adequate vitamin and mineral intake is also important, in particular calcium and iron.

Menstruating women generally require twice the daily iron intake of men – about 15 mg per day. Endurance athletes of both sexes frequently have haemoglobin and iron levels below reference range and this is, in part, due to the haemodilution in response to aerobic training. Some athletes, however, will have true iron deficiency either from low intake or absorption of iron, or from a postulated haemolysis from the repeated microtrauma of training. Amenorrhoeic athletes often have poor iron intake as part of their general malnutrition. Hence female endurance athletes, in particular, should ensure adequate iron levels or risk possible fatigue and poor performance. Serum ferritin is probably the best indicator of iron stores and a level below 30 ng/mL should be treated. Meat is the best source of iron and should be eaten daily, although vegetarians can manage to maintain iron stores with a careful diet. Total daily nutrition should exceed 2000 kcal (8300 kJ) and include fortified cereals and bread, green vegetables, and fruit. It is useful to remember that vitamin C improves iron absorption, while phytic acid (found in fibrous cereals) and tannic acid (found in tea and coffee) bind iron in the gut and hence limit absorption. In practice, overt iron deficiency often requires supplementation under medical control. Many athletes find the gastrointestinal disruption of oral iron too debilitating and, if anaemia persists, intramuscular iron in small doses may be necessary.

All women need adequate calcium intake and regular weightbearing exercise to ensure optimal bone density. Current guidelines suggest a recommended daily intake (RDI) of 800 mg per day for young (menstruating) women and 1500 mg per day for postmenopausal women, and it is likely that amenorrhoeics require similar intake. In practice this may be difficult to achieve from diet alone. Athletes must be encouraged not to avoid dairy products, the main source of dietary calcium. Low-fat cheese, milk and yoghurt are excellent nutritional choices for sportswomen. Half a litre of low-fat milk and 300 g of low-fat plain yoghurt will meet the daily calcium needs of the amenorrhoeic athlete. High-protein, tea, and coffee ingestion have a negative effect on calcium status because of increased renal excretion.

Any increase in body weight for the amenorrhoeic athlete should be slow and integrated with alterations in training to ensure that lean mass (muscle and bone) rather than excess fat is laid down. Some sessions of aerobic work could be replaced for light resistance work, core stability training or skill acquisition. It is important that there is adequate rest and recuperation and that 'quality' replaces unnecessary 'quantity' in the programme. Reduction of stress in the athlete's life is important and may require the input of a psychologist.

In practice total weight increase may require only a few kilos but, with improved nutrition and more targeted training, menses usually restart over 3–4 months. If this is not successful serious consideration must be given to a more formal break from training over 3–6 months during an 'off-season' to establish a normal menstrual pattern. Often, if this is not done, injury intervenes and the athlete is forced to take an unscheduled break from their sport that is likely to be more disruptive.

The medical management of exercise-related amenorrhoea is not well researched or understood and assumptions have been made relating to the use of oestrogen replacement as a parallel to the treatment of the post-menopausal woman. Low oestrogen levels are only one factor in the endocrine picture and, as low bone formation rather than bone resorption appears to be responsible for lower bone density, it is unlikely to be the most significant change. There is no good evidence that oestrogen administration improves bone density or heals stress fractures in the amenorrhoeic athlete (Hergonroeder 1995). Indeed, therapeutic oestrogen could, theoretically, decrease bone formation and repair further by limiting osteoclastic activity that stimulates bone repair. Hence, oestrogen, as hormone replacement therapy or the oral contraceptive, is not indicated in exercise-related amenorrhoea.

There are currently several new drugs becoming available for the management of osteoporosis that may have relevance to the young population of amenorrhoeics in the near future. However, it is preferable for the holistic health of the athlete that those factors responsible for amenorrhoea are reversed and training is optimized.

Coaches, athletes and their family need to understand the ramifications of the problem and be prepared to alter a programme for the long-term health and success of the athlete. In practice this is often very difficult to achieve. There may be a need for long-term cultural change within a sport. The sport of gymnastics in particular has addressed the problem over the past decade, increasing the minimum competitive age to 16, and allowing the gymnasts to assume a more healthy physique. Hopefully, as the understanding of the interrelationship of health, nutrition, exercise and performance increases in the sporting community, more women will be able to enjoy the health benefits of sport.

## KEY POINTS

1. Exercise has both general and reproductive health benefits.
2. Exercise results in significant endocrine changes which, in the presence of chronic energy drain, may cause hypothalamic dysfunction and subsequent amenorrhoea.
3. These changes are reversible with good nutrition and training programmes.
4. Prolonged amenorrhoea from negative energy balance is associated with infertility, poor bone health and a high incidence of injury.
5. Athletes can suffer other serious medical conditions that may present with amenorrhoea and require formal medical diagnosis.

## THE ATHLETE'S HEART

## LEARNING OBJECTIVES:

This section is intended to ensure that the reader:

1. Appreciates the physiological adaptation of the heart to training.
2. Appreciates the physiological mechanism underpinning cardiac enlargement.
3. Is able to recall the upper normal limits of left ventricular wall thickness and cavity size.
4. Recognizes the causes of sudden cardiac death in young and aged athletes.
5. Recognizes the types of arrhythmia observed in athletes and their importance.
6. Appreciates the nature of syncope in athletes and recognizes causes of syncope.
7. Recognizes the role of emergency care for athletes

## INTRODUCTION

Regular physical training is associated with a number of unique structural and functional adaptations that enhance cardiac output during exercise. Hypertrophy of the ventricles, increase in cardiac chamber size and enhanced ventricular filling in diastole result in an increased stroke volume at rest and throughout exercise. Athletes also have reduced resting heart rate (bradycardia) at rest and for a given submaximal workload, in response to an increased vagal tone possibly associated with the functional effect of an increased stroke volume. A large heart and slow heart rate are well-recognized features of athletes' hearts and manifest as a displaced and forceful cardiac apical impulse on physical examination, large QRS complexes, sinus bradycardia, first and second-degree heart block on the 12-lead ECG, and an increased cardiothoracic ratio on plain chest radiographs (Sharma et al 1997) (Summary box 9.1). These physiological adaptations may, however, mimic pathology. Differentiation of physiological and pathologic changes of the heart is important given the incidence of sudden cardiac death in young athletes.

## CARDIAC STRUCTURE AND FUNCTION IN HIGHLY TRAINED ATHLETES

Training-induced adaptations in cardiac structure have been traditionally divided into two main types depending upon the specific nature of the haemodynamic load placed upon the heart. Endurance training imposes an increased preload on the heart associated with a sustained increase in venous return combined with a mild to moderate increase in blood pressure resulting in an increased afterload. As a result of this increased preload and afterload, left ventricular cavity dilatation with minor increases in wall thickness occurs. Resistance training, in contrast, leads to dramatic elevations in blood pressure as a result of simultaneous muscular contraction and valsalva manoeuvre. This increased afterload results in an increased left ventricular wall thickness and a relatively normal sized left ventricular cavity dimension (Fig. 9.2). Training rarely conforms to this rigid dichotomy of cardiovascular responses, however, with most programmes utilizing a combination of endurance and strength training. Thus, the literature supporting a simple division of endurance and strength athletes does not exist. In the vast majority of athletes the cardiac adaptations exhibited tend to reflect a combination of responses to increased preload and afterload. Indeed, the largest athletic hearts are observed in those athletes that combine elements of strength and endurance exercise during training, often undertaking high resistance exercise for prolonged periods e.g. rowing, cycling, swimming and rugby (Pelliccia et al 1991, Whyte et al 2004b) (Fig. 9.2).

Cardiac dimensions in athletes are slightly increased compared with non-athletic matched controls and a large overlap is often observed. While the difference is small it does reach statistical significance and amounts to a 15–20% larger left ventricular wall thickness and 10% larger left ventricular cavity size compared with non-athletes. The modest increases in left ventricular wall thickness and left ventricular cavity size result in a marked increase in left ventricular mass in the region of 50% (Maron 2002).

The vast majority of athletes have cardiac dimensions within normal limits for the general population, i.e. a left ventricular wall thickness <12 mm and left ventricular

---

**Summary box 9.1**

Characteristics of the athlete's heart.
- Training results in a reversible increase in left ventricular muscle mass (LVM)
- The largest hearts are observed in athletes participating in events requiring a combination of both endurance and strength/power.
- Adaptations are similar between males and females and junior and seniors; however, males exhibit larger hearts than females, and seniors larger hearts than juniors
- Upper normal limits of left ventricular wall thickness for males and females are 14 mm and 12 mm respectively
- Upper normal limits of left ventricular cavity for males and females are 65 mm and 60 mm respectively
- Diastolic and systolic function are normal or enhanced in the athletes' heart

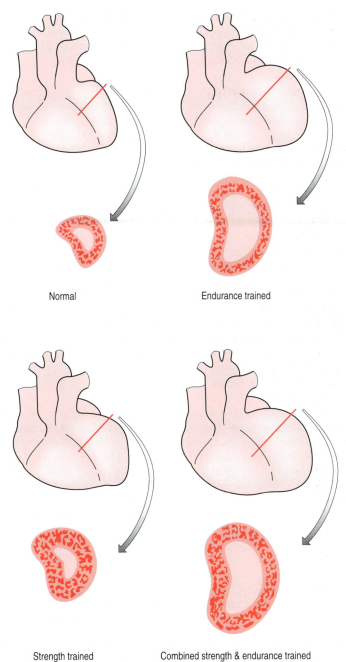

Normal

Endurance trained

Strength trained

Combined strength & endurance trained

**Figure 9.2**   The athlete's heart.

cavity size <55 mm. A small proportion of athletes, however, have a left ventricular wall thickness and more commonly a left ventricular cavity size exceeding predicted normal limits. In this group of athletes cardiac dimensions may be similar to those seen in patients with morphologically mild hypertrophic and dilated cardiomyopathy respectively (Pelliccia et al 1991, Sharma et al 2002, Whyte et al 2004b). The differentiation between physiological cardiac enlargement (athlete's heart) and cardiomyopathy is crucial when one considers that the cardiomyopathies are the commonest cause of exercise-related sudden death (Sharma et al 1997).

Studies have identified upper normal limits for left ventricular wall thickness in adult and adolescent athletes (Pelliccia et al 1991, Sharma et al 2002, Whyte et al 2004b). Upper wall thickness limits for adult male and female athletes are 14 mm and 12 mm respectively. In adolescent athletes a left ventricular wall thickness >12 mm warrants further investigation. Left ventricular cavity size in athletes more commonly exceeds normal limits with upper limits for male and female athletes of 66 mm and 60 mm respectively (Whyte et al 2004b). Values in excess of these should be viewed with caution and should prompt further investigation to identify the underlying cause.

Normal or enhanced indices of left ventricular systolic and diastolic function are observed in the athlete's heart despite significant increases in left ventricular mass (Whyte et al 2004b, c).

## THE ELECTROCARDIOGRAM (ECG)

Common ECG manifestations of the athlete's heart include sinus bradycardia, sinus arrhythmia, voltage criteria for left ventricular enlargement and early repolarization changes such as tall T-waves and concave ST segment elevation. Incomplete right bundle branch block (possibly reflecting right ventricular enlargement) is also relatively common. First-degree heart block and Mobitz type I second degree AV block are also recognized findings; however, higher degrees of AV block are rare. Minor T-wave inversions are observed and usually confined to the right chest leads (V1, V2, V3) but ST segment depression or deep (> 0.3 mV) T-waves are uncommon. Pathological Q-waves and left bundle branch block are not features of the athlete's heart.

## SUDDEN CARDIAC DEATH (SCD)

Sudden cardiac death in a young athlete is considered a non-traumatic, non-violent, unexpected death due to cardiac causes. Sudden death can occur during exercise or at rest. The time course of death remains equivocal ranging from during or immediately post-exercise to 24 hours post-exercise. Despite this lack of consensus agreement previous studies have reported a tenfold increase in the incidence of cardiovascular events in individuals with cardiovascular disease during exercise (Seto 2003). The sudden death of a young athlete is an uncommon event with an estimated prevalence between 1:100 000 and 1:300 000, with death rates five times higher in males than females (Maron et al 1996, van Camp et al 1995). Data from the National Federation of State High School Associations (USA) estimates 10–25 deaths in young individuals (<30 years) occur per year (van Camp 1992). The exact prevalence of sudden cardiac death remains unclear due to the paucity of well controlled studies. Most studies to date have relied upon self-reporting of physicians and media accounts of deaths. Despite the relatively low prevalence, the sudden death of an athlete has a profound effect not only on the athlete's immediate family but also on their team mates, the local community and the sport as a whole. Indeed, the sudden cardiac death of a young athlete is often highly publicized leading to ramifications nationally and internationally.

The causes of sudden cardiac death in young (<35 years) athletes are associated with a small number of congenital cardiac diseases. The most common cause is hypertrophic cardiomyopathy accounting for about 50% of sudden deaths (Maron et al 1996). Other causes include arrhythmogenic right ventricular cardiomyopathy, anomalous coronary arteries, the ion channelopathies (Brugada's and Long QT), W-P-W, Marfan's syndrome and myocarditis (Sharma et al 1997). Physical training results in cardiac adaptations that may mimic pathology (Sharma et al 1999, Whyte et al 2004b). To avoid false-positive and false-negative diagnosis the differentiation of physiological and pathological changes in cardiac structure and function is fundamental. The congenital nature of sudden cardiac death together with the increased incidence of events during exercise indicates adequate cardiovascular screening and evaluation are important to identify individuals with underlying cardiovascular disease prior to the commencement of rigorous training and competition.

In 1996 the American Heart Association (AHA) developed consensus recommendations for the cardiovascular screening of student athletes as part of a comprehensive pre-participation physical examination. This was incorporated into the pre-participation physical evaluation guidelines in the USA (Smith et al 1997). This system of pre-participation screening does not exist for sport in the UK. Indeed, because of the large differences in design and content of pre-participation screening among sports in the UK (Batt et al 2004) a national standard for pre-participation medical evaluation, including cardiovascular screening would enhance the quality of care offered to athletes. While limited evidence from the Italians suggests that pre-participation screening reduces the incidence of sudden cardiac death (Thiene et al 1999), the efficacy of such programmes remain to be fully elucidated due to the absence of systematic cardiovascular screening programmes in other countries, including the UK.

The content of pre-participation cardiovascular screening remains an area of much debate. In general, a full cardiovascular screen will include family history, medication and drug use history, blood pressure, pulse, recognition of Marfan's syndrome, auscultation of the heart (unnecessary when echocardiography is employed), ECG and echocardiography. A 12-lead integrated cardiopulmonary stress test may be a valuable tool in a differential diagnosis and is often part of an athletes support programme (Whyte et al 1999)(Fig. 9.3). Financial constraints may dictate the inclusion of ECG and echocardiography in the pre-participation screen. Indeed, finance is often used as the main factor precluding cardiovascular screening of the athlete. To date, however, limited evidence exists supporting or refuting the efficacy of pre-participation cardiovascular screening for athletes making discussions regarding the financial viability of such programmes problematic.

The incidence of sudden death in older athletes (>40 years) has been reported as 1 death per 396 000 man-hours jogging (Thompson et al 1980), but appears to be lower for men with higher levels of habitual physical activity (American College of Sports Medicine 1995). No evidence currently exists for death rates in women. Coronary artery disease is the most common condition leading to exercise related sudden cardiac death. The increased metabolic and physiological demands experienced during exercise lead to an increased risk of a cardiac event. Sudden death is often observed in highly conditioned older athletes due to occult coronary atheroma. Those older athletes at higher risk often have more than one recognized risk factors including smoking, a family history of myocardial infarction under the age of 55 years, hypertension and hypercholesterolaemia.

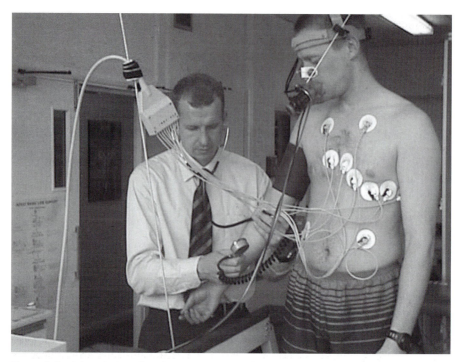

**Figure 9.3** Integrated cardiopulmonary stress testing.

Education programmes for older athletes should be aimed at increasing aware-ness of warning symptoms, including chest pain, palpitation, and syncope (faint-ing). Severe exercise should be undertaken cautiously in patients over the age of 40 years, particularly those with risk factors. Older individuals intending on com-mencing training for the first time or following a prolonged period of inactivity should seek medical advice before doing so. Older individuals presenting with symp-toms suggestive of coronary artery disease during exercise should be fully evalu-ated prior to re-commencing training.

Another mechanism for SCD in individuals free of cardiac disease is blunt chest impact produced either by a projectile or by collision with another athlete (com-motio cordis). Three determinants of a commotio cordis have been identified: (1) rel-atively low-energy chest impact located directly over the heart; (2) precise timing of the blow to a narrow 15-millisecond segment of the cardiac cycle vulnerable to poten-tially lethal ventricular arrhythmias, just prior to the T wave peak, and (3) a nar-row, compliant chest wall, typical of young children. The majority of commotio cordis events are fatal; however, a small number of athletes survive, supporting the impor-tance of early recognition and prompt institution of CPR and defibrillation (Maron 2002).

## ARRHYTHMIAS AND THE ATHLETE

Cardiac arrhythmias in athletes range from the benign and asymptomatic to the symptomatic and potentially life threatening. Supraventriuclar and ventricular extrasystoles are common and are usually of no clinical significance. The high vagal

## Summary box 9.2

Causes of exercise-related sudden cardiac death in young athletes. Adapted from Sharma S, Whyte G & McKenna WJ (1997) Sudden cardiac death in young athletes – fact or fiction? *British Journal of Sports Medicine* 31(4):269–276.

| Common | Uncommon |
|---|---|
| Hypertrophic cardiomypathy (HCM)* | Myocarditis |
| Coronary artery anomalies (CAA) | Coronary artery disease (CAD) |
| Arrhythmogenic right ventricular | Long QT/Brugada's syndrome |
| Cardiomypathy (ARVC)** | Marfan's |
| | Mitral valve prolapse (MVP) |
| | Wolf-Parkinson-White (W-P-W) |
| | Aortic stenosis |

\* Most common cause of ERSCD

\*\* Most common cause of ERSCD in Northern Italy

tone associated with physical training may result in athletes being more susceptible to certain bradyarrhythmias. Asymptomatic bradyarrhythmias such as sinus brady-cardia, nodal bradycardia and Mobitz second degree AV block (Mobitz I) are common among athletes and are due to the high vagal tone associated with intense physical training. Higher degrees of AV block and supraventricular arrhythmias are uncommon in athletes. In a small number of athletes high vagal tone may predispose to atrial fibrillation (Whyte et al 2004a).

Potentially life-threatening ventricular arrhythmias are uncommon in athletes and are generally associated with underlying structural heart disease, coronary artery disease or ion channnelopathies. In these circumstances participation in sport of high and moderate intensities is contraindicated. In a few cases, ventricular tachycardia may occur in the absence of these predisposing substrates and be amenable to treatment with electrophysiological radiofrequency ablation.

## SYNCOPE AND THE ATHLETE

Unexplained syncope in an athlete is a potentially ominous symptom that requires a thorough cardiovascular evaluation. The most frequent cause is neurocardiogenic (vasovagal) syncope, commonly associated with neurally mediated mechanisms but may be compounded by dehydration. The vast majority of cases occur in the absence of an underlying cardiac cause; however, structural heart disease and other causes should be eliminated before considering neurocardiogenic syncope as the aetiology (Summary box 9.3). Integrated cardiopulmonary stress testing is useful and should be performed while recording the ECG during the sport in which the athlete participates (Whyte et al 1999) (Fig. 9.3). Athletes with syncope associated with exercise who have a fully negative cardiac evaluation can safely participate in sport of all types and intensities. The exception to this rule are individuals with recurrent syncope who participate in sporting disciplines where even transient loss of consciousness may be hazardous, i.e. high-speed or water-based sports.

Traditional pharmaco-therapy for vasovagal syndrome includes $\beta_1$-andrenergic blocking agents, anti-arrhythmics and plasma volume expanders. These groups of

## Summary box 9.3

Causes of syncope. Adapted from Wang D, Sakaguchi S & Babcoack M (1997) Exercise induced vasovagal syncope. *Physician Sports Med* 25:64–74.

**Neurally mediated (vasovagal)**
Emotional faint
Carotid sinus syncope
Coughing
Swallowing, defecation, micturation
Airway stimulation

**Orthostatic and vascular**
Idiopathic orthostatic hypotension
Shy-Drager syndrome
Diabetic neuropathy with orthostatic hypotension
Drug-induced orthostasis

**Cardiac arrhythmia**
Sinus node dysfunction
Atrioventricular conduction system disease
Paroxysmal supraventricular tachycardia
Paroxysmal ventricular tachycardia
Cardiac implant malfunction

**Structural cardiac disease**
Vascular disease
Myocardial infarction
Obstructive cardiomyopathy
Subclavian steal syndrome
Pericardial disease
Pulmonary embolus
Primary pulmonary hypotension

**Neurological**
Cerebrovascular (i.e. vertebrobasilar disease)
Central nervous system substrate disorder (i.e. seizure disorder, subarachnoid haemorrhage)

**Non-cardiovascular**
Hypoglycaemia
Volume depletion
Hypoxaemia
Hyperventilation
Panic attack
Hysteria

drugs are currently prohibited by international governing bodies of sport. In addition, care must be taken when prescribing drugs that posses negative inotropic actions. Strategies to reduce/eliminate vaso-vagal symptoms are targeted at maintaining blood pressure and venous return post-exercise including warm-down, coughing, muscle tensing and leg crossing (Krediet et al 2002).

## EMERGENCY MEDICAL CARE AND ATHLETE EVALUATION

Sudden cardiac death in sport is preventable. Unfortunately most athletes collapsing during or immediately after sport die because cardio-pulmonary resuscitation is delayed. Facilities to deal with cardiac events should be available at training and competition venues. These facilities should include personnel trained in basic/advanced life support and the provision of external automated cardiovertor defibrillators. Personnel responsible for athletes during training and competition should also receive training in basic/advanced life support.

## KEY POINTS

1. Athlete's heart (AH) is characterized by left ventricular enlargement, resting bradycardia, conduction anomalies and additional heart sounds.
2. Upper normal limits of LV wall thickness and LV cavity diameter for male athletes is 14 mm and 65 mm and for female athletes is 12 mm and 60 mm.
3. Diastolic and systolic function are normal or enhanced in AH.
4. Differentiation of AH and pathological cardiovascular disease is crucial in preventing possible fatalities.
5. The causes of sudden cardiac death in young (<35 years) athletes are associated with a small number of congenital cardiac diseases. In older athletes (>35 years) sudden death is most commonly linked to coronary artery disease.
6. Unexplained syncope in an athlete is a potentially ominous symptom that requires a thorough cardiovascular evaluation.
7. Facilities to deal with cardiac events should be available at training and competition venues including: personnel trained in basic/advanced life support and the provision of external automated cardiovertor defibrillators.

## THE UNEXPLAINED UNDERPERFORMANCE SYNDROME (UUPS)

## LEARNING OBJECTIVES:

This section is intended to ensure that the reader:

1. Recognizes what underperformance syndrome is and how it is caused.
2. Is able to recall the prevalence of underperformance syndrome.
3. Appreciates the symptoms of underperformance syndrome.
4. Recognizes precipitating factors to underperformance syndrome.
5. Appreciates the tools used to identify athletes with underperformance syndrome.
6. Appreciates the ways in which underperformance syndrome can be prevented.
7. Comprehends the management and rehabilitation of an athlete with underperformance syndrome.

## INTRODUCTION

It is common for athletes to suffer from a short period (<2 weeks) of relative underperformance at times of hard training. This reversible decrement in performance is termed over-reaching (see Ch. 1). Sometimes underperformance persists for more than 2 weeks despite adequate rest. A reduction in performance for >2 weeks despite adequate recovery has been termed unexplained underperformance syndrome (UUPS). Other common terms employed to describe UUPS include burnout, staleness, overtraining syndrome, chronic fatigue in athletes, sports fatigue syndrome or under-recovery syndrome (Budgett et al 2000). Up to 10% of elite endurance athletes per year may suffer from UUPS (Budgett 1998). Any athlete training hard, however, is vulnerable. Indeed, Morgan et al (1987) reported 10% of collegiate swimmers in the USA are identified as 'burning out' each year.

It is important to differentiate UUPS from possible pathological conditions. Exclusion of underlying illness is achieved with an appropriate history and examination. A full blood count with measurement of iron stores and thyroid function may identify unexpected causes, otherwise routine blood screening is rarely helpful, unless indicated by the history and examination (Budgett 1998, Lac & Maso 2004). No specific medical cause is found in the majority of athletes suffering from UUPS.

## SYMPTOMS

The predominant symptoms in athletes suffering from UUPS are fatigue, heavy muscles and depression (Varlet-Marie et al 2003). Some athletes suffer from frequent minor infections breaking down with an upper respiratory tract infection (URTI) every 3–4 weeks due to immunosupression (Lakier-Smith 2003). Many athletes commonly describe increased lightheadiness (postural hypotension) and a raised resting pulse rate (Hedelin et al 2000). There is often a loss of motivation and an increased emotional lability, anxiety and irritability. A loss of appetite leading to weight loss is often observed. Direct questioning reveals sleep disturbance with difficulty getting to sleep, nightmares, waking during the night or prolonged sleep but waking un-refreshed (Lac & Maso 2004) (see Summary box 9.4).

Performance symptoms often manifest as athletes describing an ability to keep up at the beginning of a race but being unable to lift the pace or sprint for the line. This inability to increase exercise intensity may be associated with a reduced ability to recruit type II muscle fibres for maximum power output (Koutedakis et al 1995). This may be related to an increase in type I and reduction in type II muscle fibres, a myopathy type state (Steinacher et al 2004).

## DIAGNOSIS

Distinguishing UUPS from normal training fatigue (over-reaching) is difficult and can only be achieved once an athlete has failed to recover. Many athletes will be

---

**Summary box 9.4**

Symptoms of UUPS.
1. Underperformance
2. Depression with loss of motivation, competitive drive and libido
3. Increased anxiety and irritability
4. Sleep disturbance
5. Loss of appetite and weight
6. Fatigue
7. Frequent minor infections, particularly of the upper respiratory tract
8. Raised resting pulse rate
9. Increase symptoms of postural hypotension

fatigued, irritable, anxious and depressed with increased resting pulse rate and minor infections, but nevertheless recover quickly once the training volume has been reduced. The challenge for doctors, sports scientists and coaches is to develop reliable measures of recovery so that athletes can train as hard as possible but not so hard that they break down for many weeks with UUPS. No diagnostic tests currently exist for UUPS and the diagnosis is often made on the history and objective underperformance alone (Urhausen & Kindermann, 2002).

## PRECIPITATING FACTORS

Many athletes break down when they switch from low-intensity winter training to high-intensity summer training with intensive interval work. The stress of competition and selection pressures may also be a contributory factor in the development of UUPS.

Athletes rarely break down after less than 2 weeks of hard training provided that they then rest and allow themselves to recover afterwards. This is what happens with normal tapering after a typical hard training camp. In some sports, however, training is heavy and monotonous and lacks much periodization (see Ch. 1). This may result in a lack of programmed recovery resulting in a difficulty recovering from heavy periods of training. Large volumes of training, however, are generally well tolerated as long as the intensity is low enough.

While inadequate recovery is likely to be the critical factor, other stressors, including exams and other life events, glycogen depletion due to poor diet and dehydration will reduce the ability to recover from, or respond to, heavy training (Kentta et al 2001, MacKinnon 2000).

Very hard training may cause immunosuppression associated with raised serum cortisol concentrations, lowering serum glutamine concentrations, lowering salivary IgA concentrations and saliva volume, and reducing T helper/T suppressor cell ratios (Lakier-Smith 2003). An increased catabolism of amino acids as an energy substrate may explain many of the biochemical changes observed in athletes with so called 'endurance overtraining' (Petibois et al 2003).

## INVESTIGATION

A diagnosis of UUPS is often poorly accepted by athlete and coach. This situation has led to the development of some basic screening to convince the athlete/coach that there is no undiagnosed illness. The history and examination should guide the doctor in deciding whether further investigations might be helpful. Some serious diseases have presented as UUPS, such as viral myocarditis, cardiac abnormalities or hypothyroidism, but this is rare. Prolonged glycogen depletion sometimes due to disordered eating (or even eating disorders such as anorexia or bulimia) is a more common cause of fatigue and underperformance (Costill et al 1988, Snyder 1998). Anaemia may occur particularly in female endurance athletes due to poor diet and/or blood loss. Allergic rhinitis and atopy may present as recurrent upper respiratory tract infections (Budgett 1994).

## HOSPITAL TESTS

Laboratory tests are occasionally helpful but cannot be used to make a diagnosis of UUPS.

## FULL BLOOD COUNT

Haemoglobin concentrations and packed cell volume may decrease as a normal response to heavy training associated with a concomitant increase in plasma volume. This relative haemodilution may be misinterpreted as anaemia in the absence of a performance decrement (Budgett 1998).

## IRON STORES

Low iron stores reflected in a low serum ferritin concentration can cause fatigue in the absence of anaemia. Serum ferritin levels may be affected by concurrent illness. The majority of menustruating endurance athletes have ferritin levels of less than 30 ng.L$^{-1}$ which may contribute to fatigue, and iron stores are particularly important if they are considering altitude training. Many sports and exercise medicine doctors recommend giving oral iron (often a liquid preparation as this seems to be better tolerated), and vitamin C to help absorption, to most female endurance athletes who are menustruating.

## VIRUSES

Viral titres may be shown to rise or the Paul Bunell test may be positive, strongly suggesting glandular fever. Identifying a specific virus, however, does not change the management, so is of limited value (Bailey et al 1997).

## TRACE ELEMENTS AND VITAMINS

It has not been possible to show any link between vitamins, trace elements and UUPS or chronic fatigue syndrome in non-athletes. The widespread use of supplements by athletes does not offer protection from fatigue and underperformance and should be discouraged due to the risks of contamination. Dietary advice should be sought by all athletes and they must be given strong reassurance that a varied diet with sufficient calories negates the need for supplements except in specific cases under medical and dietetic advice (Costill et al 1988).

## PREVENTION AND EARLY DETECTION

Athletes can tolerate different levels of training and competition stress. Excessive training for one athlete may be insufficient training for another. Each athlete's tolerance level will also change through the season so training must be individualized and varied and should be reduced at times of stresses such as exams. Unfortunately, athletes are exhausted most of the time, unless they are tapering for a competition, so it is difficult for them to differentiate early UUPS from over-reaching. Investigators have tried to identify strategies for early detection with limited success (Urhausen & Kindermann 2002).

## PSYCHOLOGICAL PROFILING

In American college swimmers a 10% incidence of burn out was reduced to zero by daily mood monitoring with a profile of mood state (POMS) questionnaire, and by reducing training whenever mood deteriorated and increasing it when mood improved (Morgan et al 1987).

## HEART RATE

Many athletes monitor their early morning heart rate. A 10 beat per minute rise is non-specific but does provide objective evidence that something is wrong. A more sophisticated measure is heart rate variability which has been used for decades by the Eastern bloc to monitor the training status of athletes. Changes in the balance of the activity of the sympathetic and parasympathetic nervous systems occur with hard training and then recovery (with high parasympathetic drive after successful tapering). This may be reflected in heart rate variability giving an objective guide to the extent of recovery (Hedelin et al 2000, 2001, Mourot et al 2004). Unfortunately the changes in athletes with UUPS are very variable and so heart rate variability cannot be used to make a reliable diagnosis (Park et al, personal observation). The heart rate variability seems to change unpredictably as athletes go through fatigue, exhaustion, de-training and recovery (Bosquet et al 2003). Nevertheless it is possible that by profiling individual athletes across time a reliable pattern may be obtained.

## OTHER FACTORS

Underperformance after a taper is probably most significant so performance should be monitored carefully. Serial measurements of blood concentrations of haemoglobin and creatine kinase are unlikely to help (Urhausen & Kindermann 2002). In some athletes immune parameters may change with low serum glutamine concentrations (Castell 2003), and changes in salivary IgA and serum cortisol concentration. Nevertheless, there is still no reliable objective test to predict which athletes are going to break down after a period of hard training

Prevention requires good diet, full hydration and rest between training sessions. Coaches and athletes must realize that sports people with full-time jobs and other commitments will not recover as quickly as those who can relax after training. Correct periodization of training should ensure recovery.

## MANAGEMENT

Following the diagnosis of UUPS the whole support team must work with the coach and athlete to agree a recovery programme. The most important task is to persuade both coach and athlete of the diagnosis and that prolonged recovery is needed. Athletes will benefit from a multidisciplinary approach and should seek the support of a performance nutritionist and sports psychologist where available. Physiologists can also help by confirming underperformance, monitoring recovery and helping to set training levels. During this time, rest and regeneration strategies are essential to recovery.

## THERAPEUTIC EXERCISE

There is evidence that a very low level of exercise will help athletes with UUPS to recover (Fulcher & White 1997). Athletes with UUPS show improvement in both performance and mood state with 5 weeks of relative rest (Koutedakis et al 1995). Athletes are advised to exercise aerobically at a level well below lactate threshold (see Ch. 4) for a few minutes each day and slowly build this up over many weeks. The starting level and speed of increase in training volume will depend on the clinical picture and rate of improvement. Recovery generally takes 6–12 weeks (Budgett 1998). Unless held strictly to a recovery programme, many athletes make the mistake of trying to recommence a normal training session when feeling a little better, suffering from severe fatigue for several days before partially recovering and repeating the same pattern. Cross-training may be the only way to avoid the tendency to increase the intensity too fast.

Once athletes can tolerate 20 minutes of light exercise each day then it is useful to introduce short sprints of less than 10 seconds with at least 3 minutes recovery between each sprint (Summary box 9.5).

There is a close link between UUPS and depression (Armstrong & van Heest 2002, Uusitalo et al 2004). If an athlete is severely depressed there is evidence that a graded exercise programme will be less effective unless the depression is treated (Wearden et al 1998). Psychological intervention and antidepressants can be used.

Athletes are often surprised at the performance they can produce after 12 weeks of extremely light exercise. It is then that care must be taken to avoid increasing training too fast. On return to normal training, it is helpful to consider alternate hard and light training days. As they return to full training athletes are advised to train hard but make sure that they rest and recover completely at least once a week to optimize training adaptation (Budgett 1998).

## CONCLUSIONS

Unexplained underperformance syndrome is common in elite endurance athletes and is difficult to prevent and reliably identify. Once a definitive diagnosis is made and other medical causes have been excluded then a graded exercise programme over many weeks normally leads to full recovery. This will be most effective with the support of a multidisciplinary team and if there is full co-operation of the coach and athlete with the programme and regeneration strategies.

## KEY POINTS

1. A reduction in performance for >2 weeks despite adequate recovery has been termed unexplained underperformance syndrome (UUPS).
2. Up to 10% of elite endurance athletes per year may suffer from UUPS.
3. UUPS symptoms include: fatigue, heavy muscles, depression, frequent minor infections, lightheadiness (postural hypotension), raised resting pulse rate, loss of

---

**Summary box 9.5**

Typical rehabilitation programme for an athlete suffering from UPS.

| | |
|---|---|
| Week 1: | 20 minutes light exercise at 120 pulse rate per day |
| | 7 × 10 seconds sprints or weights 3 times per week |
| Week 2: | 30 minutes light exercise including 10 × 10 seconds sprint |
| Week 3: | 40 minutes light exercise including 10 × 10 seconds sprint |
| Week 4: | 50 minutes light exercise including 10 × 10 seconds sprint |
| Week 5: | 60 minutes light exercise including 10 × 10 seconds sprint |
| Week 6: | 60 minutes light exercise including 2 × 2 minutes normal intensity |
| Weeks 6–10: | Build-up normal intensity within 60 minutes to full 60 minutes at normal intensity |
| Weeks 10–12: | Add second session. Increase to normal training |

motivation, increased emotional lability, anxiety, irritability, loss of appetite, and sleep disturbance.

4. Distinguishing UUPS from normal training fatigue (over reaching) is difficult and can only be achieved once an athlete has failed to recover.
5. No diagnostic tests currently exist for UUPS and the diagnosis is often made on the history and objective underperformance alone.
6. Following the diagnosis of UUPS the whole support team must work with the coach and athlete to agree a recovery programme.

# ASTHMA AND EXERCISE-INDUCED ASTHMA

## LEARNING OBJECTIVES:

This section is intended to ensure that the reader:

1. Recognizes what asthma is and how it is caused.
2. Is able to recall the prevalence of asthma in sporting and non-sporting populations.
3. Appreciates the mechanisms that underlie the triggering of exercise-induced asthma and the potential long-term implications of airway drying.
4. Appreciates the time course of the airway response to exercise in susceptible individuals.
5. Appreciates the mechanisms by which asthma may limit exercise performance.
6. Recognizes the cardinal signs and symptoms of exercise-induced asthma, as well as the methods used for diagnosis.
7. Comprehends the ways in which exercise-induced asthma can be managed.

## WHAT IS ASTHMA?

Asthma is the most common chronic condition affecting the sporting population. Asthma is defined as 'a chronic inflammatory disorder of the airways' (Global Initative for Asthma 1995), the cardinal symptoms of which are wheezing, breathlessness, chest tightness and cough. These symptoms are the result of airway inflammation and narrowing in response to an inflammatory trigger. Acute airway narrowing occurs via a complex cascade of events that start with the release of inflammatory mediators and culminate in the contraction of smooth muscle around the airways. The resulting airway narrowing is called bronchoconstriction. Details of this cascade are beyond the scope of this chapter, and the reader is referred to Rundell & Jenkinson (2002) for further information. In addition to the airway narrowing induced by smooth muscle contraction, narrowing can become a chronic event due to the inflammation-induced swelling and incursion of the airway lining into the lumen of the airway, as well as the build-up of mucus. These events reduce the internal diameter of the airways, inducing the symptoms described above.

The trigger factors that induce bronchoconstriction vary enormously between individuals, but common triggers include animal dander, house dust mite, pollen, cigarette smoke and air pollution. In addition, colds, influenza and other viral infections can trigger bronchoconstriction. Less common triggers are moulds and fungi, and certain foods, for example, dairy products, fish, shellfish, yeast products, nuts, and some food colourings and preservatives. A small proportion of asthmatics also respond adversely to some common drugs such as aspirin, ibuprofen and paracetamol. This is particularly relevant to people with asthma who are regular exercisers, as these medications are often used to treat musculoskeletal injuries or strains.

Perhaps the most common trigger of bronchoconstriction is exercise. In about 90% of people with allergic asthma, and some people without allergic asthma, exercise is a potent bronchoconstrictor (Lacroix 1999). The severity of exercise-induced asthma (EIA) varies between individuals and peaks at about 10 minutes after stopping exercise (Beck et al 1999). The bronchoconstriction is accompanied by cough, airway inflammation and mucus production. Because airway responsiveness to exercise may occur in people who do not have allergic asthma, the term exercise-induced bronchoconstriction (EIB) has been suggested as a more precise definition of the condition (Anderson & Henricksen 1999).

## PREVALENCE IN THE SPORTING POPULATION

The prevalence of asthma in the general population varies between nations, being highest in the developed, Western countries such as the UK, where 8% of the adult population and 12–15% of children are diagnosed with asthma (National Asthma Campaign 2001). New Zealand has the highest rates of asthma internationally, with 15% of adults affected (ISAAC 1998). Rundell & Jenkinson (2002) suggest that the prevalence of EIA in elite athletes is between 10 and 50%, depending upon the sport in question. Winter sports athletes are reported to have the highest prevalence rates, especially those engaged in endurance events. For example, Wilbur et al (2000) reported the prevalence of asthma in cross-country skiers to be 50% and 21% in figure skaters. Other endurance-based events with high prevalence rates include cycling and triathlon (Helenius & Haahtela 2000). In addition, certain indoor environments are also associated with high prevalence rates for asthma, for example, swimming (Helenius & Haahtela 2000).

Data obtained as part of routine screening of Team GB athletes prior to the Athens Olympics confirms the relatively high prevalence of asthma/EIA/EIB in high-performance athletes (Dickinson et al 2005). The recorded prevalence for Team GB across all sports was 21%, which is more than double the prevalence rate in the UK's general population (see below). These data were the first to systematically assess prevalence across sports using rigorous, quantitative International Olympic Committee (IOC) criteria (see Diagnosis below). The two sports with the highest prevalence rates were swimming and cycling (both over 40%).

Generally, the consensus is that the prevalence of asthma is higher in the sporting population than it is in the general population (Nystad et al 2000). Recent insight into the aetiology of EIA and EIB have helped to shed light on the reasons for the variations in prevalence rates between sports, and between sports people and the sedentary population (see The pathophysiology of EIA and EIB, below). The higher than expected prevalence rates in some sports demands further research in order that the respiratory health of sports people can be protected.

## THE PATHOPHYSIOLOGY OF EIA AND EIB

Many people with asthma find the severity of EIA is greater in cold weather. However, this effect is not thought to be due to cold per se, but rather to the fact that cold air is dryer than warm air (Hahn et al 1984). Data from Anderson et al (1982) have demonstrated a dose–response relationship between water loss from the airways and the severity of EIB, suggesting that dry air, whether warm or cold, is a more potent stimulus to EIB than humid air. More recent research has confirmed that the severity of EIA is proportional to the water content of the inspired air (Eschenbacher et al 1992). Furthermore, bronchoconstriction is attenuated, or even abolished, if the inspirate is hot and humid (Anderson et al 1979).

Thus, the current consensus regarding the aetiology of EIA centres around one major trigger, airway drying (Rundell & Jenkinson 2002). The high ventilatory flow rates associated with exercise are thought to induce a cascade of responses that begin with water loss from the airway surface liquid, and a consequential change in the osmotic potential of the airway lining cells. When exercise stops, the rate of water loss from the airway returns to normal, and there is a restoration of normal osmolarity within the airway lining cells. However, this re-equilibration is accompanied by the release of inflammatory mediators from the affected cells, which trigger constriction of airway smooth muscle, causing bronchoconstriction.

The greater prevalence rates of EIA in cold weather sports are thought to be due to the chronic influence of airway drying and resulting inflammation, which induce airway remodelling (Karjalainen et al 2000). This remodelling leads to a condition known as airway hyper-reactivity or hyper-responsiveness, such that the athlete may become sensitized to the effects of airway drying. Under these conditions, the athlete has EIB, rather than EIA. Other environmental stimuli may also exacerbate EIA, as well as being responsible for the development of hyper-reactivity, e.g. vehicle exhaust gases, chlorine (swimming pools), and ice-resurfacing machine pollutants (Rundell 2004).

A recent 10-year follow-up study of three cross-country skiers suggests that their participation in their sport had led to permanent, detrimental remodelling of their respiratory systems (Verges et al 2004). These changes were associated with an obstructive pattern of lung disease and associated flow limitation. Further systematic research is needed before clear linkages can be identified, but the fact that repeated episodes of airway drying may lead to airway remodelling and the development of EIB is of growing concern. If a causal relationship is established, future research must seek to identify methods of minimizing the potentially damaging effects of airway drying and air pollution upon the respiratory health of sports people.

## THE TIME COURSE OF EIA AND EIB

The zenith of the EIA and EIB response generally occurs within 10–15 minutes of the cessation of exercise (Beck et al 1999). Previously, the literature has contained contradictory evidence regarding the occurrence of bronchoconstriction during exercise. However, it is now generally accepted that the bronchoconstrictor response does not occur until after the cessation of exercise (Beck et al 1999). These observations are consistent with a mechanism for EIA and EIB based upon airway water loss during exercise, followed by a recovery of osmolarity and the induction of inflammatory mediators post-exercise.

The fact that broncoconstriction does not occur during continuous exercise, but does occur during intermittent exercise has implications for athlete management. For endurance athletes, symptoms are unlikely to occur until they cease training or competition. During training, however, endurance athletes may experience symptoms during interval training. In contrast, athletes from repeated sprint sports are likely to experience symptoms during training and competition. Surprisingly, it is not uncommon for sprint and power athletes with EIA/EIB to remain undiagnosed. This is most likely because they perceive the symptoms of breathlessness that they experience between bouts of intense exercise to be a normal part of exercise, and therefore do not report them.

## DO EIA AND EIB LIMIT EXERCISE PERFORMANCE?

The human lung is traditionally thought to be overbuilt relative to the rest of the oxygen transport system (Dempsey & Babcock 1995). However, it has been known for some time that there are some highly trained endurance athletes for whom this is not true (Dempsey & Babcock 1995); these athletes exhibit arterial hypoxaemia during heavy exercise, indicating a diffusion limitation to oxygen transport. Two of the underlying mechanisms proposed to explain exercised-induced arterial hypox-aemia (EIAH) may also have relevance to athletes with EIA and EIB. First, there is evidence linking EIAH to hypoventilation due to a mechanical ventilatory limitation (Johnson et al 1992), and second to a diffusion limitation due to interstitial pulmonary oedema (Hopkins et al 1998). The inflammation and increased airways resistance that accompany asthma, EIA and EIB induce both a mechanical ventilatory limitation and an increase in the diffusion distance. Thus, in theory at least, it is conceivable that asthma, EIA and EIB may limit exercise performance.

The impairment of expiratory flow generating capacity that accompanies asthma (see Fig. 9.4) may not only induce hypoventilation (and EIAH), it also generates a condition known as 'dynamic hyperinflation'. This forces breathing into the inspiratory

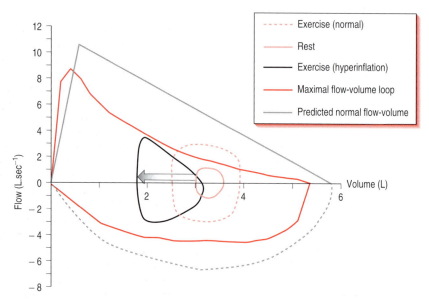

**Figure 9.4** Dynamic hyperinflation: comparison of the response of the exercise tidal flow volume in a person with asthma (solid red lines), compared with that predicted for someone with normal lungs (grey lines). Note that in the presence of expiratory flow limitation the person with asthma must encroach upon their inspiratory capacity in order to increase minute ventilation (flow volume loop shifts to the left). The person with normal lungs is able to increase minute ventilation by utilizing both their inspiratory and expiratory reserve volumes.

reserve volume, towards total lung capacity (a shift to the left of the flow–volume envelope). This is a region where the work of breathing is raised by an increased elastic load, which increases the requirement for inspiratory muscle work. The main symptom of hyperinflation and increased inspiratory muscle work is a heightened sensation of respiratory effort, or breathlessness (Lougheed et al 1993). It is the intensification of respiratory effort sensation that limits the degree to which dynamic hyperinflation develops, i.e. hyperinflation is limited by effort sensation. Because breathlessness contributes significantly to total body effort sensation, the consequence of dynamic hyperinflation is an increased overall sense of effort during exercise. Most athletes rely upon effort sensation as a means of pacing; the consequences of dynamic hyperinflation and increased airways resistance for an athlete's ability to achieve and maintain a given pace are therefore self-evident. It is also possible that the increased inspiratory muscle work may exacerbate inspiratory muscle fatigue, which would intensify respiratory effort sensation further. It is currently unknown whether respiratory effort sensation and/or inspiratory muscle fatigue are greater in athletes with EIA or EIB.

As well as performance impairment due to mechanical changes, it is also reasonable to suggest that inflammation within the respiratory endothelium may impair gas exchange by increasing the diffusion distance (as occurs in interstitial pulmonary oedema) thereby inducing a potential diffusion limitation. However, confirmation that either ventilatory flow limitation or diffusion limitation impair performance in athletes with EIA/EIB awaits experimental verification.

## DIAGNOSIS

Until relatively recently, the diagnosis of asthma for the purposes of using asthma medications during competition was made almost exclusively on the basis of symptoms. However, this has been shown to be very unreliable. For example, Rundell et al (2001) demonstrated that the proportion of their athlete sample reporting two or more symptoms was the same for athletes with a spirometrically-confirmed diagnosis of EIA as it was for those who were EIA-negative (39% versus 41%). This suggests that diagnosis on the basis of symptoms is no better than flipping a coin. These observations are supported to some extent by those of Dickinson et al (2005) who screened 84 members of Team GB prior to participation in the Athens Olympics. Sixty-two of these had a previous diagnosis of asthma (either by questionnaire or spirometry), while a further 15 athletes reported symptoms, but had no formal diagnosis. Thirteen (21.0%) of the 62 athletes with a previous diagnosis of asthma tested negative using International Olympic Committee criteria (IOC; see below). Seven of the 15 athletes with no previous diagnosis of asthma tested positive. Though not quite as bad as flipping a coin, these data support the notion that accurate diagnosis requires more than just a symptom-based approach.

The cardinal sign of asthma is 'reversible airways obstruction'. Diagnosis of airways obstruction is most commonly made using electronic spirometry (see Fig. 9.5). By plotting flow against volume during a maximal expiratory and inspiratory manoeuvre, a flow–volume loop is constructed. Abnormalities are confined primarily to the expiratory loop, and Figure 9.6 illustrates the typical findings in an athlete with EIA or EIB. At baseline, lung function typically appears normal (black line), or even superior to normal (as denoted by the measured loop being outside the loop predicted for the athlete's age and body size). However, following exercise, abnormalities of the expiratory loop become apparent, with evidence of a characteristic concavity to the expiratory flow profile (red line). The single diagnostic index that is derived from

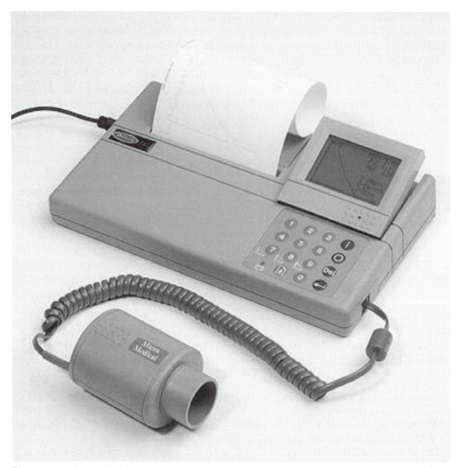

**Figure 9.5** An electronic spirometer.

these measurements is most commonly the forced expiratory volume in 1 second ($FEV_1$). This is the volume of air that is exhaled during the first second of a force expiratory manoeuvre, and it is normalized to the individual's forced vital capacity (FVC). 'Normality' of $FEV_1$ is represented by an $FEV_1$/FVC ratio of >80%.

The International Olympic Committee (IOC) guidelines for the diagnosis of EIA require the use of 'spirometric' methods, i.e. the production of a flow–volume loop using an electronic spirometer (see Fig. 9.6). The IOC rules make provision for two methods of diagnosis: (1) response to inhaled bronchodilator medication ($\beta_2$-agonists), and (2) response to a bronchoprovocation challenge.

The criteria for a positive response differ depending upon which test is undertaken. For test 1, the IOC accepts a 15% increase in the $FEV_1$ within 10 minutes of taking a bronchodilator as a positive test for the presence of asthma. However, athletes may have very little ongoing airway inflammation, and consequently, no ongoing bronchoconstriction, particularly if they have EIB (airway

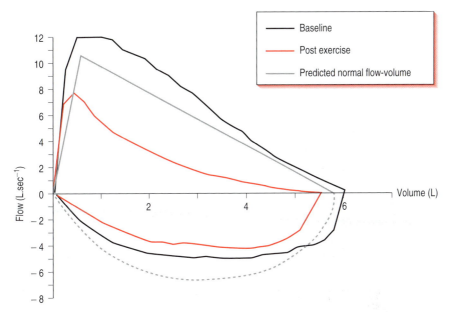

**Figure 9.6**   EIA-positive provocation challenge: Typical flow–volume loops generated before and after a bronchoprovocation challenge. The grey line represents the predicted normal flow–volume loop (based upon the subject's age, weight and height); the black line is the baseline loop; the red line is the post-challenge loop showing characteristic changes (lower peak expiratory flow rate, concave expiratory flow profile, reduced vital capacity due to airway closure).

hyper-responsiveness) and not EIA. Thus, the IOC also accepts the results of 'bronchoprovocation' challenges.

Bronchoprovocation challenges are of three main types, the simplest of which is a straightforward exercise test. In order to provoke a response in a susceptible individual, the exercise must be high intensity (>85% maximum heart rate) and last for at least 6 minutes; this ensures that the ventilatory requirement is sufficient to provoke airway drying. The main problem with an exercise challenge is that it is difficult to control environmental variables and the environmental conditions may not favour a positive response, e.g. it may be a warm humid day. The second type of test is a somewhat artificial, but very standardized method of inducing airway drying. This test is known as 'eucapnic voluntary hyperpnoea' (EVH), and requires the athlete to hyperventilate for 6 minutes into an apparatus that supplies dry air. This challenge has been shown to have high specificity and sensitivity for EIA and EIB (Rundell et al 2004). The third challenge involves the inhalation of a substance that triggers an inflammatory response in the airways of susceptible individuals (e.g. saline, mannitol, methacholine or histamine). The IOC regulations for diagnosis on the basis of an inhalation challenges are complex, involving reference to the dose–response of the athlete. For this reason these challenges are not the preferred method of diagnosis, although the use of a mannitol challenge may become so. The specificity and sensitivity of mannitol has recently been shown to be at least as good as EVH (Holzer et al 2003).

In the case of exercise and EVH, the IOC requires a fall of 10% in $FEV_1$ within 30 minutes of the provocation challenge, for a positive demonstration of EIA. In all of these tests, the athlete must have ceased taking any prescribed medication as follows:

- short-acting $\beta_2$-agonists 12 hours prior;
- long-acting $\beta_2$-agonists 48 hours prior;
- corticosteroids (anti-inflammatory) 72 hours prior.

Because athletes must be removed from their medication, EIA provocation challenges should only be conducted by appropriately qualified individuals, and under conditions where medical support is available.

## MANAGEMENT

The management of EIA is dependent upon whether an athlete is in competition, and therefore bound by the doping regulations of their governing body. If in doubt, athletes should refer to the rules of their governing body for up-to-date guidance on permissible pharmacological management of EIA.

The goal of any management strategy is to minimize symptoms, reduce the risk of exacerbations, and to optimize the athlete's ability to compete to the limits of their potential. The 'traditional' method of managing asthma is under the supervision of a GP or chest physician using medication (pharmacological management). For athletes who are in competition, however, this requires a thorough understanding of the doping regulations for their sport, and it is inadvisable to take any prescribed medication without first referring to the most recent version of the doping regulations for the sport in question.

Assuming that the regulations governing the use of asthma medications have been met, the following pharmacological treatment options are available:

## PHARMACOLOGICAL MANAGEMENT

Pharmacological management of EIA must be undertaken under the supervision of a physician. There are large inter-individual variations in EIA, which necessitate a highly individualistic approach to its management (Rundell & Jenkinson 2002). The most commonly used pharmacological agents are:

### Bronchodilators ($\beta_2$–agonists)

Frequently known as 'reliever' medication, $\beta_2$-agonists relax the muscles around the airways, dilating them and reducing their resistance to airflow. Short-acting $\beta_2$-agonists can be used up to four times daily, and are most effective when taken prophylactically immediately prior to exercise, or in response to the development of acute EIA. If EIA is mild and infrequent, this may be the only pharmacological treatment required. However, if it is not, then it may be necessary to supplement with inhaled corticosteroids.

### Corticosteroids

Known as 'preventer' medication, corticosteroids suppress the chronic inflammation that is associated with asthma, or frequent bouts of EIA. Reducing inflammation will improve pre-exercise lung function, as well as reducing the sensitivity of the airways to EIA. For athletes with mild EIA, a once-daily dose of inhaled corticosteroid may be the only medication required to manage EIA effectively.

Increasingly, pharmaceutical companies are providing so-called 'combination' therapies that combine a $\beta_2$-agonists and a corticosteroid in a single inhaler.

## NON-PHARMACOLOGICAL MANAGEMENT

Both athletes and the general public are increasingly turning to non-pharmacological methods of managing chronic conditions such as asthma. Furthermore, there may be a small number of athletes who have noticeable symptoms but whose airway responsiveness to provocation falls short of the minimum criteria required for use of $\beta_2$-agonists during competition. Accordingly, it is relevant to consider the range of non-pharmacological methods that exist to manage EIA and EIB.

### Warm-up

About half of the people with asthma experience what is known as a 'refractory period' following a 10- to 15-minute bout of moderate intensity exercise (50–60% maximum heart rate), or 'warm up'. For up to 2 hours after the 'warm up', asthmatics can exercise (even intensely) and not experience EIA (McKenzie et al 1994). The precise mechanisms for refractoriness remain unknown, but it can be used to good effect in those who show refractoriness.

### Dietary modification

The relationship between diet and the severity of EIA has only recently been the subject of systematic research, but the results to date appear promising.

One of the earliest dietary components to be linked to exacerbation of asthma was dietary salt. A high-sodium diet has been found to worsen post-exercise falls in $FEV_1$ (Gotshall et al 2000). In contrast, recent evidence suggests that restricting salt intake reduces (by about two-thirds) the severity of the post-exercise decline in lung function in people with asthma, after as little as 1 week of restriction (Gotshall et al 2003). The effective range of sodium intake for EIA attenuation is 1000–1800 mg.day$^{-1}$. This is considerably lower than the recommended daily allowance for reducing hypertension (2400 mg.day$^{-1}$), but it is nonetheless, readily achievable.

Consumption of fish oils also appears to alleviate EIA. Fish oils are rich sources of omega-3 poly-unsaturated fatty acids (PUFAs), which have been implicated in the reduction of inflammatory responses. The link between fish oils and asthma was made by the observation that the prevalence of asthma is very low in Eskimo populations who have high intakes of fish oils (Mickleborough & Gotshall 2003). A recent study has demonstrated a positive effect of 3 weeks of supplementation with fish oils capsules on the severity of EIA in elite athletes. The double-blind, randomized, cross-over design compared a normal diet with a placebo diet and a fish-oil-supplemented diet. The fish oil supplementation reduced the post-exercise fall in $FEV_1$ from 17% on the normal diet to just 3% on the supplemented diet (Mickleborough et al 2003).

Asthma is an inflammatory disease, and inflammatory cells produce oxidants; thus, the role of antioxidants in EIA has been investigated. The principle antioxidant vitamins studied are C and E, and recent studies have demonstrated beneficial effects of both upon asthma. Preliminary data from Murphy et al (2003) suggest that a 3-week supplementation with a combination of vitamin C (500 mg/day) and vitamin E (33 IU/day) reduced the post-exercise fall in $FEV_1$ by 10%. An earlier study examined the effect of vitamin C alone, and with a much shorter supplementation period; just 90 minutes. Schachter & Schlesinger (1982) showed a halving of the post-exercise fall in $FEV_1$ from 20% to 10% after the acute supplementation with 500 mg of vitamin C; they saw no effect of a placebo in the same subjects.

## Inspiratory muscle training (IMT)

The principal symptom of bronchoconstriction is an increased sense of respiratory effort, or breathlessness. There is a strong relationship between the strength of the inspiratory muscles and the sense of respiratory effort (see McConnell & Romer 2004a for a review), and this has been demonstrated directly for people with asthma. Weiner and colleagues (1992) have conducted a number of studies examining the influence of specific inspiratory muscle resistance training upon symptoms, respiratory effort and consumption of medication in asthmatics. They made some impressive observations, with subjects showing huge reductions in their consumption of both $\beta_2$-agonists, and their ratings of breathlessness (Weiner et al 1992, 2002). No studies have yet examined the influence of IMT upon EIA per se, but it is very unlikely that IMT has a direct effect upon the severity of bronchoconstriction. However, it appears that IMT ameliorates the principal symptoms of bronchoconstriction (breathlessness), as well as providing an ergogenic effect (see McConnell & Romer 2004b for a review).

The mainstay of asthma management continues to be pharmacological. However, for those athletes who have mild symptoms, or for those wishing to optimize management using all means available, the approaches described above offer evidence-based alternatives or additions to traditional pharmacological management.

## SUMMARY

Unfortunately, asthma, EIA and EIB continue to increase in prevalence in both the athletic and general populations. A major cause for concern is the higher prevalence rate for EIA in elite athletes, especially when evidence begins to point to a causal relationship between participation in some sports, and the development of EIA/EIB. Careful diagnosis and management are essential for optimal care of the athlete, as well as to ensure that she/he achieves their full performance potential. Future research must clarify the relationship between sports participation and the development of EIA/EIB, as well as identifying methods of protecting the respiratory health of athletes.

## KEY POINTS

1. Asthma and EIA are inflammatory disorders of the lung airways.
2. EIA occurs in approximately 90% of people with allergic asthma.
3. Asthma, EIA and EIB are more prevalent in the sporting population than in the general population (e.g. UK prevalence data = 21% versus 8%, respectively).
4. EIA occurs through mechanism(s) linked to airway drying during exercise.
5. EIA is more prevalent in endurance- and cold-weather athletes.
6. EIA develops only after exercise has ceased, reaching a maximum about 10 minutes after exercise has ceased.
7. It is possible that EIA and EIB may limit exercise performance, but this awaits experimental verification.
8. The diagnosis of EIA can be made accurately only by using spirometry in conjunction with standardized bronchoprovocation challenges.
9. The mainstay of asthma management is pharmacological, but a number of evidence-based non-pharmacological approaches do exist.

# References

## Reproductive health in exercising women

Bale P, Doust J, Dawson D 1996 Gymnasts, distance runners, anorexics body composition and menstrual status. Journal of Sports Medicine and Physical Fitness 36:49–53

Bennell KL, Malcolm SA, Thomas SA et al 1995 The incidence and distribution of stress fractures in competitive track and field athletes. A twelve-month prospective study. American Journal of Sports Medicine 24 (2):211–217

Carbon RJ, Sambrook PN, Deakin V et al 1990 Bone density of elite female athletes with stress fractures. Medical Journal of Australia 153:373–376

Drinkwater BL, Nilson K, Ott S, Chestnut CH 1996 Bone mineral density after resumption of menses in amenorrhoeic athletes. Journal of the American Medcial Association 256:380–382

Hergonroeder AC 1995 Bone mineralization, hypothalamic amenorrhoea, and sex steroid therapy in female adolescents and young adults. Journal of Paediatrics 26:683–689

Kaiserauer S, Snyder A, Sleeper M, Zierath J 1989 Nutritional, physiological, and menstrual status of distance runners. Medicine and Science in Sports and Exercise 21:120–125

Kaufman BA, Warren M, Dominguez J et al 2002 Bone density and amenorrhoea in ballet dancers are related to a decreased resting metabolic rate and lower leptin levels. Journal Clinical Endocrinology and Metabolism 87:2777–2783

Lloyd T, Triantafyllou S, Baker E et al 1986 Women athletes with menstrual irregularity have increased musculoskeletal injury. Medicine and Science in Sports and Exercise 18:1246–1250

Loucks AB, Laughlin GA, Mortola JF et al 1992 Hypothalamic–pituitary–thyroidal function in eumenorrhoeic and amenorrhoeic athletes. Journal of Clncial Enodocrinology and Metabolism 75:514–518

Musey VC, Goldstein S, Farmer PK et al 1993 Differential regulation of IGF-1 and IGF binding protein-1 by dietary composition in humans. American Journal of the Medical Sciences 305:131–138

Stacey E, Korkia P, Hukkanen MVJ et al 1998 Decreased nitric oxide levels and bone turnover in amenorrhoeic athletes with spinal osteopenia. Journal of Clinical Endocrinology and Metabolism 83(9):3056–3061

Wolman RL, Clark P, McNally E et al 1990 Menstrual state and exercise as determinants of spinal trabecular bone density in female athletes. British Medical Journal 301:516–518

Zanker CL, Swaine IL 1998 Relation between bone turnover, oestradiol, and energy balance in women distance runners. British Journal of Sports Medicine 32:167–171

## The athlete's heart

American College of Sports Medicine 1995 Benefits and risks associated with exercise. Guideline for exercise testing and prescription, p. 3–11. Williams and Wilkins, Baltimore

Batt ME, Jaques R, Stone M 2004 Preparticipation examination (screening): practical issues as determined by sport: a United Kingdom perspective. Clinical Journal of Sport Medicine 14(3):178–182

Krediet P, van Dijk N, Linzer M et al 2002 Management of vasovagal syncope: controlling or aborting faints by leg crossing and muscle tensing. Circulation 106:1684–1689

Link M, Homoud M, Wang P, Estes M 2001 Cardiac arrhythmias in the athlete. Cardiology Reviews 9:21–30

Maron BJ 2002 The young competitive athlete with cardiovascular abnormalities: causes of sudden death, detection by preparticipation screening, and standards for disqualification. Cardiac Electrophysiology Review 6:100–103

Maron BJ, Shirani J, Poliac LC et al 1996 Sudden death in young competitive athletes. Clinical, demographic and pathological profiles. Journal of the American Medical Association 276:199–204

Pelliccia A, Maron BJ, Spataro A et al 1991 The upper limits of physiologic cardiac hypertrophy in highly trained athletes. New England Journal of Medicine 324:295–301

Sharma S, Whyte G, McKenna WJ 1997 Sudden cardiac death in young athletes – fact or fiction? British Journal of Sports Medicine 31(4):269–276

Sharma S, Whyte G, Elliott PM et al 1999 Electrocardiographic changes in 1000 highly trained elite athletes. British Journal of Sports Medicine 30:319–324

Sharma S, Elliott PM, Whyte G et al 2002 Physiologic limits of left ventricular hypertrophy in elite junior athletes: relevance to differential diagnosis of athlete's heart and hypertrophic cardiomyopathy. Journal of the American College of Cardiology 40(8):1431–1436

Smith DM, Kovan JR, Rich BS et al 1997 Preparticipation physical evaluation, 2nd edn. McGraw-Hill, Minneapolis MN

Seto CK 2003 Preparticipation cardiovascular screening. Clinics in Sports Medicine 23:23–35

Thiene G, Basso G, Basso C et al 1999 Sudden death in the young and in the athlete: causes, mechanisms and prevention. Cardiologica 126:99–105

Thompson P, Funk E, Charlton R, Sturner W 1980 The incidence of death during jogging in Rhode Island from 1975 through 1980. Journal of the American Medical Association 247:2535–2538

van Camp SP 1992 Sudden death. Clinics in Sports Medicine 11:273–289

van Camp SP, Bloor CM, Mueller FO et al 1995 Non-traumatic sports death in high school and college athletes. Medicine and Science in Sports and Exercise 27:641–647

Wang D, Sakaguchi S, Babcoack M 1997 Exercise induced vasovagal syncope. Physician and Sports Medicine 25:64–74

Whyte G, George K, Sharma S, McKenna WJ 1999 Exercise gas exchange response in the differentiation of physiologic and pathologic left ventricular hypertrophy. Medicine and Science in Sports and Exercise 31(9):1237–1241

Whyte G, Stephens N, Budgett R et al 2004a Spontaneous atrial fibrillation in a freestyle skier. British Journal of Sports Medicine 38(2):230–232

Whyte G, George K, Sharma S et al 2004b The upper limit of physiologic cardiac hypertrophy in elite male and female athletes. The British Experience. European Journal of Applied Physiology 31:592–597

Whyte GP, George K, Nevill A et al 2004c Left ventricular morphology and function in female athletes: a meta-analysis. International Journal of Sports Medicine 25:380–383

## The unexplained underperformance syndrome (UUPS)

Armstrong LE, van Heest JL 2002 The unknown mechanism of the overtraining syndrome: clue from depression and psychoneuroimmunology. Sports Medicine 32(3):185–209

Bailey DM, Davies B, Budgett R, Gandy G 1997 Recovery from infectious mononucleosis after altitude training in an elite middle distance runner. British Journal of Sports Medicine 31(2):153–154

Bosquet L, Papelier Y, Leger L, Legros P 2003 Night heart rate variability during overtraining in male endurance athletes. Journal of Sports Medicine and Physical Fitness 43(4):506–512

Budgett R 1994 The overtraining syndrome. British Medical Journal 309:465–468

Budgett R 1998 Fatigue and underperformance in athletes: the overtraining syndrome. British Journal of Sports Medicine 32:107–110

Budgett R, Newsholme E, Lehmann M et al 2000 Redefining the overtraining syndrome as the unexplained underperformance syndrome. British Journal of Sports Medicine 34:67–68

Castell L 2003 Glutamine supplementation in vitro and in vivo, in exercise and in immunodepression. Sports Medicine 33(5):323–345

Costill DL, Flynn MG, Kirwan JP et al 1988 Effects of repeated days of intensified training on muscle glycogen and swimming performance. Medicine and Science in Sports and Exercise 20:249–254

Fulcher KY, White PD 1997 Randomised controlled trial of graded exercise in patients with chronic fatigue syndrome. British Medical Journal 314:1647–1652

Hedelin R, Kentta Gm, Wiklund U et al 2000a Short-term overtraining: effects on performance, circulatory responses, and heart rate variability. Exercise and Sports Science Reviews 32:1480–1484

Hedelin R, Wiklund U, Bjerle P et al 2000b Cardiac autonomic imbalance in an overtrained athlete. Medicine and Science in Sports and Exercise 32(9):1531–1533

Hedelin R, Bjerle P, Henriksson-Larsen K 2001 Heart rate variability in athletes: relationship with central and peripheral performance. Medicine and Science in Sports and Exercise 33:1394–1398

Kentta G, Hassmen P, Raglin JS 2001 Training practices and overtraining syndrome in Swedish age group athletes. International Journal of Sports Medicine 22(6):460–465

Koutedakis Y, Frischknecht R, Vrbova G et al 1995 Maximal voluntary quadriceps strength patterns in Olympic overtrained athletes. Medicine and Science in Sports and Exercise 27(4):566–572

Lac G, Maso F 2004 Biological markers for the follow-up of athletes throughout the training season. Pathology Biology (Paris) 52(1):43–49

Lakier-Smith L 2003 Overtraining, excessive exercise, and altered immunity: this T helper-1 versus T helper-2 lymphocyte response? Sports Medicine 33(5):347–364

MacKinnon LT 2000 Special feature for the Olympics: effects of exercise on the immune system: overtraining effects on immunity and performance in athletes. Immunology and Cell Biology 78(5):502–509

Morgan WP, Brown DR, Raglin JS et al 1987 Psychological monitoring of overtraining and staleness. British Journal of Sports Medicine 21(3):107–114

Mourot L, Bouhaddi M, Perrey S et al 2004 Decrease in heart rate variability with overtraining: assessment by the Poincare plot analysis. Clinical Physiology and Functional Imaging 24(1):10–18

Petibois C, Cazorla G, Poortmans JR, Deleris G 2003 Biomechanical aspects of overtraining in endurance sports: the metabolism alteration process syndrome. Sports Medicine 33(2):83–94

Snyder AC 1998 Overtraining and glycogen depletion hypothesis. Medicine and Science in Sports and Exercise 30:1146–1150

Steinacker JM, Lormes W, Reissnecker S, Liu Y 2004 New aspects of the hormone and cytokine response to training. European Journal of Applied Physiology 91(4):382–391. Epub Nov 8 2003

Urhausen A, Kindermann W 2002 Diagnosis of overtraining: what tools do we have? Sports Medicine 32(2):95–102

Uusitalo AL, Valkonen-Korhonen M, Helenius P et al 2004 Abnormal serotonin reuptake in an overtrained, insomnic and depressed team athlete. International Journal of Sports Medicine 25(2):150–153

Varlet-Marie E, Gaudard A, Mercier J et al 2003 Is the feeling of heavy legs in overtrained athletes related to impaired hemorheology? Clinical Hemorheology Microcirculation 28(3):151–159

Wearden AJ, Morris RK, Mullis R et al 1998 A randomised, double blind, placebo controlled treatment trial of fluoxetine and a graded exercise programme for chronic fatigue syndrome. British Journal of Psychiatry 172: 485–490

## Asthma and exercise-induced asthma

Anderson SD, Henricksen JM 1999 Management of exercise-induced asthma. In: Carlsen K-H, Ibsen T (eds) Exercise-induced asthma and sports in asthma. Munksgaard, Copenhagen, p 99–108

Anderson SD, Daviskas E, Schoeffel RE, Unger SF 1979 Prevention of severe exercise-induced asthma with hot humid air. Lancet ii(8143):629

Anderson SD, Schoeffel RE, Follet R et al 1982 Sensitivity to heat and water loss at rest and during exercise in asthmatic patients. European Journal of Respiratory Disease 63(5):459–471

Beck KC, Hyatt RE, Mpougas P, Scanlon PD 1999 Evaluation of pulmonary resistance and maximal expiratory flow measurements during exercise in humans. Journal of Applied Physiology 86(4):1388–1395

Dempsey JA, Babcock MA 1995 An integrative view of limitations to muscular performance. Advances in Experimental Medical Biology 384:393–399

Dickinson JW, Whyte GP, McConnell AK, Harries M 2005 The impact of changes in the IOC-MC asthma criteria: a British perspective. Thorax (British perspective paper)

Eschenbacher WL, Moore TB, Lorenzen TJ et al 1992 Pulmonary responses of asthmatic and normal subjects to different temperature and humidity conditions in an environmental chamber. Lung 170(1):51–62

Global Initiative for Asthma 1995 Global strategy for asthma management and prevention. In US. Department of Health and Human Sciences. Public Health Service, National Heart, Lung & Blood Institute, ed. NHLBI/WHO workshop report, 1–8. Bethesda, Maryland: Medical Communications Resources

Gotshall RW, Mickleborough TD, Cordain L 2000 Dietary salt restriction improves pulmonary function in exercise-induced asthma. Medicine and Science in Sports and Exercise 32(11):1815–1819

Gotshall RW, Fedorczak LJ, Rasmussen JJ 2003 One week versus two weeks of a low salt diet and severity of exercise-induced bronchoconstriction [abstract]. Medicine and Science in Sports and Exercise 35(5):S10

Hahn A, Anderson SD, Morton AR 1984 A reinterpretation of the effect of temperature and water content of the inspired air in exercise-induced asthma. American Reviews of Respiratory Disease 130(4):575–579

Helenius I, & Haahtela T 2000 Allergy and asthma in elite summer sport athletes. Journal of Allergy Clinical Immunology 106(3):444–452

Holzer K, Anderson SD, Chan HK, Douglass J 2003 Mannitol as a challenge test to identify exercise-induced bronchoconstriction in elite athletes. American Journal of Respiratory Critical Care Medicine 167(4):534–753

Hopkins SR, Gavin TP, Siafakas NM 1998 Effect of prolonged, heavy exercise on pulmonary gas exchange in athletes. Journal of Applied Physiology 85(4):1523–1532

ISAAC 1998 Lancet 351 (9111):1225–1232

Johnson BD, Saupe KW, Dempsey JA 1992 Mechanical constraints on exercise hyperpnea in endurance athletes. Journal of Applied Physiology 73(3):874–886

Karjalainen EM, Laitinen A, Sue-Chu M et al 2000 Evidence of airway inflammation and remodeling in ski athletes with and without bronchial hyperresponsiveness to methacholine. American Journal of Respiratory Critical Care Medicine 161(6):2086–2091

Lacroix VJ 1999 Exercise-induced asthma. Physician and Sports Medicine 27:75–92

Lougheed MD, Lam M, Forkert L et al 1993 Breathlessness during acute bronchoconstriction in asthma. Pathophysiologic mechanisms. American Reviews of Respiratory Disease 148(6 Pt 1):1452–1459

McConnell AK, Romer LM 2004a Dyspnoea in health and obstructive pulmonary disease: the role of respiratory muscle function and training. Sports Medicine 34(2):117–132

McConnell AK, Romer LM 2004b Respiratory muscle training in healthy humans: resolving the controversy. International Journal of Sports Medicine 25(4):284–293

McKenzie DC, McLuckie SL, Stirling DR 1994 The protective effects of continuous and interval exercise in athletes with exercise-induced asthma. Medicine and Science in Sports and Exercise 26:951–956

Mickleborough T, Gotshall R 2003 Dietary components with demonstrated effectiveness in decreasing the severity of exercise-induced asthma. Sports Medicine 33(9):671–681.

Mickleborough TD, Murray RL, Ionescu AA, Lindley MR 2003 Fish oil supplementation reduces severity of exercise-induced bronchoconstriction in elite athletes. American Journal of Respiratory Critical Care Medicine 168(10):1181–1189

Murphy JD, Ferguson CS, Brown KR et al 2003 The effect of dietary antioxidants on lung function in exercise-induced asthmatics [abstract]. Medicine and Science in Sports and Exercise 34:S115

National Asthma Campaign 2001 www.asthma.org.uk/pros/publications.php

Nystad W, Harris J, Borgen JS 2000 Asthma and wheezing among Norwegian elite athletes. Medicine and Science in Sports and Exercise 32(2):266–270

Rundell KW 2004 Pulmonary function decay in women ice hockey players: is there a relationship to ice rink air quality? Inhalation Toxicology 16(3):117–123

Rundell KW, Jenkinson DM 2002 Exercise-induced bronchospasm in the elite athlete. Sports Medicine 32(9):583–600

Rundell KW, Im J, Mayers LB et al 2001 Self-reported symptoms and exercise-induced asthma in the elite athlete. Medicine and Science in Sports and Exercise 33(2):208–213

Rundell KW, Anderson SD, Spiering BA, Judelson DA 2004 Field exercise vs laboratory eucapnic voluntary hyperventilation to identify airway hyperresponsiveness in elite cold weather athletes. Chest 125(3):909–915

Schachter EN, Schlesinger A 1982 The attenuation of exercise-induced bronchospasm by ascorbic acid. Annals of Allergy 49(3):146–151

Verges S, Flore P, Blanchi MP, Wuyam B 2004 A 10-year follow-up study of pulmonary function in symptomatic elite cross-country skiers – athletes and bronchial dysfunctions. Scandinavian Journal of Medicine and Science in Sports 14(6):381–387

Weiner P, Azgad Y, Ganam R, Weiner M 1992 Inspiratory muscle training in patients with bronchial asthma. Chest 102(5):1357–1361

Weiner P, Magadle R, Massarwa F et al 2002 Influence of gender and inspiratory muscle training on the perception of dyspnea in patients with asthma. Chest 122(1):197–201

Wilber R, Rundell K, Szmedra L et al 2000 Incidence of exercise-induced bronchospasm in Olympic winter sport athletes. Medicine and Science in Sports and Exercise 32 (4):732–737

## Further reading

### Reproductive health in exercising women

Harries M, Williams C, Stanish W, Micheli L (eds) 2000 Oxford textbook of sports medicine. Oxford University Press, Oxford

Landry G, Bernhardt D (eds) 2005 Essentials of primary care sports medicine. Human Kinetics, Champaign IL

Whyte G, Harries M, Williams C (eds) 2005 The ABC of sports medicine, 3rd edn. BMJ Books, London

### The athlete's heart

Harries M, Williams C, Stanish C (eds) 2000 Oxford textbook of sports medicine. Oxford University Press, Oxford

Landry G, Bernhardt D (eds) 2005 Essentials of primary care sports medicine. Human Kinetics, Champaign IL

Whyte G, Harries M, Williams C (eds) 2005 The ABC of sports medicine, 3rd edn. BMJ Books, London

### The unexplained underperformance syndrome (UUPS)

Harries M, Williams C, Stanish C (eds) 2000 Oxford textbook of sports medicine. Oxford University Press, Oxford

Landry G, Bernhardt D (eds) 2005 Essentials of primary care sports medicine. Human Kinetics, Champaign IL

Whyte G, Harries M, Williams C (eds) 2005 The ABC of sports medicine, 3rd edn. BMJ Books, London

### Asthma and exercise-induced asthma

Cotes JE 1993 Lung function, 5th edn. Blackwell, London

Rundell KW, Wilder RL, Lemanske RF (eds) 2002 Exercise-induced asthma. Human Kinetics, Champaign IL

West JB 2001 Pulmonary physiology and pathophysiology. Lippincott, Williams & Wilkins, London

# Glossary

**Acclimatization:** The adaptation of physiological systems and processes to environmental stressors leading to an enhanced functional capacity in that environment.

**Asthma:** A chronic inflammatory disorder of the airways. Symptoms include: wheezing, breathlessness, chest tightness and cough. These symptoms are the result of airway inflammation and narrowing (bronchoconstriction) in response to an inflammatory trigger.

**Adenosine triphosphate (ATP):** The hydrolysis of ATP (catalysed by the enzyme ATPase) is the primary source of energy. The store of ATP in skeletal muscle is very small (5 mmol.kg$^{-1}$ of muscle).

**Athlete's Heart (AH):** The adaptation of the heart to physical training characterized by resting bradycardia, cardiac remodelling, ECG changes and additional heart sounds.

**ATP/CP system:** The system used to produce energy from the hydrolysis of endogenous intra-muscular stores of the high energy phosphates ATP and CP. The ATP-CP system is the dominant energy pathway in short-duration, high-intensity sports of less than 10 seconds

**Anaerobic capacity:** It is this capacity that determines an athlete's ability to sustain high-intensity exercise associated with the finite capacity for anaerobic energy production. The term 'anaerobic endurance' is synonymous with 'anaerobic capacity'

**Anaerobic glycolysis:** An anaerobic process comprising 10 enzymatically controlled chemical reactions that catabolize muscle glycogen or glucose to provide energy for ATP resynthesis.

**Anaerobic endurance training:** The aim of anaerobic endurance training is to maximally stress anaerobic energy systems (ATP-CP, anaerobic glycolysis). As a consequence of the intensity of training and the resultant fatigue, exercise bouts will be of short-duration (<3 min), therefore training is normally divided into repeated bouts or intervals of short duration with variable work:rest ratios.

**Anaerobic endurance training (short-duration):** The repetition of short-duration maximal intensity exercise bouts (≤ 15 seconds) with a work:rest ratio in the region of 1:10. This type of training increases the capacity of the ATP-CP energy pathway and enhances muscular power.

**Anaerobic endurance training (long-duration):** The repetition of maximal intensity exercise of 1–3 minutes duration with a work:rest ratio in the region of 1:4. This type of training places significant demands on the anaerobic glycolysis energy system.

**Anaerobic endurance training (Lactate Tolerance Training):** The repetition of short-duration (20–120 sec) maximal intensity exercise bouts interspersed with short duration rest periods with a work : rest ratios of 1 : 1.

**Circuit training:** A training session composed of a number of specific exercises targeted at specific muscle groups (and often skills) involved in the target activity.

**Creatine phosphate (CP):** The hydrolysis of CP (catalysed by the enzyme creatine kinase, CK) provides an immediate supply of energy for the rapid resynthesis of ATP. Intramuscular stores of CP are approximately 15 mmol.kg$^{-1}$ of muscle

**Cross-training:** Defined in a number of ways: (1) the simultaneous training for 2 or more events (i.e. triathlon); (2) the cross-transfer of training effects from one sport to another; (3) the conveyance of training effects from one limb to the contralateral or ipsilateral limb.

**Endurance performance:** For the purpose of this text endurance performance is defined as continuous activity beyond 5 minutes, but less than 4 hours in duration. Whilst this represents a wide spectrum of sporting endeavors the predominant source of ATP is via aerobic processes.

**Exercise economy:** The oxygen uptake required to produce a specific power output or speed.

**Exercise induced asthma:** Where exercise is the inflammatory trigger responsible for an asthma response (see above). In around 90% of people with allergic asthma, and some people without allergic asthma, exercise is a potent bronchoconstrictor.

**Fatigue:** A term often used to describe the general feeling of tiredness. In relation to sports performance, it is the decline in muscular power output and thus performance.

**Flexibility:** The ability to move a joint smoothly through its entire range of motion.

**Form:** The practice of implementing recommended movement patterns, maintenance of postural control, use of full range of motion and regulation of breathing.

**Fractional utilization:** The % of $\dot{V}O_2$max that can be sustained whilst exercising at race pace, and is dependent upon both the training status and exercise duration.

**Glycogen supercompensation:** The use of carbohydrate loading regimes resulting in supra-normal amounts of muscle glycogen storage.

**Hypertrophy:** An increase in muscle fibre cross-sectional area associated with an addition of contractile proteins (actin and myosin) to the periphery of the myofibril. In this process, a larger myofibril is formed since packing density and cross bridge spacing is left unchanged

**Interval training:** The repetition of exercise bouts with defined periods of recovery to develop aerobic endurance capacity. The repetition of intervals allows the athlete to undertake a greater volume of training at the appropriate intensity in a single training session.

**Interval training – High Intensity Interval Training (HIT):** Short duration (30 seconds to 5 minutes) repetitions performed at an intensity above an athlete's $\dot{V}O_2$max, with rest intervals typically lasting 15–120 seconds.

**Jet lag:** A lack of synchrony between the body clock and the outside world. Symptoms include: general feeling of fatigue, loss of concentration, loss of appetite, headache, dizziness, nausea and constipation. A decline in performance of activities involving complex mental activity, reduced hand grip and leg strength, reduced maximum performance, and a general loss of motivation is often observed in athletes suffering from jet lag.

**Lactic acid:** Considered the primary cause of muscular fatigue during high-intensity exercise, lactic acid rapidly dissociates to lactate and hydrogen ions ($H^+$). It is the accumulation of $H^+$ that causes metabolic acidosis. During high-intensity exercise when $H^+$ accumulates in the cytosol, intracellular proteins provide buffering of some of the excess acidity; in addition, hydrogen ions efflux from the cell are buffered by extracellular bicarbonate.

**Lactate threshold:** The velocity, power, heart rate, or $\dot{V}O_2$max resulting in a sustained increase in blood lactate above baseline values.

**Long Slow Distance training (LSD):** LSD training sessions are performed at very conservative intensities (<70% $\dot{V}O_2$max), for prolonged periods that greatly exceed the duration of exercise performed during competition.

**Maximal Accumulated Oxygen Deficit (MAOD):** A method for estimating the anaerobic energy contribution during supramaximal exercise. This procedure requires the calculation of the individual's submaximal oxygen consumption-power relationship, which can be attained from an incremental submaximal exercise test. This relationship is then applied to the power output achieved during an exhaustive supramaximal exercise of 2–3 minutes duration in which the anaerobic capacity is fully utilized. The difference between this estimated oxygen cost and the total oxygen consumed is termed the MAOD.

**Maximal oxygen consumption ($\dot{V}O_2$max):** The highest rate at which oxygen can be extracted, transported and consumed, in the process of aerobic ATP synthesis. Measured in litres of oxygen consumption per minute ($L.min^{-1}$) it is typically expressed in millilitres of oxygen per kilogram of body weight per unit of time (i.e. $ml.kg^{-1}.min^{-1}$).

**Menstrual cycle:** The cycle of the female reproductive system regulated by periodic changes in the secretion of follicular-stimulating hormone (FSH) and luteinizing hormone (LH). The normal menstrual cycle (eumenorrhea) lasts 28–35 days. There are a number of disorders of the menstrual cycle including: dysmenorrhoea (painful periods), menorrhagia (heavy bleeding), amenorrhoea (loss of menses for a minimum of 6 months), oligomenorrhoea (cycles longer than the normal 28–35 days), polymenor-rhoea (unusually short cycle).

**Muscle fibre types:** Muscle fibres differ according to their contractile and metabolic proportion, and can accordingly be broadly categorized into three types; fast contracting fibres with a predominantly glycolytic metabolism (type IIb fibres); fast contracting fibres with a more oxidative metabolism (type IIa fibres) and slow contracting, oxidative fibres (type I fibres). A fourth type (type IIc fibres) are thought to be fibres in transition from type II to type I, and are uncommon except in muscle undergoing intensive training, or in young developing muscle. Most human muscles are made up of the two main fibre types, I and IIb

**Overload:** An increase in training volume above that normal imposed achieved by increasing the intensity and/or duration of the training stimulus. The overload event acts as a discrete stimulus for the biological mechanisms of adaptation.

**Over-reaching:** A reversible decrement in performance associated with a period of high training volume.

**Periodization:** The purposeful variation of a training programme over time, so that the athlete attains optimal adaptive potential just prior to an important event.

**Plyometrics:** A specialist exercise aimed at improving power output arising from the stretch shortening cycle.

**Power (P):** The rate of force production calculated as work done (force [f] × distance [d]) divided by velocity (v); $[P = (f.d)/v]$.

**Repetition maximum (RM):** The maximum number of repetitions per set that can be performed at a given resistance with correct exercise technique and form.

**Resistance training:** A physical stimulus for the musculoskeletal system to respond by reordering the control and architecture of active tissues resulting in an advancement of maximal force expression.

**Reversibility:** A de-conditioning process caused by the reduction or cessation of optimal training stimuli often termed 'detraining'.

**Specificity:** The use of training stressors that optimally stress the physiological systems associated with performance. Three components of specificity exist: (1) skill specificity, (ii) muscle group specificity, and (iii) energy system specificity.

**Strength:** The ability to produce force, generated isotonically, isometrically, or isokinetically. Strength is often measured by a set of repetitions at a given load performed to momentary voluntary muscular fatigue or failure (repetition maximum).

**Supercompensation cycle:** The association between training load and regeneration characterized by four distinct elements; exercise, fatigue, recovery and adaptations

**Tapering:** A specialized exercise training technique designed to reverse training-induced fatigue without a loss of the training adaptations, often termed as 'peaking'.

**Threshold training:** Typically lasting 30–90 minutes at an intensity associated with lactate threshold (LT).

**Training principles:** A number of basic principles which, when appropriately applied, result in optimal adaptation and performance, they include: individuality, reversibility, progression, overload (progressive overload), periodization and specificity.

**Travel fatigue:** Characterized by a group of transient negative effects associated with prolonged periods of time spent in transit, irrespective of time zone changes. Travel fatigue generally lasts 1–2 days.

**Unexplained Under Performance Syndrome (UUPS):** A reduction in performance for >2 weeks despite adequate recovery. Other, common terms employed to describe UUPS include: burnout, staleness, overtraining syndrome, chronic fatigue in athletes, sports fatigue syndrome or under-recovery syndrome.

# Index

Note: page numbers in *italics* refer to figures, tables and boxes